Model-Based Approaches in Biomedical Engineering

Online at: https://doi.org/10.1088/978-0-7503-4016-8

IPEM–IOP Series in Physics and Engineering in Medicine and Biology

About the Series

The series in Physics and Engineering in Medicine and Biology will allow the Institute of Physics and Engineering in Medicine (IPEM) to enhance its mission to 'advance physics and engineering applied to medicine and biology for the public good'.

It is focused on key areas including, but not limited to:
- clinical engineering
- diagnostic radiology
- informatics and computing
- magnetic resonance imaging
- nuclear medicine
- physiological measurement
- radiation protection
- radiotherapy
- rehabilitation engineering
- ultrasound and non-ionising radiation.

A number of IPEM–IOP titles are being published as part of the EUTEMPE Network Series for Medical Physics Experts.

A full list of titles published in this series can be found here: https://iopscience.iop.org/bookListInfo/physics-engineering-medicine-biology-series.

Model-Based Approaches in Biomedical Engineering

Ean Hin Ooi and Yeong Shiong Chiew
Mechanical Engineering Discipline, School of Engineering, Monash University Malaysia,
Jalan Lagoon Selatan, Bandar Sunway, 47500 Selangor, Malaysia

IOP Publishing, Bristol, UK

Permission to make use of IOP Publishing content other than as set out above may be sought at permissions@ioppublishing.org.

Ean Hin Ooi and Yeong Shiong Chiew have asserted their right to be identified as the authors of this work in accordance with sections 77 and 78 of the Copyright, Designs and Patents Act 1988.

ISBN   978-0-7503-4016-8 (ebook)
ISBN   978-0-7503-4014-4 (print)
ISBN   978-0-7503-4017-5 (myPrint)
ISBN   978-0-7503-4015-1 (mobi)

DOI   10.1088/978-0-7503-4016-8

Supplementary material is available for this book from https://doi.org/10.1088/978-0-7503-4016-8.

Version: 20230401

IOP ebooks

British Library Cataloguing-in-Publication Data: A catalogue record for this book is available from the British Library.

Published by IOP Publishing, wholly owned by The Institute of Physics, London

IOP Publishing, No.2 The Distillery, Glassfields, Avon Street, Bristol, BS2 0GR, UK

US Office: IOP Publishing, Inc., 190 North Independence Mall West, Suite 601, Philadelphia, PA 19106, USA

~ Declare the past, diagnose the present and foretell the future ~

—Hippocrates, 400 BC

Contents

Preface

The idea for this book came about in 2020 when we were planning the contents of a course to introduce undergraduate engineering students to biomedical engineering. During the process, we discovered that many of the existing biomedical engineering textbooks do not emphasise the modelling approaches. As such, we have taken up the challenge of introducing readers to the two-leading model-based approaches, namely mechanistic modelling and physiological modelling, and their applications in biomedical engineering. This is achieved through careful selection of topics that showcase the role of computational modelling in biomedical engineering. These topics include bioheat transfer, haemodynamics, drug delivery, glucose–insulin system, respiratory system, and cardiovascular system.

We have prepared this book in such a way that each chapter is standalone. The majority of the chapters are accompanied by case studies that cover a broad range of specialisation to facilitate better understanding among the readers. Solutions of these case studies were demonstrated though the use of the computational package MATLAB® and COMSOL Multiphysics®, and the source files for each are provided as supplementary material to aid readers (available at https://doi.org/10.1088/978-0-7503-4016-8). When writing this book, we assumed the readers to already have some prior knowledge in computer programming, finite element method, calculus, and partial differential equations. Having said that, we have endeavoured to provide as much supplementary information and clarification as possible to help readers who may not be as well-equipped with pre-assumed knowledge.

The advancement of high-performance computing and technology has benefited various disciplines including healthcare. The enhanced computational capabilities have helped biomedical engineers in reaching practical solutions to sophisticated and complex biophysical and physiological problems. Successful simulation of computational models can assist physicians in the early diagnosis and treatment of health-related problems. Key to the success is the modelling strategy employed in describing the different biophysical and physiological problems that are involved. As such, we hope that this book will become a valuable source of information for readers of all levels (novices and experts) who wish to explore model-based approaches in biomedical engineering and their applications in healthcare systems.

Ean Hin Ooi and Yeong Shiong Chiew
March 2023

Acknowledgments

The completion of this book is made possible by the following people. Firstly, I would like to thank the co-author, Dr Yeong Shiong Chiew for accepting the invitation to collaborate and work on this book. Needless to say, this book would not have been possible without his participation. I am forever grateful to my wife Joy, whose motivation and sacrifices in the past two years have allowed me to focus my time on writing and completing this book. I would also like to thank William Tze Hau Lim for his help in proofreading early drafts of this book, and Michael Slaughter from IOP Publishing Ltd for his assistance throughout the publication process. A special thank you goes to Emeritus Professor Kwan Hoong Ng from University of Malaya for recommending me to IOP Publishing Ltd, which ultimately led to the publication of this book. Last but not least, to my parents for their unconditional love and support.

Ean Hin Ooi
March 2023

I would like to thank several people who supported me throughout the completion of the book chapter. First, I would like to thank my collaborators and mentors for their invaluable advice and guidance. To the members of the Centre of BioEngineering at the University of Canterbury, GIGA Cardiovascular Science at the University of Liege, the Institute of Technical Medicine at Furtwangen University, and the Department of Control Engineering and Information Technology at Budapest University of Technology and Economics, who have unselfishly shared their time and knowledge with me. Their encouragement and dynamic ideas enabled me to prepare the book's chapter. Next, to my family, friends and my loving wife for their support and encouragement during book preparation. Last but not least, I would like to thank the principal author, Associate Professor Dr Ean Hin Ooi, for his invitation and collaboration in this book.

Yeong Shiong Chiew
March 2023

Editor biographies

Ean Hin Ooi

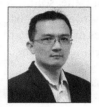

Dr Ean Hin Ooi is an Associate Professor at the Mechanical Engineering Discipline, School of Engineering, Monash University Malaysia, where he leads the Biomedical Engineering Modelling and Simulations (BEMS) group. He obtained his bachelor's degree in mechanical engineering from Universiti Teknologi Malaysia and his PhD in engineering from Nanyang Technological University, Singapore. His research experience includes research positions in School of Clinical and Experimental Medicine, University of Birmingham, Wessex Institute of Technology and the Institute of Biomedical Engineering, University of Oxford, where he worked on research projects funded by the European Commission. He has more than 10 years of experience working in biomedical engineering research, specialising in the application of computational modelling techniques to solve problems in healthcare and medicine. He is an Associate Editor for the journal *Computer Methods and Programs in Biomedicine* and is a technical consultant for Ascend Technologies Ltd in the United Kingdom. Dr Ooi's primary research interests are in thermal ablation therapy for cancer treatment, and ocular and soft tissue biomechanics. He also retains an interest in the development of mesh reduction numerical methods.

Yeong Shiong Chiew

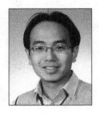

Dr Yeong Shiong Chiew graduated from Universiti Teknologi Malaysia with a Bachelor of Engineering Mechanical-Automotive and a Masters of Engineering in Mechanical Engineering. He obtained his PhD at the University of Canterbury, New Zealand. He worked as a postdoctoral fellow at the Centre for Bioengineering at the University of Canterbury in a range of research, investigating model-based mechanical ventilation for patients with respiratory failure, including leadership of a large randomised controlled trial. He is currently a Senior Lecturer at Monash University Malaysia, pioneering in model-based clinical mechanical ventilation trials in Malaysia and Singapore hospitals. His work spans from developing physiological models, model development, algorithm and system identification methods, and creating unique clinical decision metrics, to conducting clinical trials. Dr Chiew leads the Data Analytics team in the Biomedical Engineering Modelling and Simulations (BEMS) group. He is a chartered member of the IMechE United Kingdom and a member of the IFAC TC 8.2. Biological and Medical System. He is an editorial board member in the *BMC Pulmonary Medicine* journal, and he also serves as an academic editor in the *BioMed Research International* journal.

Foreword

I congratulate both Associate Prof Dr Ean Hin Ooi and Dr Yeong Shiong Chiew for taking up the challenge to produce such a practical guidebook that focuses on the application of engineering concepts to biomedical engineering and the solution strategies. Both are active researchers and passionate teachers from Monash University Malaysia. They explain two main model-based approaches in biomedical engineering, namely mechanistic modelling and physiological modelling, and their various applications in healthcare.

The book is useful for those who are just starting as well as those who wish to explore further. It covers a wide range of topics in biomedical engineering including thermal therapy, drug delivery, blood flow, respiratory mechanics, cardiovascular system and glucose–insulin system.

I like the way the book is organized—each chapter is standalone, and is accompanied by case studies and applications. As healthcare moves toward digitalization, computational modeling is expected to play a larger role in the advancement of medicine through the development of digital twins and virtual patients. As a result, this book is timely and will serve as an excellent learning tool and resource.

Emeritus Professor Kwan Hoong Ng
PhD, DABMP, FASc, FIOMP, FIUPESM, FTWAS
Department of Biomedical Imaging
Faculty of Medicine
Universiti Malaya
Kuala Lumpur
Malaysia

IOP Publishing

Model-Based Approaches in Biomedical Engineering

Ean Hin Ooi and Yeong Shiong Chiew

Chapter 1

Introduction

1.1 Early developments of biomedical engineering

Mankind has always been fascinated with the human body and how it works. In 400 BC, Hippocrates, who is known as the Father of Medicine, was the first to describe body illnesses as the result of naturally occurring phenomena, and not divine intervention or mystical forces. The first attempt at applying concepts of physics and engineering to describe the human body can be traced back to the 15th century, through the various works of the famous Italian engineer Leonardo da Vinci. His contributions to the knowledge of human anatomy and physiology through numerous drawings and sketches have resulted in Leonardo da Vinci being credited as the first medical physicist (Kron and Krishnan 2019) and the first bioengineer (Armentano and Kun 2019). It must be stressed that Leonardo da Vinci's contributions to the understanding of the human body are far more inclusive than just his drawings and sketches. His concept of addressing many interacting systems in a complex and nonlinear fashion has laid the foundation for many interdisciplinary studies today, with biomedical engineering being a prime example.

Biomedical engineering is a multidisciplinary engineering field that applies the knowledge from various sub disciplines of engineering to the study of biology, medicine, and healthcare. In essence, biomedical engineering is a diverse field of study, including but not limited to biomaterials, bioinstrumentation, bioinformatics, biomechanics, medical imaging, and medical devices. Each field of study may involve one or more engineering disciplines, such as mechanical, chemical, electrical and mechatronics, just to name a few. Biomedical engineering continues to be a relevant field of study today and for the foreseeable future, a fact that is spurred by the utilisation of technology in healthcare. For example, many of the surgical procedures currently in practice, such as laparoscopic surgery, are reliant on engineering. The dawn of the Fourth Industrial Revolution (IR4.0) has also led to the use of artificial intelligence in healthcare to assist in decision making and diagnosis. Therefore, there is a continuous demand for biomedical engineers and

doi:10.1088/978-0-7503-4016-8ch1

many universities today are offering undergraduate and graduate degree programs that centre on biomedical engineering.

1.2 Modelling in biomedical engineering

A model is a representation of the actual system. As such, all models are incomplete and therefore inaccurate. This is because of the various assumptions and approximations that must be made to make the models practical and numerically tractable. A model that accounts for all the factors and parameters may be more complete but is impractical due to the difficulty in solving them. On the other hand, a model that makes numerous assumptions and approximations may be oversimplified and cannot represent accurately the actual system.

Despite these shortcomings, mathematical and computational modelling play an important role in the study of biomedical engineering. Models allow complex physical processes of the human body and their interactions to be described through elegantly derived mathematical formulations and equations, albeit with underlying assumptions and approximations. These mathematical models have not only led to better understanding of biological systems, but also the ability to predict the outcome of a given system. The latter is particularly useful in disease diagnosis and protocol planning of various treatments.

There are several advantages of using mathematical and computational modelling in biomedical engineering. Firstly, experimental studies involving the human body are very difficult if not impossible to conduct. This procedure is often complicated by the requirement for human ethics approval before any experimentation can begin. Secondly, variability in the anatomy and physiology among different individuals can complicate the results analysis, making the process of identifying patterns and trends extremely tricky. In contrast, modelling is not affected by these restrictions. Thirdly, computational models provide users with better control of all the variables of interest, which is important for the reproducibility and repeatability of the numerical results. These variables can be altered to understand the causality between the variables and the outcome, thus making computational models useful prediction tools. Fourthly, mathematical and computational modelling allow the isolation of subsystems from the entire system. This can be done at both the macro- and microscale. Lastly, model-based studies are less costly than their experimental-based counterparts. This is especially true in biomedical engineering, where specialised equipment may be required to carry out different types of measurements needed for a particular experiment.

It is worth pointing out that numerically solving complex mathematical models is no longer a critical issue today compared to how it was a decade ago. The advancement in computational technology, and the advent of high-performance computers have allowed complex and sophisticated models to be solved within reasonable time. Furthermore, improvements in the computational capabilities of domestic computers have allowed more researchers to venture into this field without the financial burden that comes with securing large and powerful workstations. As a result, mathematical and computational modelling is now regarded as a well-established technique that complement experimental and clinical studies in biomedical engineering.

1.3 Modelling approaches in biomedical engineering

There are two approaches one may take when modelling problems in biomedical engineering, namely, (1) mechanistic modelling and (2) physiological modelling. Mechanistic models describe the physical processes within a biological system using well-established principles of physics, engineering and biology. The domain of interest is often localised to a small region of the tissue and, in some cases, form a subset of a larger biological system (Baker *et al* 2018). Physiological models describe the physiological processes of a biological system, such as the respiratory system and the cardiovascular system, by partitioning it into a series of compartments, where each compartment interacts with the others through an established set of mathematical relationships (Clairambault 2013).

There is a common misconception on whether physiological and phenomenological models represent the same thing. Phenomenological models are models that seek to describe the relationship of the variables within a data set (Clairambault 2013). In most cases, the models are derived empirically to best describe the relationship without strict adherence to the fundamental laws of nature, unlike mechanistic and physiological models. In the context of this book, phenomenological models are not the same as physiological models.

Both mechanistic and physiological models can be constructed to describe the same system inside the human body. For example, a mechanistic model of the cardiovascular system may choose to isolate the specific regions of interest such as the aorta to model blood flow in these regions (Benim *et al* 2011, Pirola *et al* 2017). This is illustrated in figure 1.1(a). Physiological models on the other hand, may

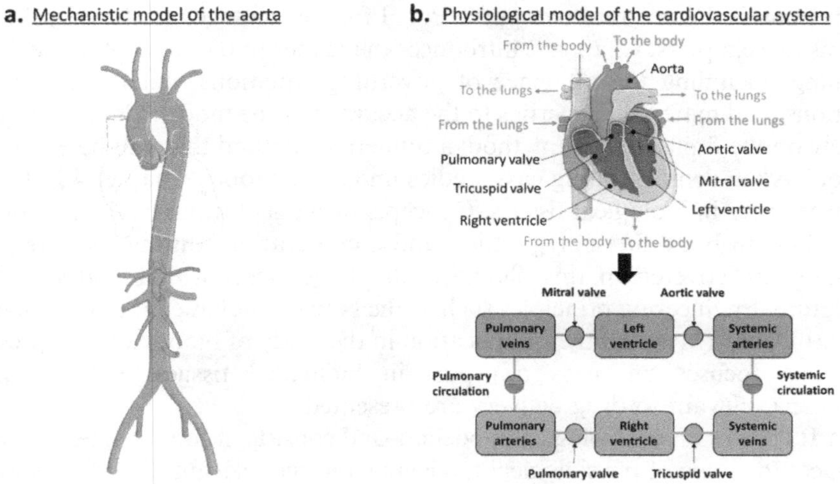

Figure 1.1. Comparison between (a) a mechanistic model of the aorta and (b) a physiological model of the cardiovascular system. Both models describe the cardiovascular system but differently. The mechanistic model in this case isolates the aorta from the heart for blood flow analysis. The physiological model describes flow through the entire cardiovascular system. Copyright © smart.servier.com. The figure was partly generated using Servier Medical Art, provided by Servier, licensed under a Creative Commons Attribution 3.0 unported license.

choose to compartmentalise the cardiovascular system into several blocks, where the variables of interest are defined at specific points called nodes (Shi *et al* 2018, Zheng *et al* 2018). Each block can represent a single element, a cardiac chamber or vascular resistance. This is shown in figure 1.1(b).

It is clear from the example above that mechanistic and physiological models describe very differently the physical processes that occur within the same biological system, in this case, the cardiovascular system. Hence, a question that is of relevance is:

'When should a mechanistic model be chosen over a physiological model and vice versa?'

Unfortunately, there is no straightforward answer. The choice between a mechanistic and a physiological model is circumstantial and ultimately depends on the system that is to be represented. Both mechanistic and physiological modelling contribute equally to the study of biomedical engineering. As such, when discussing model-based approaches in biomedical engineering, it is important to consider both modelling approaches and how they are applied within the context. Whether a mechanistic model is more accurate than a physiological model is a moot point since both models describe biological systems very differently.

The purpose of this book is therefore to present the two abovementioned model-based approaches and their applications in biomedical engineering. These modelling approaches are conveyed through the consideration of various topics in biology and medicine. Each topic is conveyed through the ordinary and partial differential equations that describe the problem, and their solutions are demonstrated through the utilisation of appropriate numerical strategy.

This book is divided into two parts. Part I focuses on mechanistic modelling and contains five chapters. Chapter 2 introduces the reader to the concept of mechanistic modelling, including the influence of governing equations, initial and boundary conditions, and material properties to the accuracy of the model. Chapter 3 presents a review on the finite element method; a numerical method that will be employed in this book when demonstrating case studies under each topic. Chapter 4 is dedicated to heat transfer in biological tissues. Concepts of bioheat transfer, the role of blood flow in human body thermoregulation and considerations during bioheat transfer modelling are covered in this chapter. Chapter 5 deals with blood flow in the vasculature. Engineering principles such as the Navier–Stokes equations, Poiseuille's flow and Darcy's law, and their application in the study of blood flow are presented. Chapter 6 focuses on mass transport in biological tissues. Solute transport phenomena relevant to drug delivery are presented.

Part II focuses on physiological modelling and consists of four chapters. Chapter 7 introduces the topic of physiological modelling and the relevant disciplines surrounding it. The chapter continues with fundamental theories required to perform model fitting. Examples of model identification with data presentation, data analytics and interpretation will be presented. Chapter 8 focuses on human glucose–insulin system. It dives into human endocrine system, metabolism, followed by blood glucose level regulation. The minimal model and other complex modelling of the human glucose–insulin interaction are presented. At the end of the chapter, modern medical technology, and treatment capable of regulating diabetic patients' glucose level are presented. Chapter 9 deals with the human respiratory system. Gas transport and the diffusion process into blood are presented and modelled via the compartment model. The effect of impaired respiratory system, and the need of breathing apparatus, such as a mechanical ventilator to support the patient's work of breathing will be presented. Chapter 10 introduces readers to the human cardiovascular system, with an overview of the three-chamber and six-chamber models. The chapter then follows through with technology used to monitor and regulate the health of the human cardiovascular system. An overview of ethics and biosafety, two important concepts in biomedical engineering, is provided in chapter 11.

References

Armentano R L and Kun L 2019 Leonardo da Vinci—the first bioengineer: educational innovation to meet his desire for knowledge and promote his concept of interdisciplinarity *Creat. Educ.* **10** 1180–91

Baker R E, Peña J-M, Jayamohan J and Jérusalem A 2018 Mechanistic models versus machine learning, a fight worth fighting for the biological community? *Biol. Lett.* **14** 20170660

Benim A C, Nahavandi A, Assmann A, Schubert D, Feindt P and Suh S H 2011 Simulation of blood flow in human aorta with emphasis on outlet boundary conditions *Appl. Math. Model.* **35** 3175–88

Clairambault J 2013 Phenomenological vs physiological modeling ed W Dubitzky, O Wolkenhauer, K H Cho and H Yokota *Encyclopedia of Systems Biology* (New York: Springer)

Kron T and Krishnan P 2019 Leonardo da Vinci's contributions to medical physics and biomedical engineering: celebrating the life of a 'Polymath' *Australas. Phys. Eng. Sci. Med.* **42** 403–5

Pirola S, Cheng Z, Jarral O A, O'Regan D P, Pepper J R, Athanasiou T and Xu X Y 2017 On the choice of outlet boundary conditions for patient-specific analysis of aortic flow using computational fluid dynamics *J. Biomech.* **60** 15–21

Shi Y, Lawford P and Hose D R 2018 Construction of lumped-parameter cardiovascular models using the CellML language *J. Med. Eng. Technol.* **42** 525–31

Zheng D, Yin M, Fan X, Yang X and Luo X 2018 A patient-specific lumped-parameter model of coronary circulation *Sci. Rep.* **8** 874

IOP Publishing

Model-Based Approaches in Biomedical Engineering

Ean Hin Ooi and Yeong Shiong Chiew

Chapter 2

Mechanistic modelling

2.1 Background

Mechanistic modelling in biomedical engineering is defined as the model representation of one or more physical processes within a biological system. These models
are described using mathematical formulations and analytical expressions that are
typically derived based on fundamental laws of physics and biology, and through
observations of the physical mechanisms of interest (Baker *et al* 2018). For example,
different bioheat transfer models have been derived based on physical observations
of tissue anatomy and their contribution to heat transfer in biological tissues.
Upon validation, these models can be used as predictive tools to investigate how
certain variables respond to changes in the input parameters (Stalidzans *et al* 2020).
Mechanistic models are particularly useful in studies where experiments are too
difficult or costly to execute. They can be as simple as having one differential
equation that describes the output variable in response to an input variable, or one
that is highly complex such that the model is governed by multiple variables and
parameters. The latter is typically the case when the biophysical mechanisms to be
described are of a highly sophisticated nature.

An example of a biophysical model is the thermal damage model of Henriques Jr
and Moritz (1947); an ordinary differential equation (ODE) that relates the rate of
thermal damage formation ($d\Omega/dt$) with three input parameters, namely temperature, T (K), frequency factor, A (s^{-1}) and activation energy, ΔE (J mol^{-1}). This
model is mathematically expressed as:

$$\frac{d\Omega}{dt} = A\exp\left(-\frac{\Delta E}{RT}\right), \tag{2.1}$$

where R (J (mol·K)$^{-1}$) is the universal gas constant. As pointed out above, the
relationships described using mechanistic models are based on natural laws, and in
the case of equation (2.1), is based on the Arrhenius first order reaction kinetics.

Knowing the values of A and ΔE for a particular cell line allows one to use equation (2.1) to predict the rate of thermal damage formation at a given temperature T.

Of course, mechanistic models can be more complicated than what is shown in equation (2.1), even when describing the same physical process. For example, the three-state cell death model derived by O'Neill *et al* (2011), which is described by the pair of ODEs:

$$\frac{dA}{dt} = -\overline{k}_\text{f}\exp\left(\frac{T}{T_\text{k}}\right)A(1 - A) + k_\text{b}(1 - A - D), \tag{2.2}$$

$$\frac{dD}{dt} = -\overline{k}_\text{f}\exp\left(\frac{T}{T_\text{k}}\right)(1 - A)(1 - A - D), \tag{2.3}$$

also describes the formation of thermal damage; however, it is more complicated than the model of Henriques Jr and Moritz (1947). In this case, the model defined by equations (2.2) and (2.3) relates two output variables A and D with four input variables $\overline{k}_\text{f}$ (s^{-1}), k_b (s^{-1}), T (°C) and T_k (°C).

Equation (2.1), and equations (2.2) and (2.3) represent two of the many examples illustrating how a physical process can be described using different mechanistic models. The choice on the level of complexity of the model depends on various factors including the degree of accuracy required and the availability of resources that are needed to solve the model.

2.2 Fundamentals of mechanistic modelling

The typical steps involved in the development of a mechanistic model may be generalised based on the flow chart illustrated in figure 2.1. Each step will be explained in the subsections below.

2.2.1 Problem definition

The first step in any mechanistic model development is to define the problem that is to be solved. Details including the objective(s) of why the model is needed should be made clear. This is because such information is important in determining the complexity of the model required.

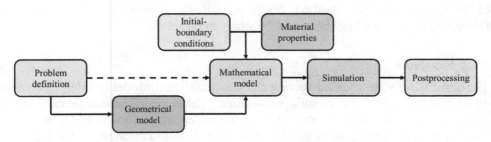

Figure 2.1. Flow chart depicting the general steps involved in mechanistic modelling.

2.2.2 Geometrical model

Once the problem is defined, the user can proceed to construct the geometrical model to represent the problem. As pointed out earlier, the complexity of the model will depend on the problem and the degree of accuracy required. A model that is very intricate can be difficult to solve, while a model that is oversimplified may not accurately represent the actual problem. Consequently, a very clear definition of the problem is required to balance the requirement for model complexity and accuracy. For example, if the objective is to determine the flow profile of blood within the aorta, then one may choose to construct only the model of the aorta and not the entire heart. In this case, the simplification of the model geometry to only the aorta reduces its complexity while at the same time, not significantly sacrificing on the accuracy.

It is worth mentioning that a geometrical representation is not always required. For instance, the cell death models presented in equations (2.1)–(2.3) do not require a geometry to be defined because the unknown variables are independent of space. In this case, this step is skipped, and one may proceed to the next step (see dashed arrow in figure 2.1).

2.2.3 Mathematical model

The equations describing the physics of the problem are selected in this step. The type of equation depends on the nature of the problem. A problem that centres around heat transfer in biological tissues can be described using the bioheat transfer equation, while one that centres around fluid flow phenomena will likely involve the Navier–Stokes equations. As demonstrated in section 2.1, the same problem can be described using different governing equations.

Once the governing equation(s) is selected, the initial and boundary conditions pertaining to the problem are prescribed. Initial conditions are mathematical expressions that describe the initial state of the problem. Boundary conditions are mathematical expressions that define the conditions at the boundary of the model. Different problems may require different initial and boundary conditions, even if the model geometry and the governing equations are identical. The last component of the mathematical model step is to input values of all relevant material properties that describe the governing equations and the boundary conditions.

It is important to point out that the accuracy of a model depends on the accuracy of the imposed initial condition, boundary conditions and the selected material properties in representing the actual problem to be solved.

2.2.4 Simulation

The simulation step involves solving the computational model (model, governing equations, and initial and boundary conditions) developed. This can be carried out using various numerical methods, such as finite element method (FEM), boundary element method (BEM), finite volume method (FVM) and meshless method, among others. Depending on the problem, it may be more advantageous to use one numerical method over another. Nevertheless, FEM is one of the most established numerical methods for solving engineering problems computationally and will be the main numerical method adopted in this book. Implementation of the numerical method can be carried out using self-written codes or using commercial software, such as COMSOL Multiphysics, ANSYS and ABAQUS.

2.2.5 Post-processing

Upon completion of the numerical simulation, visualisation of the results can be carried out in the post-processing step.

2.3 Ocular heat transfer: an illustrative example

To demonstrate the steps in section 2.2, an example based on the study of ocular heat transfer is presented. The considerations taken in each of the steps outlined in figure 2.1 with respect to the study of ocular heat transfer will be elaborated in detail.

2.3.1 Problem definition

We wish to describe the steady state temperature distribution across the human eye under resting conditions.

2.3.2 Geometrical model

A model of the human eye is constructed for this purpose. Since we are interested only in the temperature distribution inside the eye, we may assume the eyeball to be isolated from the human head. Inside the eye, we may choose to include only the major ocular components, such as the cornea, aqueous humour, lens, iris, vitreous, retina and sclera. One may opt to construct the model in 3D (Ooi *et al* 2009); however, to help reduce the requirement for computational resources, a 2D axisymmetry model with the pupillary axis representing the axis of symmetry can also be developed (Ooi *et al* 2008). The shape and the dimensions of the eye can be derived from the literature. Alternatively, a model reconstruction based on the medical images such as MRI and CT scans can be employed. Figure 2.2 illustrates the model of the human eye in 3D and in 2D axisymmetry. Note that the rotation of the 2D geometry around the pupillary axis results in the 3D geometry of the human eye.

2.3.3 Mathematical model

Once the model has been developed, we proceed to select the governing equations that describe the heat transfer process inside the eye. Since the problem involves heat transfer in biological tissues, we may choose the bioheat transfer equation. Several bioheat transfer models are available, such as the Pennes model, Wulff model, Klinger model and porous medium model[1]. The choice of which model to use can be decided based on how appropriate these models are in describing the problem.

---

[1] The different bioheat transfer models will be discussed in chapter 4.

3D model

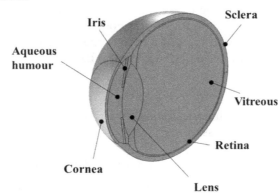

2D axisymmetry model

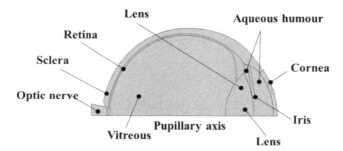

Figure 2.2. Model of the human eye in 3D (only half the model is shown) and in 2D axisymmetry. A 1D representation in this case is also possible and would be the representation of the different eye components along the pupillary axis.

In this case, we will choose the Pennes model due to the simplicity of its formulation. In steady state, the Pennes model is given by:

$$k_t \nabla^2 T_t + \rho_b c_b \omega_b (T_b - T_t) + \dot{Q}_m = 0, \qquad (2.4)$$

where T (K) is temperature, k_t (W (m·K)$^{-1}$) is tissue thermal conductivity, ρ_b (kg m^{-3}) is blood density, c_b (J (kg·K)$^{-1}$) is blood specific heat, ω_b (s^{-1}) is blood perfusion rate, T_b (K) is arterial blood temperature, and $\dot{Q}_m$ (W m^{-3}) is the rate of volumetric heat generated due to tissue metabolic activity. Note that the second term on the left-hand side of equation (2.4) vanishes in components of the human eye that are avascular (lacks blood supply), such as the cornea, aqueous humour, lens, vitreous and sclera, since $\omega_b = 0$ in these tissues.

Once the governing equation has been determined, the initial condition and boundary conditions that describe the problem are prescribed. The initial condition describes the condition at the start of simulation. Here, it is reasonable to assume that the temperature of the human eye is uniform at 37 °C.[2] Boundary conditions depend on the conditions assumed for the model. Let us assume that the corneal surface is exposed to the ambient that has a temperature lower than that of the corneal surface. Assuming heat transfer from the corneal surface to the ambient occurs via convection, radiation, and tears evaporation, we obtain (Ng and Ooi 2006):

$$-k_t \frac{\partial T_t}{\partial n} = h_{amb}(T - T_{amb}) + \varepsilon\sigma(T^4 - T_{amb}^4) + E_{vap}, \qquad (2.5)$$

where $\partial T_t/\partial n$ (K m^{-1}) is the tissue temperature gradient in the outward direction normal to the surface, h_{amb} (W (m^2·K)$^{-1}$) is the ambient convection heat transfer coefficient, T_{amb} (K) is ambient temperature, ε (dimensionless) is the corneal surface emissivity, σ (W (m^2·K^4)$^{-1}$) is the Stefan–Boltzmann constant and E_{vap} (W m^{-2}) is the heat loss from the corneal surface to the ambient due to tears evaporation.

To describe the boundary condition across the scleroid surface, we assume the eyeball, except for the corneal surface, to be embedded in an anatomically homogeneous surrounding that is at body temperature to mimic its position inside the eye socket. Convection heat transfer between the surrounding and the scleroid surface is assumed, such that (Lagendijk 1982):

$$-k_t \frac{\partial T_t}{\partial n} = h_{bl}(T - T_{body}), \qquad (2.6)$$

where h_{bl} (W (m^2·K)$^{-1}$) is the convection heat transfer coefficient between the homogeneous surrounding and the scleroid surface, and T_{body} (K) is the body temperature. Equations (2.5) and (2.6) represent the boundary conditions needed to complete the mathematical formulation.

Next, values of the material properties, such as thermal conductivity, density, specific heat, and the other parameters that describe equations (2.4)–(2.6) must be obtained and supplied to the model. At this point, it is important to recall from section 2.2.3 that the accuracy of the model developed depends on the initial condition, boundary conditions and the material properties. This is evident from how equations (2.5) and (2.6) were obtained, which were based on assumptions of the physical processes that occur at the respective surfaces. Hence, a poorly approximated boundary condition can lead to models that do not accurately mimic the actual problem.

2.3.4 Simulation

The model geometry, the governing equation, and the initial and boundary conditions can be solved using any of the numerical methods mentioned in section 2.2.4. FEM represents a practical choice due to its capability in handling models with irregular geometries such as the human eye (Tiang and Ooi 2016, Loke *et al* 2018). Nevertheless, other types of numerical methods have also been used in the

---

[2] The initial condition does not really matter in a steady state simulation but is included here for completeness.

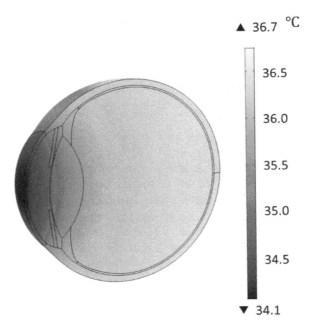

Figure 2.3. Contours of temperature (°C) across the human eye obtained from solving equations (2.4)–(2.6) utilising values of material properties sourced from the literature.

study of the human eye, including BEM (Ooi *et al* 2008, Ooi and Ng 2011), FVM (Kumar *et al* 2006, Wang *et al* 2016) and the coupled BEM-meshless method (Ooi and Popov 2014).

2.3.5 Post-processing

Once the model has been solved, the results can be presented, visualised, and analysed as part of the post-processing step. Figure 2.3 illustrates the temperature distribution across the human eye obtained using a 3D representation of the actual human eye.

2.4 Important considerations in mechanistic modelling

As with all computational models, the result obtained from the predictions of a mechanistic model is only an approximation of the actual physical phenomenon. This is due to the assumptions made during the modelling process, which may include those made when specifying the initial and boundary conditions, and when selecting values of the material properties. This aspect of modelling should be kept in mind when interpreting the results obtained from the simulations.

For the ocular heat transfer example presented above, it should be noted that the temperature profile illustrated in figure 2.3 is only an approximation of the temperature distribution inside the actual human eye due to the several assumptions that were made when constructing the model. By considering only the eyeball and the components inside, we have neglected the effects of eyelids on the heat loss from the corneal surface to the ambient. Furthermore, a steady state representation of heat transfer inside the eye meant that the thermal effects due to blinking were not considered. Despite these assumptions, the results obtained from the model showed very good agreement when compared against experimentally obtained temperatures on the corneal surface.

It is impossible to avoid making assumptions when modelling biophysical processes. The goal is therefore to ensure that the assumptions made are reasonable and justifiable within the context of the problem, and one way to substantiate this is by performing model validation against experimental studies whenever possible. If a one-to-one model validation is not possible, then a model verification study that can support the accuracy of the physics and the reliability of the model prediction should be carried out.

2.5 Summary

This chapter demonstrates the fundamental steps involved in constructing a mechanistic model for the study of biological systems and their processes. As we will show in subsequent chapters of this book, the construction of biophysical models will adopt similar steps as those presented in this chapter. As with all computational models, mechanistic models represent only an approximation to the actual phenomena, with the accuracy determined by the assumptions made specifically to the boundary conditions and the material properties employed. Experimental validation and verification of the mechanistic models are important steps that should be carried out to raise confidence in the accuracy and reliability of the models and numerical results.

References

Baker R E, Peña J-M, Jayamohan J and Jérusalem A 2018 Mechanistic models versus machine learning, a fight worth fighting for the biological community? *Biol. Lett.* **14** 20170660

Henriques F Jr and Moritz A 1947 Studies of thermal injury: I. The conduction of heat to and through skin and the temperatures attained therein. A theoretical and an experimental investigation *Am. J. Pathol.* **23** 530–49

Kumar S, Acharya S, Beuerman R and Palkama A 2006 Numerical solution of ocular fluid dynamics in a rabbit eye: parametric effects *Ann. Biomed. Eng.* **34** 530–44

Lagendijk J J W 1982 A mathematical model to calculate temperature distributions in human and rabbit eyes during hyperthermic treatment *Phys. Med. Biol.* **27** 1301–11

Loke C Y, Ooi E H, Salahudeen M S, Ramli N and Samsudin A 2018 Segmental aqueous humour outflow and eye orientation have strong influence on ocular drug delivery *Appl. Math. Model.* **57** 474–91

Ng E Y K and Ooi E H 2006 FEM simulation of the eye structure with bioheat analysis *Comput. Methods Programs Biomed.* **82** 268–76

O'Neill D P, Peng T, Stiegler P, Mayrhauser U, Koestenbauer S, Tscheiliennssnigg K and Payne S J 2011 A three-state mathematical model of hyperthermic cell death *Ann. Biomed. Eng.* **39** 570–9

Ooi E H, Ang W T and Ng E Y K 2008 A boundary element model of the human eye undergoing laser-thermokeratoplasty *Comput. Biol. Med.* **38** 727–37

Ooi E H, Ang W T and Ng E Y K 2009 A boundary element model for investigating the effects of eye tumor on the temperature distribution inside the human eye *Comput. Biol. Med.* **39** 667–77

Ooi E H and Ng E Y K 2011 Effects of natural convection within the anterior chamber on the ocular heat transfer *Int. J. Numer. Meth. Biomed. Eng.* **27** 408–23

Ooi E H and Popov V 2014 An efficient hybrid BEM–RBIE method for solving conjugate heat transfer problems *Comput. Math. Appl.* **66** 2489–503

Stalidzans E *et al* 2020 Mechanistic modelling and multiscale applications for precision medicine: theory and practice *Netw. Syst. Med.* **3** 36–56

Tiang K L and Ooi E H 2016 Effects of aqueous humor hydrodynamics on human eye heat transfer under external heat sources *Med. Eng. Phys.* **38** 776–84

Wang W, Qian X, Song H, Zhang M and Liu Z 2016 Fluid and structure coupling analysis of the interaction between aqueous humor and iris *Biomed. Eng. Online* **15** 133

Chapter 3

Review of the finite element method

3.1 Introduction

Numerical method plays an important role in the modelling of biomedical engineering problems. This is largely due to the irregular geometry of biological organs (see the human eye model developed in chapter 2 for example) and the mathematical complexity of the governing equations, which prevent the problem from being solved analytically. Among the various numerical methods that are available, the finite element method (FEM) is one of the most well-known and established, with many commercial software, such in ANSYS, ABAQUS and COMSOL Multiphysics adopting this technique as their numerical solvers. The solutions to the case studies presented in this book were obtained using FEM, which were implemented using COMSOL Multiphysics. Therefore, the purpose of this chapter is to provide some background information on FEM to facilitate readers in transitioning from the theories and concepts introduced in subsequent chapters to their applications in COMSOL Multiphysics.

The general idea behind FEM is to discretize the model into smaller domains known as *finite elements*. The governing equation(s) is then re-casted into its weak form and is expressed for each element in terms of unknown nodal values. Unknown variables across each element are approximated using basis functions that are defined across the nodes of the element. The equations from all elements are then assembled into a system of equations along with the initial and boundary conditions that define the problem. This system of equations can be solved to yield the values of the unknown variables at all the nodes.

The steps above will be presented and discussed in more detail in the subsequent sections. As stated above, this chapter will provide only the important steps in FEM and is not meant to be a complete guide to the method. For more details, readers are advised to consult specific textbooks on the subject. The textbook by Zienkiewicz *et al* (2013) is a great starting point.

3.2 Weighted residual method

The weighted residual method is the starting point of the development of the FEM. To demonstrate the concept behind the weighted residual method, let us consider the Poisson equation given by:

$$\nabla^2 u(\mathbf{x}) = b(\mathbf{x}), \quad \text{in } \Omega \cup \Gamma \tag{3.1}$$

where u is the unknown variable to be solved, b is a known function of space, Ω represents the spatial domain that is bounded by the boundary Γ and x is the spatial coordinate. The term ∇^2 in equation (3.1) represents the Laplacian operator, which is given by:

$$\nabla^2 \equiv \frac{d^2}{dx^2} \text{ in 1D}, \quad \nabla^2 \equiv \frac{\partial^2}{\partial x^2} + \frac{\partial^2}{\partial y^2} \text{ in 2D}, \quad \nabla^2 \equiv \frac{\partial^2}{\partial x^2} + \frac{\partial^2}{\partial y^2} + \frac{\partial^2}{\partial z^2} \text{ in 3D}.$$

The following boundary conditions are applied:

$$u(\mathbf{x}) = u_0, \quad \text{in } \Gamma_1 \tag{3.2}$$

$$\frac{\partial u(\mathbf{x})}{\partial n} = q_0, \quad \text{in } \Gamma_2 \tag{3.3}$$

where u_0 and q_0 are suitably prescribed functions, and Γ_1 and Γ_2 are two non-intersecting parts of Γ such that $\Gamma_1 \cup \Gamma_2 = \Gamma$. This is shown in figure 3.1.

Let $\bar{u}(\mathbf{x})$ be the approximate solution of equation (3.1) subject to the boundary conditions in equations (3.2) and (3.3). Substituting $\bar{u}(\mathbf{x})$ into equation (3.1) and re-arranging the terms, one obtains:

$$\nabla^2 \bar{u}(\mathbf{x}) - b(\mathbf{x}) = R, \tag{3.4}$$

where R is the residual, which quantifies the error of the approximated solution. Since $\bar{u}(\mathbf{x})$ is only an approximation of the actual solution, we have $\bar{u}(\mathbf{x}) \neq u(\mathbf{x})$, such that $R \neq 0$ in Ω. However, it is possible to distribute the residual across the solution domain so that they become zero in an average sense. This can be achieved by multiplying the residual with a series of linearly independent test functions $\varphi_m(\mathbf{x})$,

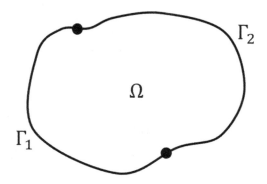

Figure 3.1. Illustration of the 2D domain Ω and the surrounding boundary Γ.

also known as the weighting functions, and integrating it over the entire domain, such that:

$$\int_\Omega \varphi_m(\mathbf{x})R \, d\Omega = 0. \tag{3.5}$$

Substituting the expression for R in equation (3.5) with the expression on the left-hand side of equation (3.4), and after some mathematical re-arrangements, one obtains:

$$\int_\Omega \varphi_m(\mathbf{x})\nabla^2\bar{u}(\mathbf{x}) \, d\Omega = \int_\Omega \varphi_m(\mathbf{x})b(\mathbf{x}) \, d\Omega. \tag{3.6}$$

Integrating by parts the left-hand side of equation (3.6) leads to:

$$\int_\Gamma [\nabla\bar{u}(\mathbf{x}) \cdot \mathbf{n}]\varphi_m(\mathbf{x}) \, d\Gamma - \int_\Omega \nabla\varphi_m(\mathbf{x}) \cdot \nabla\bar{u}(\mathbf{x}) \, d\Omega = \int_\Omega \varphi_m(\mathbf{x})b(\mathbf{x}) \, d\Omega, \tag{3.7}$$

where $\mathbf{n}$ is the unit normal vector pointing outward of the boundary Γ.

Equation (3.7) represents the weak form of equation (3.1) and is the foundation to the formulation of the FEM.

3.3 Finite element method

The starting point of FEM is to discretise the solution domain into a series of smaller subdomains known as finite elements. Supposed that the domain Ω is discretised into N number of elements, such that $\Omega = \Omega_1 \cup \Omega_2 \cup \cdots \cup \Omega_{N-1} \cup \Omega_N$. The weak form of the governing equation (see equation (3.7)) can thus be expressed for each element Ω_i:

$$\int_{\Gamma_i} [\nabla\bar{u}(\mathbf{x}) \cdot \mathbf{n}]\varphi_m(\mathbf{x}) \, d\Gamma - \int_{\Omega_i} \nabla\varphi_m(\mathbf{x}) \cdot \nabla\bar{u}(\mathbf{x}) \, d\Omega = \int_{\Omega_i} \varphi_m(\mathbf{x})b(\mathbf{x}) \, d\Omega, \tag{3.8}$$

where Γ_i is the boundary enclosing the element Ω_i, for $i=1, 2,..., N - 1, N$. The approximate solution $u(x)$ is now expressed across each element Ω_i and can be written as a linear combination of a set of trial basis functions, $\psi_j(\mathbf{x})$:

$$\bar{u}(\mathbf{x}) = \sum_{j=1}^{M} \psi_j(\mathbf{x})u_j, \tag{3.9}$$

where u_j are the values of $\bar{u}(\mathbf{x})$ evaluated at the nodes of each element (see section 3.4) and M is the number of sampling points that depends on the type and order of the element.

3.4 Finite element mesh

The type of finite element or mesh depends on the dimension of the problem. They can be lines or curves in 1D, triangles or quadrilaterals in 2D, and tetrahedrons or hexahedrons in 3D. These are shown in figure 3.2. It is noteworthy that other types

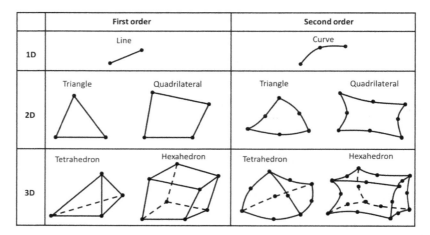

Figure 3.2. First and second order finite elements in 1D, 2D and 3D. Black circles represent nodes of each element. Note that other 3D elements such as brick, prismatic and pyramidal are also available but are not shown here.

of 3D elements not shown in figure 3.2 also exist including brick, prismatic and pyramidal elements.

Each element is defined by a set of points known as *nodes*. Nodes serve as sampling points at which the field variables of interest are calculated (see equation (3.9)). The number of nodes in each element varies depending on the type and the order of the elements. For example, a first order (linear) triangular element consists of three nodes, while a second order (quadratic) triangular element consists of six nodes. The higher the order of elements, the larger the number of nodes and the larger the number of unknowns to be solved. However, this does not imply that higher order elements should be avoided in order to conserve computational resources, as these elements typically allow curved geometries and approximations to the physical variable to be modelled more accurately than lower order elements.

Figure 3.3 shows how the same domain Ω in figure 3.1 can be discretised into first order triangular and first order quadrilateral elements. The choice between triangles and quadrilaterals in 2D, and between tetrahedrons and hexahedrons in 3D, depends on the nature of the problem. Likewise, the order of element used is influenced by the problem and the type of elements. For example, first order triangles (tetrahedrons in 3D) are known to produce very bad approximation when solving structural mechanics problems due to the constant approximation of stress and strain across each element. On the other hand, second order elements may lead to convergence issue when employed to solve problems containing convective terms (Cook *et al* 2001).

3.5 Trial basis (shape) functions

The trial basis functions, $\psi_j(\mathbf{x})$ in equation (3.9) are known as shape functions in FEM. In theory, any functions can be chosen as the trial basis functions; however, in

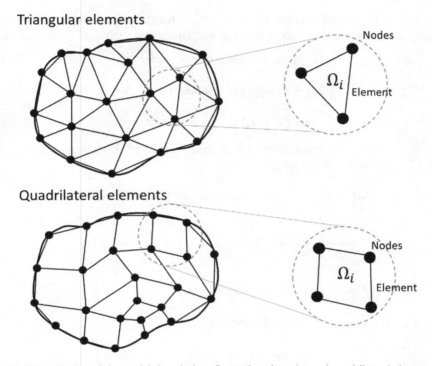

Figure 3.3. Discretisation of the model domain into first order triangular and quadrilateral elements. Each element is defined by a set of nodes.

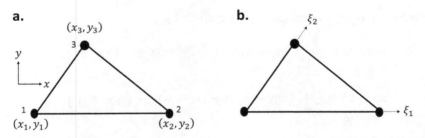

Figure 3.4. The triangular element in the (a) Cartesian coordinates (x,y) and (b) parameterised coordinates (ξ_1, ξ_2).

FEM, it is common to select polynomial basis functions. To demonstrate how these functions are derived, let us consider a first order triangular element defined by three nodes with coordinates (x_1, y_1), (x_2, y_2) and (x_3, y_3). This is shown in figure 3.4(a).

If the approximate solution $\bar{u}(\mathbf{x})$ is assumed to vary linearly across the triangular element, one has:

$$\bar{u}(x, y) = a + bx + cy, \tag{3.10}$$

where a, b and c are the coefficients of the linear function that can be determined by applying equation (3.10) to each node of the triangular element. Doing so yields:

$$u_1 = \bar{u}(x_1, y_1) = a + bx_1 + cy_1, \tag{3.11}$$

$$u_2 = \bar{u}(x_2, y_2) = a + bx_2 + cy_2, \tag{3.12}$$

$$u_3 = \bar{u}(x_3, y_3) = a + bx_3 + cy_3, \tag{3.13}$$

where u_1, u_2 and u_3 are the values of $\bar{u}$ at nodes 1, 2 and 3, respectively. Equations (3.11)–(3.13) can be solved to give:

$$a = \frac{1}{2A}\left[u_1(x_2y_3 - x_3y_2) + u_2(x_3y_1 - x_1y_3) + u_3(x_1y_2 - x_2y_1)\right], \tag{3.14}$$

$$b = \frac{1}{2A}\left[u_1(y_2 - y_3) + u_2(y_3 - y_1) + u_3(y_1 - y_2)\right], \tag{3.15}$$

$$c = \frac{1}{2A}[u_1(x_2 - x_3) + u_2(x_3 - x_1) + u_3(x_1 - x_2)], \tag{3.16}$$

where A is the area of the triangle given by:

$$A = \frac{1}{2}\left[(x_3 - x_2)y_1 + (x_1 - x_3)y_2 + (x_2 - x_1)y_3\right]. \tag{3.17}$$

Substituting equations (3.14)–(3.17) into (3.10) yields:

$$u(x, y) = \psi_1(x, y)u_1 + \psi_2(x, y)u_2 + \psi_3(x, y)u_3, \tag{3.18}$$

where $\psi_1(x, y)$, $\psi_2(x, y)$ and $\psi_3(x, y)$ are given by:

$$\psi_1(x, y) = \frac{1}{2A}\left[(x_2y_3 - x_3y_2) + (y_2 - y_3)x + (x_3 - x_2)y\right], \tag{3.19}$$

$$\psi_2(x, y) = \frac{1}{2A}\left[(x_3y_1 - x_1y_3) + (y_3 - y_1)x + (x_1 - x_3)y\right], \tag{3.20}$$

$$\psi_3(x, y) = \frac{1}{2A}\left[(x_1y_2 - x_2y_1) + (y_1 - y_2)x + (x_2 - x_1)y\right]. \tag{3.21}$$

Note that the expressions of ψ_1, ψ_2 and ψ_3 in equations (3.19)–(3.21) represent the shape functions of a linear triangular element. In deriving the shape functions above, we have adopted the Cartesian coordinate system (x, y). It is also possible to derive the shape functions using a parameterised coordinate system such as shown in figure 3.4(b). This gives rise to isoparametric elements that not only help to simplify the expressions of the shape functions, but is also a necessity when dealing with higher order triangular elements, quadrilateral elements and 3D elements. The derivations of these shape functions are beyond the scope of this book.

3.6 Galerkin finite element method

At this point, we have not mentioned about the weighting function, $\varphi_m(\mathbf{x})$ in equation (3.8). Although not necessarily a requirement, the weighting functions are typically chosen to have the same expression as the basis functions, such that:

$$\varphi_m(\mathbf{x}) = \psi_j(\mathbf{x}), \quad \text{for } m, j = 1,2, \dots, M-1, M. \tag{3.22}$$

This is known as the Galerkin method, while the finite element algorithm developed from equation (3.22) is referred to as the Galerkin FEM.

Substituting equations (3.9) and (3.22) into (3.8) yields:

$$\sum_{j=1}^{M} \int_{\Gamma_i} \left[u_j \nabla \psi_j(\mathbf{x}) \cdot n \right] \psi_m(\mathbf{x}) \, d\Gamma - \sum_{j=1}^{M} u_j \int_{\Omega_i} \nabla \psi_m(\mathbf{x}) \cdot \nabla \psi_j(\mathbf{x}) \, d\Omega$$

$$= \int_{\Omega_i} \sum_{j=1}^{M} \psi_j(\mathbf{x}) \psi_m(\mathbf{x}) \, b d\Omega, \tag{3.23}$$

where the unknowns are now expressed as u_j through the approximation made in equation (3.9).

Using equation (3.23) and applying the boundary conditions to the relevant nodes, we obtain a system of equations that can be expressed in matrix form as:

$$\mathbf{Au} = \mathbf{b}, \tag{3.24}$$

where $\mathbf{A}$ is the coefficient matrix, $\mathbf{u}$ is a column vector containing all the values of u_j and $\mathbf{b}$ is the column vector of known values. Solving equation (3.24) gives us the value of u_j that are expressed at all the nodes of the finite element mesh. To obtain the value of u at any point x, one may evaluate equation (3.9) using the known values of u_j.

3.7 Mesh convergence

The number of elements used in a finite element simulation is important not only because it controls the accuracy of the numerical solution, but also because the computation time and resources required depend on it. In theory, the larger the number of elements, the better the geometrical representation and the more accurate the results from the numerical simulations. This is demonstrated in figure 3.5, where one may observe how the ellipse at the centre of the domain is better approximated when the element number is increased. However, larger number of elements also result in larger number of unknowns to be solved, which requires longer computation time and greater computational resources.

An important concept in FEM is mesh convergence. A converged mesh is one where the numerical solutions are independent of the mesh size. This may be regarded as the most optimum mesh that balances between numerical accuracy and computational resources requirement. In every finite element simulation, it is important to carry out a mesh convergence test to ensure that the numerical solutions obtained are not influenced by the mesh size. The steps to carry out a mesh

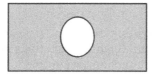 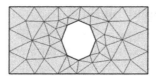 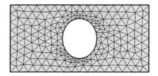

Figure 3.5. The geometrical representation of a model is more accurate as the number of elements is increased. The ellipse is poorly represented when a coarse mesh is used (middle) compared to when a fine mesh (right) is used.

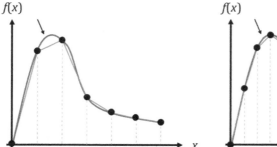 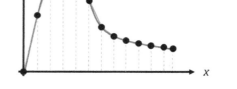

Figure 3.6. Using a refined mesh in the region with high gradients help to capture variation in the function more accurately.

convergence test varies depending on the problem; however, they may be generalised to the following:

1. Start with a particular mesh size and discretise the domain into finite elements.
2. Select the variable that will be used to determine mesh convergence. This can be the values of the physical variables at several predefined points across the domain, or the maximum (or minimum value) of the physical variable. The choice will ultimately depend on what is desired from the problem.
3. Perform the finite element simulation and evaluate the values of the variables selected in step 2.
4. Check if the percentage difference(s) in the solutions between the successive mesh setting is smaller than a given tolerance. If true, then mesh is deemed to have converged. If false, proceed to the next step.
5. Refine the mesh either by increasing the number of elements or by reducing the maximum element size and repeat step 3 until mesh convergence is achieved. Mesh refinement may be carried out globally across their entire domain or locally in regions where large solution gradients are expected.

Meshing is an art, and the ability to generate the best mesh for a given problem comes with experience. Nevertheless, there are several guidelines that one may follow during mesh refinement to improve the quality of the mesh and accuracy of the numerical model. Typically, regions with high solution gradients should be discretised using a finer mesh, while those with low solution gradients can have coarser mesh. The fine mesh is required to accurately capture the rapid change in the solution over a small distance. Figure 3.6 illustrates this concept, where one may

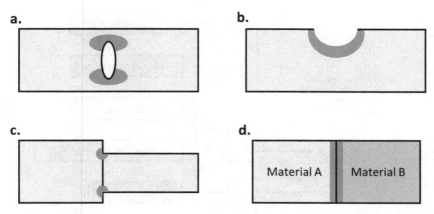

Figure 3.7. Problems where large solution gradients are expected. (a) and (b) sharply curved edges; (c) sudden change in thickness/cross-sectional area; (d) interface between two domains with different material properties. Red represents regions with high field variable gradient.

observe larger error especially in the region where the function gradient is large (see arrow) if the mesh size is not sufficiently small.

Although it is not possible to know beforehand the location of large solution gradients prior to solving the model, there are certain clues to look out for when carrying out mesh refinement. For instance, regions around corners and sharply curved edges tend to give rise to large solution gradients. Regions around domains where there is a sudden change in thickness and cross-sectional area, and the region around the interface between two domains with different material properties are also prone to large solutions gradients. These are illustrated in figure 3.7.

3.8 Finite element method with COMSOL Multiphysics

COMSOL Multiphysics (hereafter referred to simply as COMSOL) is a differential equation calculator that adopts FEM as the numerical solver. The software provides a graphical user interface that allows users to construct the model, select governing equations, impose initial and boundary conditions, carry out finite element simulation, and visualise and analyse the numerical results obtained. These are achieved without the user having to go through the daunting process of writing the numerical codes related to FEM.

As pointed out in section 3.1, other similar FEM software are also available commercially. However, we have opted to present the case studies in this book using COMSOL due to several reasons. Firstly, the ability of COMSOL to efficiently handle multiphysics problems (as the name *Multiphysics* imply), such as heat transfer, fluid flow, electric current flow, and acoustics to name a few, makes it ideal for solving multidisciplinary problems in biomedical engineering. Secondly, it is in our opinion that the interface of COMSOL is user-friendly, which is ideal for novices with very little background on computational modelling. Thirdly, the workflow in COMSOL is very similar to the flow process involved in mechanistic modelling as depicted in figure 2.1. This will be beneficial to readers when relating the contents from this book to the computational models presented in the case

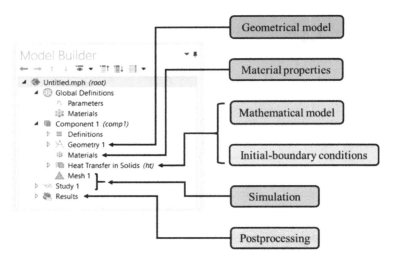

Figure 3.8. Model builder setup in COMSOL and how they relate to the steps involved in mechanistic modelling in chapter 2.

studies. Figure 3.8 shows the model builder setup in COMSOL and how it relates to the different steps involved in the development of a mechanistic model.

3.9 Summary

There are various numerical methods that can be employed to solve the computational models developed in this book. However, FEM is widely regarded as the most established, well-developed, and versatile. In this chapter, we have presented an overview of the framework related to the derivation and development of FEM, which will hopefully assist readers in the subsequent chapters of this book. Although the availability of commercial finite element software has allowed users to bypass the complexity and the tedious task of understanding and developing the numerical codes, a comprehension of the basic concept and the working principles of FEM remains crucial not only to fully exploit the functionality of the software, but also to facilitate debugging of the solvers should convergence issues arise.

References

Cook R D, Malkus D S, Plesha M E and Witt R J 2001 *Concepts and Applications of Finite Element Analysis* 4th edn (New York: Wiley)

Mohsen M F N 1982 Some details of the Galerkin finite element method *Appl. Math. Model.* **6** 165–70

Zienkiewicz O C, Taylor R L and Zhu J Z 2013 *The Finite Element Method: Its Basis and Fundamentals* 7th edn (Oxford: Butterworth-Heinemann)

IOP Publishing

Model-Based Approaches in Biomedical Engineering

Ean Hin Ooi and Yeong Shiong Chiew

Chapter 4

Heat transfer in biological tissues

4.1 Introduction

Heat transfer plays an important role in human body physiology. One example is when doctors measure the body temperature to determine if a patient is unwell. Any deviation of the body temperature from the healthy range of 36.5 °C–37.5 °C is an indication of physiological abnormality. The concept of using temperature as an indicator for human body abnormality is not new. In fact, this view has been known since the 4th century BC, when the Greek physician Hippocrates theorised that:

'Disease is to be found in parts of the body with excess heat or cold'

Today, the concept of heat and cold plays an important role in healthcare and medicine, with applications in a wide range of areas such as medical diagnosis, disease detection, treatment, and therapy. Numerous studies have demonstrated the use of abnormal thermal signatures to detect diseases such as breast cancer (Ekici and Jawzal 2020, Singh and Singh 2020), rheumatism (Gatt *et al* 2019, Tan *et al* 2020), dry eyes (Tan *et al* 2016, Su *et al* 2011), and vascular disorders (Bagavathiappan *et al* 2009, Ilo *et al* 2020). Treatment of various ailments such as thermal ablation of cancer utilises the concept of hyperthermia to induce cellular necrosis in the region of diseased tissue (Xia *et al* 2021, Chung *et al* 2021), while cryotherapy is used to speed up the recovery of muscle injury (Ramos *et al* 2016, Kwiecien and McHugh 2021).

The examples above demonstrate the role of heat transfer in biological tissues and its significance in healthcare and medicine. A good understanding of the thermal transport processes inside biological tissues is therefore important in the context of biomedical engineering, and will be the focus of this chapter. As the contents of this chapter require some background knowledge of heat transfer, readers who are not familiar may refer to appendix A for an overview of the fundamentals of heat transfer.

doi:10.1088/978-0-7503-4016-8ch4

4.2 Thermoregulation

The human body maintains a healthy body temperature of 36.5 °C–37.5 °C through a process known as thermoregulation, which is achieved through the regulation of both tissue metabolic activity and blood perfusion.

4.2.1 Tissue metabolic activity

Tissue metabolism is the process within the cells and tissues whereby useful energy is extracted from chemical bonds and converted into heat (Keener and Sneyd 2009). This process occurs continuously even when the body is at rest. When not at rest, only about 25%–30% of the energy generated from tissue metabolism is used for mechanical work, while the rest is converted to heat (Yu *et al* 1997, Febbraio 2003). This heat is transferred down the tissue temperature gradient and is carried by blood from the capillaries to the veins (Lim 2020). From here, heat is either carried through the vascular system and into the heart, where it is stored to maintain body temperature, or carried to the skin to be released to the environment. This process is shown in figure 4.1.

4.2.2 Blood perfusion

Blood perfusion also plays a significant role in the thermoregulation of the human body. Unlike tissue metabolism, blood does not produce heat. Instead, it acts as a medium that transports heat to and away from the tissue. Thermoregulation via blood perfusion is achieved through *vasodilation* and *vasoconstriction*, depending on the thermal state of the tissue.

As an example, consider the case where the skin tissue is exposed to hyperthermic conditions (conditions that raise the body temperature). In response, blood vessels dilate (vasodilation) to promote greater blood flow, which helps to carry excess heat away from the tissue. Blood perfusion in this case acts as a heat sink. This is shown in figure 4.2(a). On the other hand, when the human skin is exposed to hypothermic

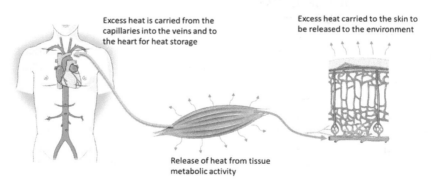

Excess heat is carried from the capillaries into the veins and to the heart for heat storage

Excess heat carried to the skin to be released to the environment

Release of heat from tissue metabolic activity

Figure 4.1. Graphical illustrate of how excess heat generated from tissue metabolism is either circulated back to the heart for heat storage or carried to the skin for release to the environment. Copyright © smart.servier. com. The figure was partly generated using Servier Medical Art, provided by Servier, licensed under a Creative Commons Attribution 3.0 unported license.

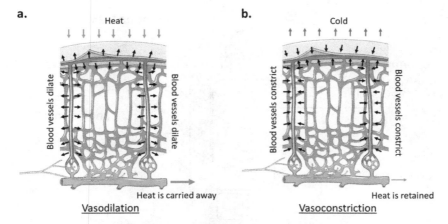

Figure 4.2. Thermoregulation through (a) vasodilation and (b) vasoconstriction in response to heat and cold, respectively. In the former, blood vessels dilate to promote greater flow of blood so that excess heat is carried away from the skin. In the latter, blood vessels constrict to retain heat inside the skin. Copyright © smart. servier.com. The figure was partly generated using Servier Medical Art, provided by Servier, licensed under a Creative Commons Attribution 3.0 unported license.

conditions (conditions that lower the body temperature), blood vessels constrict (vasoconstriction). This reduces blood flow through the skin, which helps to retain heat inside the tissue to maintain the temperature at basal level. This is shown in figure 4.2(b). Blood perfusion in this case acts as a heat source.

4.2.3 Mechanisms of heat exchange through the skin

Tissue metabolism and blood flow represent the two main physiological mechanisms that contribute to the thermoregulation of the human body. When exposed to an environment that disrupts thermoneutrality[1], four heat transfer mechanisms take place across the skin surface, namely conduction, convection, radiation, and evaporation, all of which help to maintain thermostasis[2] (Lim *et al* 2008). This is illustrated in figure 4.3.

Heat conduction takes place when there is physical contact between the skin and another object. This mode of heat transfer is ineffective and contributes to only about 3% of the total heat transfer from the skin surface. Heat convection occurs when the skin is surrounded by moving liquid (water) or gas (air). This mode of heat transfer is more effective than conduction and contributes to around 15% of the total heat transfer across the skin surface. Radiation contributes to the most heat gain/loss through the skin. Collectively, 75% of the heat gained and lost through the skin occurs via conduction, convection, and radiation. The remaining 25% occurs through heat loss via the evaporation of sweat (Arens and Zhang 2006). Whilst

---

[1] The state of an organism in an environment where it does not have to generate or lose heat (Gordon 2012).
[2] The ability of the human body to maintain a constant core body temperature.

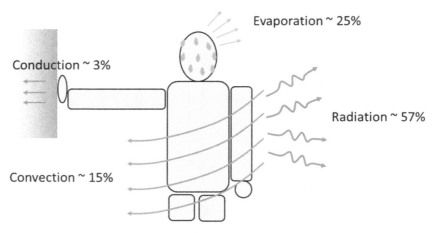

Figure 4.3. Mechanisms of heat transfer (conduction, convection, radiation and evaporation) on the skin surface.

conduction, convection and radiation can bring heat into and away from the skin, evaporation contribute only to heat loss from the skin surface.

4.3 Bioheat transfer

Bioheat transfer is the study of the thermal interaction between tissue and blood, which plays an important role in the understanding of various physiological and medical conditions related to the human body. To understand heat transfer in biological tissues, one must first look at the tissue structure. This is shown in figure 4.4. Tissue consists primarily of cells, connective tissues, and extracellular matrix that make up the interstitium, and the vasculature. At the microscale, the interstitium contains gaps that are filled with a biological liquid known as interstitial fluid. Under normal circumstances, the flow of interstitial fluid is very slow, such that its contribution to heat transfer via convection is negligible. Hence, it is common in bioheat transfer analysis to assume conduction as the dominant mode of heat transfer. Blood perfusion inside the vasculature plays an important role in bioheat transfer, as already described in section 4.2.2. The different approaches in describing the contribution of blood flow to the overall heat transfer process in biological tissues give rise to different bioheat transfer models.

Numerous bioheat transfer models have been derived and proposed over the past few decades. However, only the more prominent models will be reviewed and discussed in this section. A complete coverage of all the available bioheat transfer models will be too exhaustive and is beyond the scope of this book. It is important to point out that models that are not reviewed here are by no means an indication of their insignificance. As we will demonstrate, these bioheat transfer models are different and they account for the thermal effects of blood flow differently, each with their pros and cons.

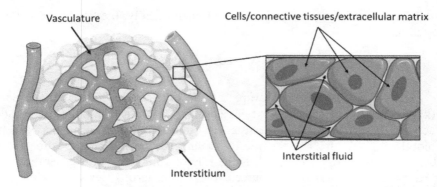

Figure 4.4. Structure of a typical biological tissue showing the tissue and vasculature. The enlarged view shows the presence of interstitial fluid among the cells, connective tissues and extracellular matrix. In bioheat transfer, the interstitial fluid is usually assumed to be stationary. Copyright © smart.servier.com. The figure was partly generated using Servier Medical Art, provided by Servier, licensed under a Creative Commons Attribution 3.0 unported license.

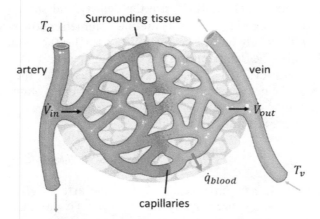

Figure 4.5. The single artery, single vein perfusion model proposed by Pennes (1948). Copyright © smart. servier.com. The figure was partly generated using Servier Medical Art, provided by Servier, licensed under a Creative Commons Attribution 3.0 unported license.

4.3.1 The Pennes model

One of the earliest and most well-known bioheat transfer model is the Pennes model, which was developed by Harry Pennes in 1948 through his landmark publication in the Journal of Applied Physiology (Pennes 1948). In the model, Pennes assumed blood to enter the tissue domain through a single artery that branches into a network of capillaries before they merge and leave the tissue via a single vein. This is shown in figure 4.5. Heat transfer between blood and the surrounding tissue is assumed to occur at the capillaries due to their large surface area to volume ratio.

According to Pennes (1948), heat conduction is the primary mode of heat transfer inside tissues. Metabolic heat generation and blood perfusion exist as volumetric contribution to the heat transfer process. Mathematically, the Pennes model can be expressed as:

$$\rho_t c_t \frac{\partial T_t}{\partial t} = \nabla \cdot (k_t \nabla T_t) + \dot{q}_{\text{blood}} + \dot{q}_{\text{met}} + \dot{q}_{\text{ext}} \qquad (4.1)$$

where T_t (K) is the tissue temperature, t (s) is time, ρ_t (kg m^{-3}) is tissue density, c_t (J (kg·K)$^{-1}$) is tissue specific heat capacity, k_t (W (m·K)$^{-1}$) is the tissue thermal conductivity, $\dot{q}_{\text{blood}}$ (W m^{-3}) is the rate of volumetric heat transfer between tissue and blood, $\dot{q}_{\text{met}}$ (W m^{-3}) is the rate of volumetric heat generation due to tissue metabolic activity, and $\dot{q}_{\text{ext}}$ (W m^{-3}) is the rate of volumetric heat generation due to tissue exposure to an external heat source. Note that the term $\dot{q}_{\text{ext}}$ exists only in problems where an external heat source is present. If a heat sink is present, then $\dot{q}_{\text{ext}} < 0$.

The rate of volumetric heat transfer between blood and tissue, $\dot{q}_{\text{blood}}$ is given by:

$$\dot{q}_{\text{blood}} = \frac{\dot{Q}_{\text{blood}}}{V_{\text{tissue}}} = \rho_b c_b \frac{(\dot{V}_{\text{in}} - \dot{V}_{\text{out}})}{V_{\text{tissue}}} (T_a - T_v), \qquad (4.2)$$

where ρ_b (kg m^{-3}) and c_b (J (kg·K)$^{-1}$) are the density and specific heat of blood, respectively, $\dot{V}_{\text{in}}$ (m^3 s^{-1}) and $\dot{V}_{\text{out}}$ (m^3 s^{-1}) are the volumetric flow rate of blood into and out of the capillary network, respectively, V_{tissue} (m^3) is the tissue volume, and T_a (K) and T_v (K) are the temperatures of blood entering the artery and vein, respectively. The term $(\dot{V}_{\text{in}} - \dot{V}_{\text{out}})/V_{\text{tissue}}$ can be expressed as the blood perfusion rate, ω_b, defined as the net volumetric flow of blood per unit volume of tissue. It has a unit of m^3 s^{-1} m^{-3} or simply s^{-1}. Replacing $(\dot{V}_{\text{in}} - \dot{V}_{\text{out}})/V_{\text{tissue}}$ with ω_b and substituting equation (4.2) into (4.1) yields:

$$\rho_t c_t \frac{\partial T_t}{\partial t} = \nabla \cdot (k_t \nabla T_t) + \rho_b c_b \omega_b (T_a - T_v) + \dot{q}_{\text{met}} + \dot{q}_{\text{ext}}. \qquad (4.3)$$

Solving equation (4.3) requires knowledge of the arterial (T_a) and venous (T_v) blood temperatures, which are usually not known. To circumvent this, Pennes assumed blood that enters the tissue to always be at a constant body temperature, such that $T_a = T_{\text{body}}$. At the capillaries, Pennes assumed heat transfer from blood to tissue occurs at a rate such that when blood exits the capillaries and into the vein, it is at thermal equilibrium with the surrounding tissue, i.e., $T_v = T_t$. With these assumptions, equation (4.3) becomes:

$$\rho_t c_t \frac{\partial T_t}{\partial t} = \nabla \cdot (k_t \nabla T_t) + \rho_b c_b \omega_b (T_{\text{body}} - T_t) + \dot{q}_{\text{met}} + \dot{q}_{\text{ext}}. \qquad (4.4)$$

Equation (4.4) represents the Pennes bioheat transfer equation, which is expressed in a form that can be solved numerically for the transient temperature distribution inside the tissue.

It is possible to use equation (4.4) to understand the thermoregulation process presented in section 4.2. In the case when tissue temperature increases beyond the body temperature ($T_t > T_{\text{body}}$), the second term on the right-hand side of equation (4.4) becomes negative. Consequently, blood flow acts as a heat sink to draw heat away from the tissue. On the other hand, when tissue temperature drops below body temperature ($T_t < T_{body}$), the term ($T_b - T_t$) becomes positive. In this case, blood flow acts as a heat source to help raise the surrounding tissue temperature.

The Pennes model is one of the most widely used bioheat transfer models due to its simplicity. Despite its popularity among researcher, there are several limitations to the Pennes model that originate from the assumptions made when deriving the model. These assumptions result in either an overestimation or underestimation of the heat source/sink effect of blood flow, and they are summarised below:

1. The assumption that arterial blood temperature is equivalent to body temperature ($T_a = T_t$) is not entirely true, especially for blood vessels of diameter larger than 300 μm (Zhu 2009).
2. The assumption that venous blood is at thermal equilibrium with the surrounding tissue ($T_v = T_t$) is valid only for blood vessels of diameter 50 μm and smaller (Zhu 2009).
3. The use of a single blood perfusion rate term ω_b to represent blood flow assumes the capillaries to be homogeneously distributed, which is not the case in actual tissues. Furthermore, the effects of directional flow cannot be accounted for using ω_b.

Despite the assumptions above, comparisons between the predictions made using the Pennes bioheat equation and experimental measurements have shown very good agreement (Zhu 2009). As such, the Pennes model continues to be adopted by many researchers when studying heat transfer in biological tissues.

4.3.2 The Wulff and Klinger models

The Wulff model (Wulff 1974) was derived to overcome some of the limitations of the Pennes model. Instead of using a global term to describe blood perfusion, Wulff (1974) proposed a localised term that accounts for the blood flow velocity within the capillaries. The Wulff model can be expressed as:

$$\rho_t c_t \frac{\partial T_t}{\partial t} + \rho_b c_b (\bar{v}_b \cdot \nabla T_b) = \nabla \cdot (k_t \nabla T_t) + \rho_b \Delta H_f (\bar{v}_b \cdot \nabla \phi) + \dot{q}_{ext}, \tag{4.5}$$

where $\bar{v}_b$ (m s^{-1}) is the local mean blood flow velocity inside the capillaries, ΔH_f (J kg^{-1}) is the specific enthalpy of reaction and ϕ (dimensionless) is the degree of reaction. The last term accounts for the heat generated due to tissue metabolic activity. Just like the Pennes model, Wulff (1974) assumed that the temperature gradient of blood is equivalent to the tissue temperature gradient such that $\nabla T_b = \nabla T_t$. Equation (4.5) can thus be rewritten as:

$$\rho_t c_t \frac{\partial T_t}{\partial t} + \rho_b c_b (\bar{v}_b \cdot \nabla T_t) = \nabla \cdot (k_t \nabla T_t) + \dot{q}_{met} + \dot{q}_{ext}, \tag{4.6}$$

where the second term on the right-hand side of equation (4.6) has been replaced with $\dot{q}_{met}$.

The Klinger model (Klinger 1974) was published in 1974 independently of the Wulff model and retains an expression that is very similar to the latter. Unlike the Wulff model, Klinger proposed the use of the local blood velocity vector field instead of a local mean to account for the directional effects of blood flow. Mathematically, the Klinger model is given by:

$$\rho_t c_t \frac{\partial T_t}{\partial t} + \rho_b c_b (\mathbf{v}_b \cdot \nabla T_t) = \nabla \cdot (k_t \nabla T_t) + \dot{q}_{met} + \dot{q}_{ext}, \tag{4.7}$$

where $\mathbf{v}_b$ (m s^{-1}) is the velocity vector field describing the flow profile inside the capillaries. Note that the assumption $\nabla T_b = \nabla T_t$ has been made when writing equation (4.7).

4.3.3 Pennes vs Wulff vs Klinger models

The main difference among the Pennes, Wulff and Klinger models is the treatment of blood perfusion and how it contributes to heat transfer inside the tissue. The Pennes model assumes blood perfusion to be represented by a global term that is expressed per unit volume of tissue. On the other hand, both the Wulff and Klinger models introduce a convective term in the bioheat transfer equation. The Wulff model adopts a local mean velocity to represent blood flow, while the Klinger model employs a spatially distributed velocity vector. A graphical representation of how blood perfusion is modelled in the Pennes, Wulff and Klinger models is shown in figure 4.6. When adopting the Wulff or Klinger models, knowledge of the blood flow velocity is required. This becomes a major hurdle to the implementation of these models as the blood capillary network is highly complex and obtaining the velocity vector field or even the local mean velocity can be problematic.

4.3.4 The Chen and Holmes model

The Chen and Holmes model (Chen and Holmes 1980) was developed in 1980 and is the first model to consider blood as a separate entity in the bioheat transfer equation. According to the Chen and Holmes model, biological tissues consist of two phases, i.e., the solid (tissue) phase and the liquid (blood) phase. Mathematically, the Chen and Holmes model is a two-equation coupled system given by:

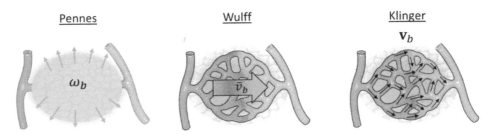

Figure 4.6. Graphical illustration comparing the treatment of the blood flow effect in the Pennes, Wulff and Klinger models. Copyright © smart.servier.com. The figure was partly generated using Servier Medical Art, provided by Servier, licensed under a Creative Commons Attribution 3.0 unported license.

$$(1 - \epsilon)\rho_t c_t \frac{\partial T_t}{\partial t} = (1 - \epsilon)\nabla \cdot (k_t \nabla T_t) + \dot{q}_{tb} + \dot{q}_{met} + (1 - \epsilon)\dot{q}_{ext}, \qquad (4.8)$$

$$\epsilon \rho_b c_b \left(\frac{\partial T_b}{\partial t} + (\mathbf{v}_b \cdot \nabla T_b) \right) = \epsilon \nabla \cdot (k_b \nabla T_b) - \dot{q}_{tb} + \epsilon \dot{q}_{ext}, \qquad (4.9)$$

where ϵ (dimensionless) is the volume fraction of the blood phase, and $\dot{q}_{tb}$ (W m^{-3}) is the rate of volumetric heat exchange between the tissue and blood phases. The opposing signs preceding the term $\dot{q}_{tb}$ ensure conservation of energy between the two phases, where heat lost from blood is gained by the tissue and vice versa. Unlike the Wulff and Klinger models, the Chen and Holmes model does not assume blood to be in thermal equilibrium with the surrounding tissue. Instead, blood temperature is now an unknown field variable that must be solved from equations (4.8) and (4.9).

Although the Chen and Holmes model avoids the need to assume thermal equilibrium between blood and tissue, solving equations (4.8) and (4.9) still requires the knowledge of $\mathbf{v}_b$ and $\dot{q}_{tb}$. In their study, Chen and Holmes (1980) estimated the value of $\dot{q}_{tb}$ for different levels of vascular branches to determine the contribution of blood to heat transfer in biological tissues.

4.3.5 The Weinbaum–Jiji model

The limitations of the Pennes model, particularly on the assumption of constant arterial blood temperature and a homogeneous and isotropic blood flow, have led to the development of the Weinbaum–Jiji model (Weinbaum *et al* 1984a, 1984b), which was conceptualised based on the anatomy of the microvasculature in skin tissue. According to the Weinbaum–Jiji model, heat transfer in skin is dominated by the transfer of energy between the artery and vein, and not to the surrounding tissue. Heat transfer from blood to tissue occurs only when a thermal gradient between the two exists. Based on their analysis, Weinbaum *et al* (1984a) proposed the following bioheat transfer equation:

$$\rho_t c_t \frac{\partial T_t}{\partial t} = \nabla \cdot (k_{eff} \nabla T_t) + \dot{q}_{met}, \qquad (4.10)$$

where k_{eff} (W (m·K)$^{-1}$) is the effective thermal conductivity that describes the contribution of blood flow to tissue heat transfer. The effective thermal conductivity depends on the blood perfusion rate and can be expressed as:

$$k_{eff} = k_t(1 + f(\omega_b)), \qquad (4.11)$$

where $f(\omega_b)$ is a function of the blood perfusion rate and local vascular geometry.

Although the Weinbaum–Jiji model provides a better description of the heat transfer process in biological tissues, the model was derived based on the anatomy of surface or superficial tissues. The main assumption behind the Weinbaum–Jiji model is that the counter-current heat transfer between artery and vein is the most dominant heat transfer process, which may not be valid when applied to tissues at deeper parts of the human body. In addition, usage of the Weinbaum–Jiji model is complicated by the need to obtain detailed information of the vascular geometry and the blood flow to accurately express the function $f(\omega_b)$ in equation (4.11) (Zhu 2009).

4.3.6 Porous medium bioheat transfer model

Unlike the bioheat transfer models presented in sections 4.3.1–4.3.5, the porous medium bioheat transfer model assumes tissue to be a porous medium. In this case, the interstitium (cells, connective tissues, and extracellular matrix) represent the solid matrix of the porous medium, while the blood vessels represent the pores. This concept is illustrated in figure 4.7. Based on this idealisation, analysis of the heat transfer phenomena inside biological tissues can be carried out using the principle of heat and fluid flow in a fluid-saturated porous medium. A rigorous mathematical derivation of the porous medium bioheat transfer model based on the volume averaging theory is available in the paper by Nakayama and Kuwahara (2008).

Two types of porous medium bioheat transfer equations are available; one where blood and tissue are assumed to be in local thermal non-equilibrium (LTNE), and one where blood and tissue are assumed to be in local thermal equilibrium (LTE).

4.3.6.1 Local thermal non-equilibrium model

The LTNE model assumes tissue and blood to not be in thermal equilibrium and was first proposed by Xuan and Roetzel (1997). The LTNE porous bioheat transfer model is a two-equation system, where one equation describes heat transfer inside the tissue, while the other describes heat transfer inside blood. Inside the tissue domain, we have:

$$(1 - \epsilon)\rho_t c_t \frac{\partial \langle T_t \rangle}{\partial t} = \nabla \cdot [(1 - \epsilon)k_t \nabla \langle T_t \rangle] + \rho_b c_b \omega_b (\langle T_b \rangle - \langle T_t \rangle)$$
$$+ h_c S_b (\langle T_b \rangle - \langle T_t \rangle), \tag{4.12}$$

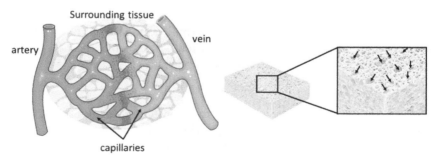

Figure 4.7. Representation of the tissue-vasculature structure as a porous medium (sponge). In this case, the solid of the sponge represents the tissue, while the pores (see black arrows) represent the complex capillary network. Copyright © smart.servier.com. The figure was partly generated using Servier Medical Art, provided by Servier, licensed under a Creative Commons Attribution 3.0 unported license.

and in the blood domain, we have:

$$\epsilon \rho_b c_b \left(\frac{\partial \langle T_b \rangle}{\partial t} + \langle \mathbf{v}_b \rangle \cdot \nabla \langle T_b \rangle \right) = \nabla \cdot [\epsilon k_b \nabla \langle T_b \rangle]$$
$$- \rho_b c_b \omega_b (\langle T_b \rangle - \langle T_t \rangle) - h_c S_b (\langle T_b \rangle - \langle T_t \rangle), \tag{4.13}$$

where h_c (W $(m^2 \cdot K)^{-1}$) is the coefficient of interfacial heat transfer between the tissue and blood domain, and S_b (m^{-1}) is the surface area per unit volume of the blood vessel wall. The bracket '$\langle \ \rangle$' represent volume averaged quantity, which is obtained by considering the length scale of blood-saturated tissue to be significantly shorter than the macroscopic characteristic length, but much larger than the microscopic characteristic length. Simply put, the control volume is small from a macroscopic point of view, and large from a microscopic (anatomical structure) point of view. The variables of interest, i.e., T_t, T_b and $\mathbf{v}_b$ are averaged over the control volume. For the sake of simplicity, the brackets '$\langle \ \rangle$' will be omitted from the variables hereafter but is implicitly understood that the variables represent volume averaged quantities.

There are similarities between the LTNE model and the Chen and Holmes model. Both models describe heat transfer in tissue and blood, and the interfacial heat transfer between the two domains. With the Chen and Holmes model, the interfacial heat transfer is described by the term $\dot{q}_{tb}$, while in the LTNE model, Newton's cooling law was used (see the last term on the right-hand side of equations (4.12) and (4.13)). Nevertheless, the LTNE model contains a volumetric blood flow effect described by the second term on the right-hand side of equations (4.12) and (4.13). This is not present in the Chen and Holmes model. These volumetric blood flow expressions are similar to the blood perfusion term in the Pennes model. In fact, the LTNE model separates the thermal effects from blood flow to an advective component and a perfusion component, as indicated by the first and second term on the right-hand side of equation (4.12) (Tucci *et al* 2021). The advective component is not accounted for in the Pennes model. By separating the blood flow effect into the advective and perfusion components, the value assigned to ω_b in equations (4.12) and (4.13) would be smaller than the value assigned to the Pennes model in equation (4.4) (Nakayama and Kuwahara 2008).

4.3.6.2 Local thermal equilibrium model
Unlike the LTNE model, the LTE model assumes thermal equilibrium between the tissue and blood, i.e., $T_t = T_b$. Setting this equilibrium temperature to T and combining equations (4.12) and (4.13), one obtains:

$$\rho_e c_e \frac{\partial T}{\partial t} + \epsilon \rho_b c_b (\mathbf{v}_b \cdot \nabla T) = \nabla \cdot (k_e \nabla T), \tag{4.14}$$

where ρ_e (kg m^{-3}), c_e (J $(kg \cdot K)^{-1}$) and k_e (W $(m \cdot K)^{-1}$) are the effective density, specific heat, and thermal conductivity, respectively, given by:

$$\rho_e = (1 - \epsilon)\rho_t + \epsilon \rho_b, \tag{4.15}$$

$$c_e = (1 - \epsilon)c_t + \epsilon c_b, \tag{4.16}$$

$$k_e = (1 - \epsilon)k_t + \epsilon k_b. \tag{4.17}$$

Note that in equation (4.14), the only contribution from blood flow comes in the form of the advective term, as thermal equilibrium results in a zero-perfusion term, since $T_t = T_b$, such that $T_t - T_b = 0$.

4.3.7 Initial-boundary conditions

Solutions to the bioheat transfer equations presented in sections 4.3.1–4.3.6 require initial and boundary conditions to be prescribed. When prescribing the initial and boundary conditions, care should be taken to ensure that they represent as close as possible the actual problem. Some of the initial and boundary conditions that are typically used in bioheat transfer analysis are summarised in table 4.1.

4.3.8 Summary

The models presented in sections 4.3.1–4.3.6 represent some of the major works on bioheat transfer. As stated at the beginning of this section, other variations of bioheat transfer models exist, such as the model of Keller and Seiler (1971), the counter-current bioheat transfer model of Mitchell and Myers (1968), and the dual- and triple-phase lag bioheat transfer models (Xu *et al* 2008, Choudhuri 2007). It is not possible to cover every bioheat transfer model in the literature within the scope of this book. Interested readers may refer to the source material listed above for more information.

The choice of which bioheat model to use is a difficult one, as each model comes with its pros and cons. Despite its simplicity and the crude assumptions on the effects of blood flow, the Pennes model continues to be used regularly by numerous researchers when investigating heat transfer in biological tissues (Hall *et al* 2014, Cheong *et al* 2021, Ooi and Ooi 2021) even to this day. It is perhaps the simplicity of the model and the ability to produce predictions that generally agree with experimental data that have led to the continuous adoption of the Pennes model. The lack of a practical alternative is likely a secondary factor.

In the study by Chen and Holmes (1980), they showed that different levels of the vasculature can lead to different thermal effects of blood flow. In other words, blood flow in arteries and veins may contribute to bioheat transfer differently from that in arterioles and venules. Investigations into the thermal significance of the vasculature at different levels were carried out by Peng *et al* (2011) using a dimensionless number known as the thermal significance coefficient. They found that large vessels such as arteries have thermal significance coefficient greater than one, suggesting that blood in these large vessels holds a constant temperature. On the other hand, for small vessels such as the capillaries, the thermal significance coefficient becomes significantly smaller than one, indicating that the blood is in continuous equilibrium with tissue temperature.

Table 4.1. Thermal boundary conditions that complement the heat equation.

Condition	Expression	Remarks
Body temperature	$T = T_{\text{body}}$	• Sets the temperature at the boundary to the body temperature T_{body}. • T_{body} is usually set to 37 °C. • Used to represent the temperature at a far-field boundary, where thermoregulation of the surrounding tissue is assumed to be able to maintain the temperature at the boundary to be at body temperature. • This is also typically set as the initial condition, which represents the initial tissue temperature at body temperature.
Convective heat flux (blood flow)	$-k\nabla T \cdot \mathbf{n} = h_{\text{bl}}(T - T_{\text{bl}})$	• Used to describe the heat transfer on boundaries representing blood vessel wall. • Typically used for large blood vessel. • h_{bl} (W (m²·K)⁻¹) represents the convective heat transfer coefficient and T_{bl} (K) is blood temperature that is typically set to 37 °C.
Heat transfer to the environment	$-k\nabla T \cdot \mathbf{n} = h_{\text{amb}}(T - T_{\text{amb}})$ $+ \, \varepsilon\sigma(T^4 - T_{\text{amb}}^4) + E_{\text{vap}}$	• Used to describe heat transfer from the boundary to the environment. • Heat transfer occurs via convection, radiation, and evaporation. • h_{amb} (W (m²·K)⁻¹) is the ambient convection coefficient, T_{amb} (K) is ambient temperature, ε (dimensionless) is surface emissivity, σ (W (m²·K⁴)⁻¹) is the Stefan–Boltzmann constant and E_{vap} (W m⁻²) is the heat flux due to evaporation of sweat. • Any process that is not present in the problem can be conveniently removed from the right-hand side.
Thermal insulation/ heat outflow	$-k\nabla T \cdot \mathbf{n} = 0$	• Used to describe boundary where heat flux is zero. • For models with fluid flow, this condition can also be used to describe the outflow of heat from the domain through the boundary.

Meanwhile, several recent studies have demonstrated that the porous medium bioheat transfer model is able to produce temperature predictions during thermal ablation treatment of liver cancer that agree better with *in vivo* experimental measurements when compared to the Pennes model (Andreozzi *et al* 2019, Tucci *et al* 2021)

Perhaps a universal bioheat transfer model that can account for the blood flow effects from all levels of vasculature in all types of tissue does not exist. Consequently, the selection of which bioheat transfer model to use should ultimately depend on the problem and the type of tissue to be analysed. The model that best describes heat transfer in tissues dominated by arteries and veins may be different from the one used for tissues dominated by arterioles, venules, and capillaries. In such a case, an understanding of the thermal significance of blood flow at different levels of the vasculature can help with the selection of the best bioheat transfer model to address a given problem. This will be explored in case study 4.1.

4.3.7.1 Case study 4.1: thermal significance of blood flow at different vasculature level

This case study[3] is adapted from the work of Peng *et al* (2011), where we will examine the thermal significance of blood flow at the different levels of the vasculature vessel and their role in describing heat transfer in biological tissues. This will be accomplished using the model of Chen and Holmes. Consider the 1D tissue domain defined by $x \in [-0.05, 0.05]$ m. The Chen and Holmes model, when expressed in 1D, is given by:

$$(1 - \epsilon)\rho_\mathrm{t} c_\mathrm{t}\frac{\partial T_\mathrm{t}}{\partial t} = (1 - \epsilon)k_\mathrm{t}\frac{\partial^2 T_\mathrm{t}}{\partial x^2} + h_\mathrm{tb}S_\mathrm{b}(T_\mathrm{b} - T_\mathrm{t}) + (1 - \epsilon)\dot{q}_\mathrm{ext}, \qquad (4.18)$$

$$\epsilon\rho_\mathrm{b} c_\mathrm{b}\left(\frac{\partial T_\mathrm{b}}{\partial t} + \left(u_\mathrm{b} \cdot \frac{\partial T_\mathrm{b}}{\partial x}\right)\right) = \epsilon k_\mathrm{b}\frac{\partial^2 T_\mathrm{b}}{\partial x^2} - h_\mathrm{tb}S_\mathrm{b}(T_\mathrm{b} - T_\mathrm{t}) + \epsilon\dot{q}_\mathrm{ext}, \qquad (4.19)$$

where u_b (m s^{-1}) is the one-dimensional velocity of blood flow, and $\dot{q}_\mathrm{ext}$ is the volumetric heat generated due to an external heat source. One may notice that the expression $\dot{q}_\mathrm{tb}$ (W m^{-3}) in the original Chen and Holmes model (see equations (4.8) and (4.9)) has been replaced by $h_\mathrm{tb}S_\mathrm{b}(T_\mathrm{b} - T_\mathrm{t})$, which shares a similar expression to the one used in the LTNE porous bioheat transfer model. This follows from the works of Peng *et al* (2011). In this case, h_tb (W (m^2·K)$^{-1}$) is the convection heat transfer coefficient quantifying the interfacial heat transfer between tissue and blood, and S_b (m^{-1}) is the surface area of the capillaries per unit volume of tissue. Within the domain, there is a spatially varying heat source given by:

$$\dot{q}_\mathrm{ext} = Q_\mathrm{o}\exp\left(-\frac{x^2}{0.05^2}\right), \qquad (4.20)$$

---

[3] Source files for case study 4.1 are available at https://doi.org/10.1088/978-0-7503-4016-8.

where Q_o (W m^{-3}) is the magnitude of the heat source chosen in this study to be 500 000 W m^{-3}.

To determine the value of S_b, blood vessels inside the capillary network are assumed to be represented by bundles of vascular tubes with radius r (Peng *et al* 2011). This is shown in figure 4.8. Assuming that there are n vessels within the bundle, each with a length of ℓ, S_b can be expressed as:

$$S_b = \frac{2n\pi r\ell}{V} = \frac{2n\pi r\ell}{V}\frac{V_b}{V_b} = \frac{2n\pi r\ell}{V_b}\frac{V_b}{V}, \tag{4.21}$$

where V (m^3) is the volume of the tissue, and V_b (m^3) is the volume of blood. Recognising that $\epsilon = V_b/V$ and $V_b = n\pi r^2\ell$, equation (4.21) can be further simplified to:

$$S_b = \frac{2\epsilon}{r}. \tag{4.22}$$

The convection heat transfer coefficient h_{tb} (W (m^2 K)$^{-1}$) can be expressed as (Nakayama and Kuwahara 2008):

$$h_{tb} = \frac{\mathrm{Nu}k_b}{2r}, \tag{4.23}$$

where Nu (dimensionless) is the Nusselt number and k_b (W (m·K)$^{-1}$) is the thermal conductivity of blood. A value of Nu = 4.96 is commonly used to describe convective heat transfer between blood flow and tissue (Roetzel and Xuan 1998). Equations (4.22) and (4.23) indicate that different vessel radii, which correspond to different levels of the vasculature, can result in different values of h_{tb} and S_b that affect the interfacial heat transfer between blood and tissue.

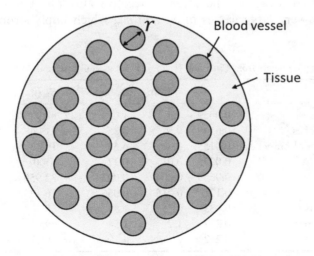

Figure 4.8. Representation of the capillary network as a bundle of blood vessels, each with radius r.

We are interested in determining the transient temperature changes inside the tissue and blood due to the external heat source in equation (4.20) for different levels of vessel generation. The vascular parameters presented by Chen and Holmes (1980) were adopted and they are summarised in table 4.2. The values of S_b and h_{tb} calculated from equations (4.22) and (4.23), respectively are also presented. Large arteries and veins are characterised by their high blood flow velocity. On the other hand, capillaries, arterioles, and venules are defined by their large surface area to volume ratio.

Values of the thermal properties used in this case study are tabulated in table 4.3. The temperatures of tissue and blood at $x = -0.05$ m was fixed at 37 °C, while thermal insulation was prescribed at $x = 0.05$ m for both domains to simulate an outflow condition. The initial tissue and blood temperatures are set to 37 °C. For the purpose of this case study, the temperature distribution during 60 s of exposure to the external heat source will be examined.

Only the results for the largest large arteries ($j = 1$) and smallest capillaries ($j = 5$) vessels from table 4.2 are presented. Figures 4.9(a) and (b) plot the transient temperature changes of tissue and blood at $x = -0.03, -0.01, 0.01$ and 0.03 m in tissues with larger arteries. Corresponding plots for tissues with capillaries are shown in figures 4.10(a) and (b). In the presence of large arteries, tissue temperature increased to an average of 40.6 °C (39.8 °C–41 °C), while the increase in blood temperature was only 0.7 °C. In the presence of capillaries, tissue and blood temperatures were identical, implying that both the tissue and blood phases are in thermal equilibrium.

These results may be explained using the values of S_b and h_{tb} shown in table 4.2. Large arteries resulted in small values of S_b and h_{tb}, which indicate weak interfacial heat transfer between tissue and blood. As such, heat generated inside the tissue cannot be effectively transferred to blood. The high blood flow velocity in large arteries also prevents the rise in blood temperature, as any heat that is generated here is quickly carried away by the large convective currents. On the other hand, capillaries have very large values of S_b and h_{tb}, which imply strong heat transfer

Table 4.2. Vascular parameters from Chen and Holmes (1980) used in case study 4.1.

j	Vessel	ϵ	r_j (mm)	u_b (cm s^{-1})	S_b (m^{-1})	h_{tb} (W (m^2·K)$^{-1}$)
1	Large arteries	0.0659	1.5	13	87.9	958.9
2	Arterial branches	0.0549	0.5	8.85	219.6	2876.8
3	Terminal arterial branches	0.0155	0.3	6.55	103.3	4794.7
4	Arterioles	0.0275	0.01	0.37	5500	143 840
5	Capillaries	0.0659	0.004	0.092	32 950	359 600
6	Venules	0.121	0.015	0.066	16 133	95 893.3
7	Terminal veins	0.033	0.75	1.31	88	1917.9
8	Venous branches	0.297	1.2	1.54	495	1198.7
9	Large veins	0.242	3	4.1	161.3	479.5

Table 4.3. Thermal properties for tissue and blood used in case study 4.1.

Parameter	Value
Tissue thermal conductivity, k_t	0.54 W $(\text{m·K})^{-1}$
Tissue density, ρ_t	1060 kg m^{-3}
Tissue specific heat, c_t	4169 J $(\text{kg·K})^{-1}$
Blood thermal conductivity, k_b	0.58 W $(\text{m·K})^{-1}$
Blood density, ρ_b	1040 kg m^{-3}
Blood specific heat, c_b	3300 J $(\text{kg·K})^{-1}$

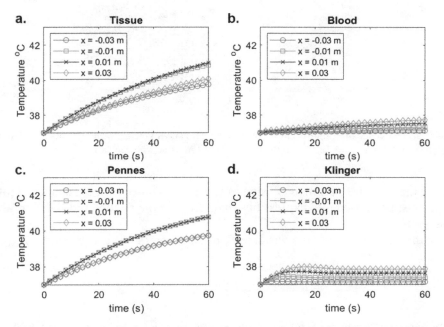

Figure 4.9. Transient temperature changes obtained using (a) and (b) the Chen and Holmes model for tissue and blood, (c) the Pennes model and (d) the Klinger model in tissue with large arteries.

between the tissue and blood. This, coupled with the very slow blood flow velocity in the capillaries, meant that any heat that is absorbed by the tissue and blood cannot be carried away from the solution domain. This led to an increase in temperature in both tissue and blood. The large interfacial heat transfer in capillaries also enhances thermal equilibrium between the two domains.

The results presented in figures 4.9(a) and (b), and figures 4.10(a) and (b), raise an interesting question on the range of applicability of some of the other bioheat transfer models, such as the Pennes and the Klinger models. Both models assume heat transfer between tissue and blood to take place at the capillary level (see sections 4.3.1 and 4.3.2). It is thus of interest to determine if this assumption holds

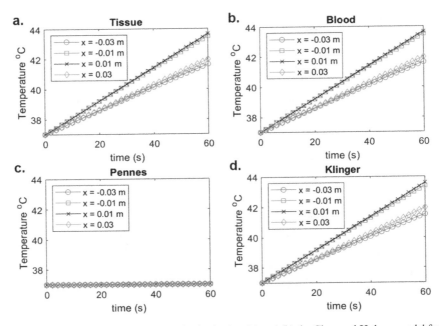

Figure 4.10. Transient temperature changes obtained using (a) and (b) the Chen and Holmes model for tissue and blood, (c) the Pennes model and (d) the Klinger model in tissue with capillaries.

true for the vascular parameters listed in table 4.2. To do so, the Chen and Holmes model must be revised into expressions that replicate the Pennes and Klinger models (Peng *et al* 2011).

For the Pennes model, the variable T_b in equation (4.18) can be set to T_{body} and rearranged to give:

$$\rho_t c_t \frac{\partial T_t}{\partial t} = k_t \frac{\partial^2 T_t}{\partial x^2} + \frac{h_{tb} S_b}{(1 - \epsilon)} \left(T_{body} - T_t \right) + \dot{q}_{ext}, \qquad (4.24)$$

where the expression $h_{tb} S_b/(1 - \epsilon)$ represents the ω_b term in equation (4.4). For the Klinger model, the second term on the right-hand side of equation (4.18) is removed and the advective term due to blood flow is added to the left-hand side, such that:

$$\rho_t c_t \frac{\partial T_t}{\partial t} + \rho_b c_b u_b \epsilon \frac{\partial T_t}{\partial x} = k_t \frac{\partial^2 T_t}{\partial x^2} + \dot{q}_{ext}. \qquad (4.25)$$

Equations (4.24) and (4.25) were solved with the same initial-boundary conditions and material properties, and the results are presented in figures 4.9(c) and (d) for tissues with large arteries, and figures 4.10(c) and (d) for tissues with capillaries.

In tissues with large arteries, the temperatures predicted using the Pennes model are almost identical to the tissue temperature predicted using the Chen and Holmes model (compare figure 4.9(a) and figure 4.9(c)). However, in tissues with capillaries, the temperatures predicted using the Pennes model remain almost constant at body temperature. This may be explained based on the use of a global perfusion term ω_b to describe blood flow across the capillaries, but a more likely reason for this could be the assumption that blood enters the tissue at a temperature of 37 °C. One may note from table 4.2 that the values of S_b and h_{tb} for capillaries are several orders of magnitude higher than those of large arteries. Hence, assuming blood temperature to be constant creates a strong artificial heat sink that draws heat away from the tissue, thus leaving the tissue temperature relatively unchanged. This observation is interesting as it contradicts the assumption made in the Pennes model on tissue-blood heat transfer occurring at the capillary level.

The predictions obtained using the Klinger model match well the Chen and Holmes model for tissues with capillaries (compare figure 4.10(a) and figure 4.10(d)) but not with large arteries (compare figure 4.9(a) and figure 4.9(d)). However, there is good agreement between the blood temperature of Chen and Holmes, and the temperature obtained from the Klinger model. This suggests that in large arteries, the strong convective effect from blood flow becomes the dominant factor in heat transfer, such that any heat that is generated inside the tissue is carried away by the convective currents. As such, the tissue temperature predicted from the Klinger model was almost unchanged by the external heat source.

Results from this case study demonstrate how tissues with different levels of vasculature can influence the prediction of bioheat transfer analysis. Comparisons between the Chen and Holmes model and the Pennes model indicate that the assumption of constant arterial blood temperature and thermal equilibrium between venous blood and tissue mimics more closely the tissue with large arteries than tissues with capillaries. The Klinger model on the other hand simulates more closely the temperature of blood phase. Hence, in tissues with capillaries, the thermal equilibrium between tissue and blood allows the Klinger model to better match the tissue temperature.

4.4 Hyperthermia

Hyperthermia is a physiological condition defined by an increase in body temperature beyond the normal range of 36.5 °C–37.5 °C. The reason for the increase in body temperature can be due to internal (increased metabolic heat) and/or external (hot weather) factors. For example, strenuous physical activity results in the production of large metabolic heat. If this heat is not released from the body fast enough through thermoregulation, which is typically the case in an environment of elevated temperature, this will cause the body temperature to rise and eventually lead to hyperthermia. Heat stroke or heat exhaustion experienced by marathon runners under gruelling running conditions is an example of hyperthermia.

4.4.1 Bioheat transfer analysis of hyperthermia

Failure in thermoregulation leading to hyperthermia can be understood from a simple bioheat transfer analysis using the Pennes model (see equation (4.4)). In the absence of an external heat source and assuming the spatial variation in tissue temperature to be negligible, the Pennes model can be rewritten into:

$$\rho_t c_t \frac{dT_t}{dt} = \rho_b c_b \omega_b (T_{body} - T_t) + \dot{q}_{met}. \tag{4.26}$$

Introducing the following dimensionless variables:

$$\theta = \frac{T_t - T_{ref}}{T_{body} - T_{ref}}, \; t^* = \frac{t}{t_{ref}}, \tag{4.27}$$

where T_{ref} (K) and t_{ref} (s) are reference temperature and time, respectively, equation (4.26) can be non-dimensionalised to give:

$$\frac{d\theta}{dt^*} = m(1 - \theta) + b, \tag{4.28}$$

where m and b are dimensionless mathematical expressions given by:

$$m = \frac{\rho_b c_b \omega_b t_{ref}}{\rho_t c_t}, \; b = \frac{\dot{q}_{met} t_{ref}}{\rho_t c_t (T_{body} - T_{ref})}. \tag{4.29}$$

The expressions for m and b describe contributions due to blood flow and metabolic heat generation, respectively.

Equation (4.28) can be solved analytically to give:

$$\theta(t^*) = 1 + \frac{b}{m} + c e^{-mt^*}, \tag{4.30}$$

where c is an unknown coefficient that can be determined from the initial condition. Assuming the initial temperature to be 37 °C (or T_{body}), such that at $t^* = 0$, $\theta(0) = 1$, then simple substitution leads to:

$$c = -\frac{b}{m},$$

which upon substitution into equation (4.30), yields:

$$\theta(t^*) = 1 + \frac{b}{m}(1 - e^{-mt^*}). \tag{4.31}$$

Contours of θ evaluated from equation (4.31) at $t^* = 0.1$, 1 and 10 for different values of b and m are shown in figure 4.11. An increase in b and m implies elevation in the metabolic heat generation and blood perfusion rate, respectively. From figure 4.11, one may observe that an increase in metabolic heat generation that is not accompanied by an increase in blood perfusion rate will cause the temperature to increase (see red arrows). To bring down the temperature, the blood perfusion rate must also increase, which helps to disperse heat from the tissue. An increase in blood perfusion rate without the increase in metabolic heat generation did not lead to an increase in temperature, which explains the role of blood as a medium of heat transfer rather than a mechanism that generates heat.

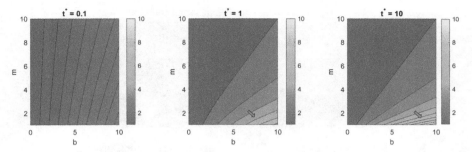

Figure 4.11. Contours of θ at $t^* = 0.1$, 1 and 10 at different values of b and m. Red arrows indicate the rise in temperature due to an increase in metabolic heat generation at a constant blood perfusion rate.

4.5 Thermal therapy

Although hyperthermia is generally viewed as a negative effect that is potentially dangerous to the human body, doctors and medical researchers have developed various treatments based on the concept of hyperthermia to eradicate unwanted or diseased tissues, such as cancer. These treatments are collectively known as thermal therapy. The main idea is to raise the temperature across the whole body, regionally or locally, to levels that are sufficient to induce cell death and thermal damage to the targeted tissue.

Whole-body and regional hyperthermia involve the delivery of energy/heat to the entire body or to a particular region of tissue (or organ), usually non-invasively. On the other hand, local hyperthermia can be invasive, minimally invasive, or non-invasive depending on the modality of treatment. With local hyperthermia, heating is localised to a specific part of the tissue, usually the part that is targeted for eradication, i.e., the cancerous tissue.

4.5.1 Whole-body and regional hyperthermia

The concept behind whole-body and regional hyperthermia is very similar. Generally, temperature of the entire body (whole-body) or a specific region of the body (regional) is raised to around 40 °C–45 °C for a duration that is sufficient to induce cell death. It is typically used to treat patients whose cancer has spread to the entire body or a specific part of the body, thus making specific targeting of these cancerous tissues difficult. The premise behind this treatment is that cancer cells are more vulnerable to heat than healthy issues. Consequently, healthy cells will be able to recover from the thermal insult, while cancer cells will die following heat exposure. Other than directly targeting cancer cells, whole-body and regional hyperthermia are also commonly used as an adjuvant therapy to other forms of cancer treatment such as radiotherapy and chemotherapy (Kok *et al* 2015).

During whole-body hyperthermia, the entire body is exposed to an external heat source that causes the temperature of the entire body to rise. This is shown in figure 4.12(a). Heating can be achieved using a variety of different approaches, such as an electromagnetic source, heating blankets and warm water immersion. In regional hyperthermia, only a region of the body is exposed to heat, see figure 4.12(b). The external heat source used to raise the tissue temperature can be

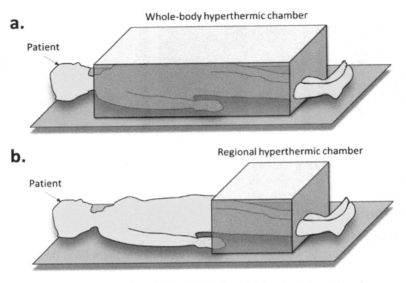

Figure 4.12. Illustration of (a) whole-body and (b) regional hyperthermia.

generated from different mechanisms, which yields different forms of heating, such as capacitive, radiative, infrared and ultrasound heating. These mechanisms have different heating size and penetration depth, and the choice of which technique to use depends on the region of the human body that is targeted for treatment.

4.5.2 Local hyperthermia

Local hyperthermia focuses on a specific region of the targeted tissue. During local hyperthermia, the temperature of the targeted tissue is raised to hyperthermic levels (40 °C–45 °C), just as in whole-body and regional hyperthermia, or to coagulative levels (>60 °C). Treatments based on the latter are known as thermal ablation treatment and they are increasingly being used in hospitals as a first line treatment option for cancer patients due to the fewer complications than surgery, fewer side effects than chemo- and radiotherapy, and its lower overall cost (Astani *et al* 2014).

Different energy sources can be used to generate heat locally within the tissue. The type of energy source used defines the type of thermal ablation treatment. Some of these thermal ablation techniques and their working principles are presented next. Focus will be given to the working principle behind each technique and the mathematical equations that describe the generation of heat inside the tissue.

4.5.2.1 Radiofrequency ablation

Radiofrequency ablation (RFA) is a thermal ablation technique that utilises electric current to increase tissue temperature through a process known as Joule heating. It is commonly used to treat liver cancers (Lee *et al* 2014, McDermott and Gervais 2013), although successful outcome in treating other forms of cancer, such as breast and prostate cancers, have also been reported (Ito *et al* 2018, Aydin *et al* 2020).

In a typical RFA procedure, the tissue forms part of an electrical circuit that consists of a needle-like metal electrode that is inserted into the cancer tissue and grounding pads that are attached to the patient thighs. This is illustrated in figure 4.13. An electric current, alternating in the frequency range of 400–550 kHz, flows from the electrode surface into the tissue and is dispersed through the grounding pads. The flow of electric current agitates the ions inside the tissue as they attempt to follow the oscillation of the alternating current (see figure 4.13). The oscillation of ions causes friction and generates heat (Joule heating) that raises the tissue temperature to levels that are sufficient to induce thermal coagulation.

The rate of volumetric heat generated inside the tissue during RFA, $\dot{q}_{rfa}$ (W m^{-3}) can be estimated using (Hall *et al* 2014):

$$\dot{q}_{rfa} = \sigma_t E^2, \tag{4.32}$$

where σ_t (S m^{-1}) is the tissue electrical conductivity and $E = \nabla V$ (V m^{-1}) is the electric field, with V (V) denoting the electric potential. The electric field distribution can be determined by solving the Maxwell equations; a set of four equations that relate the electric and magnetic fields. However, for the range of frequency used in RFA (400–550 kHz), it is possible to decouple the electric field from the magnetic field such that the tissue becomes purely resistive (Andreuccetti and Zoppetti 2006). It is also possible to adopt a quasistatic approximation since the timescale of electric current flow inside the tissue is orders of magnitude smaller than the thermal response. Under these assumptions, the Maxwell equations reduce to:

$$\nabla \cdot (\sigma_t \nabla V) = 0. \tag{4.33}$$

Two mechanisms contribute to the heating process during RFA, namely direct heating and heat conduction (Schramm *et al* 2007). This is shown in figure 4.14. Direct heating occurs in the region of tissue surrounding the surface of the electrode, where the rise in tissue temperature is caused solely by Joule heating. The region where direct heating is prominent is restricted to a few millimetres from the electrode surface. Beyond this, heating is achieved by means of heat conduction, which is

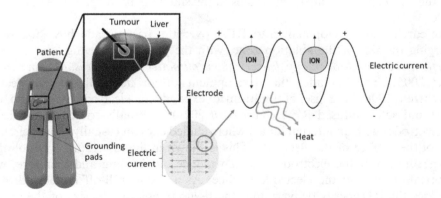

Figure 4.13. Schematic of a typical radiofrequency ablation treatment of liver cancer indicating the position of the RF electrode, the grounding pads and the oscillation of ions inside the tissue due to electric current flow.

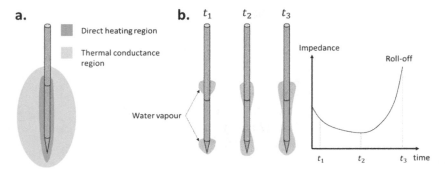

Figure 4.14. (a) Direct heating and thermal conductance region around an RF electrode. (b) Formation of water vapour and the occurrence of roll-off during RFA.

typically slower and not as efficient. The reason for the small region of direct heating may be explained using Coulomb law, which states that the magnitude of electric field is inversely proportional to the squared distance from the electrical charge. This implies that there is a large and rapid drop in the electric field magnitude as distance to the electrode surface increases. As shown in equation (4.32), a decrease in the electric field magnitude $\mathbf{E}$ results in smaller heat generation $\dot{q}_{rfa}$ inside the tissue. RFA is therefore characterised by a small ablation zone, which limits the size of tumour that can be treated using a single RF electrode in one treatment session to be smaller than 3 cm (Gao *et al* 2015).

Although the region of direct heating is small, it is sufficiently intense to raise the tissue temperature to 100 °C. At this point, water inside the tissue will vaporise. This usually occurs at the proximal and distal ends of the active tip due to heating being more intense here. As heating continues, water vapour begins to form across the entire electrode surface until they merge at the centre. This is shown in figure 4.14(b). When this happens, a rapid surge in tissue impedance occurs as the flow of electric current is impeded by the presence of water vapour surrounding the electrode. This phenomenon is known as 'roll-off' and prevents RF energy from being deposited into the tissue. Roll-off also contributes to the small ablation zone typical of that of RFA.

Research and development into RFA over the past decade have focused on enlarging the size of the ablation zone, with the goal of achieving *'one applicator insertion, one episode of energy delivery in one outpatient session, resulting in cure'* (Ni *et al* 2005). This includes the development of an internally-cooled electrode (Lorentzen 1996), the use of multi-tined expandable electrode (Costanzo *et al* 2017) and saline-infused RFA (Kho *et al* 2022). Internally-cooled electrodes are RF electrodes with an internal lumen where chilled coolant (usually saline) circulates to cool the surface of the electrode. This is shown in figure 4.15(a). By cooling the internal lumen of the electrode, one can reduce overheating and therefore, water vaporisation around the electrode surface. As a result, roll-off is delayed, which increases the RF energy delivery into the tissue to enlarge the size of the ablation zone.

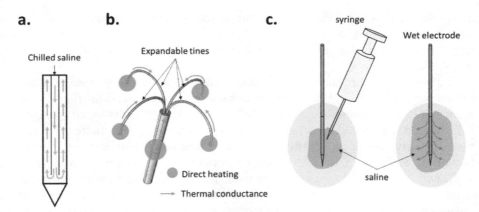

Figure 4.15. (a) Internally-cooled RF electrode, (b) multi-tined expandable electrode, (c) saline-infused RFA, with saline infusion carried out externally using a syringe and a wet electrode. In the case of the multi-tined expandable electrode, only the four tines design is shown here. Designs incorporating more than four tines are also available commercially.

Multi-tined expandable electrodes are specially designed electrodes that consist of an electrode with smaller tines that sits inside the lumen. These tines can extend outwards into the tissue, where each tine acts as a tiny electrode that helps to not only deposit RF energy at the tips of the tines, but also distribute heat to larger parts of the tissue via thermal conduction. This mechanism is illustrated in figure 4.15(b).

Saline-infused RFA involves the use of saline to alter the physical properties of tissue to enhance the ablative effects during RFA. The abundance of ions inside saline promotes a more uniform heating around the saline-saturated tissue through improved energy deposition. This is shown in figure 4.15(c). This helps to delay the occurrence of roll-off and increase the size of the ablation zone. Saline infusion can be carried out prior to or during RFA. This can be accomplished by using an infusion needle that is separate from the RF electrode or a specially designed electrode where the infusion needle is part of the RF electrode.

4.5.2.2 Microwave ablation

Microwave ablation involves the insertion of a needle-like probe into the target tissue. Electromagnetic waves in the frequency range of 0.9–2.4 GHz (microwaves), are emitted from the probe and into the tissue. Just like a domestic microwave oven, microwaves emitted from the probe into the tissue cause the water molecules inside the tissue to oscillate rapidly. The oscillation of these molecules generates frictional heating that causes tissue temperature to increase. Unlike RFA, microwaves can propagate into deep regions of the tissue. Moreover, its propagation is not influenced by the presence of water vapour. As such, there is no limiting factor when it comes to the size of the ablation zone and temperature that can be during microwave ablation. Because of this, microwave ablation is typically used to treat large cancer of the liver (typically >3 cm) and the lungs (Brace 2009).

Microwaves are emitted from a thin coaxial microwave probe, which is also known as a microwave antenna. Microwave probes can come in different variation that are differentiated by the design at the probe tip, which can include single slot, dual slot and triaxial, among others. These different designs result in different microwave emissions that influence the heating profile of the tissue. This is shown in figure 4.16.

The absence of a limiting factor in microwave ablation allows the treatment of tumours larger than 3 cm. Furthermore, it can overcome the cooling effect due to the presence of large blood vessels (Brace 2009). While this presents an advantage over RFA, the uncontrolled ablation size and temperature meant that there is a tendency for overheating to occur during microwave ablation. This can be dangerous especially if the tumour is located nearby another organ or next to a large blood vessel, such as the portal vein inside the liver. In this case, overheating can cause the nearby organ to also heat up, while in a nearby blood vessel, can cause vessel occlusion (Chiang *et al* 2016). Incidence of 'steam pop' has also been reported during microwave ablation (Qian *et al* 2020). This is a complication that arises when water vaporisation inside the tissue causes a build-up of pressure that if not relieved, will result in tissue 'explosion' or 'pop'. Figure 4.17 shows the occurrence of steam pop in a laboratory demonstration of microwave ablation on a piece of chicken breast.

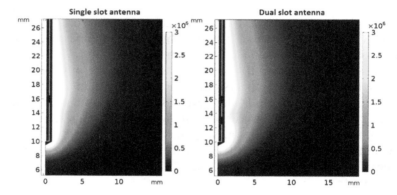

Figure 4.16. Microwave energy distribution (W m^{-3}) of a single- and dual-slot microwave antenna.

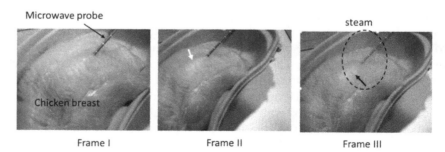

Figure 4.17. Steam pop during microwave ablation of chicken breast. White arrow indicates the formation of thermal coagulation. Black arrow in frame III indicates perforated chicken breast where steam is released (dashed circle).

Frame I depicts the position of the microwave probe inside the chicken breast. Thermal coagulation due to microwave heating is clearly demonstrated by the change in the colour of the chicken breast in frame II (see white arrow). Steam pop occurs in frame III, where perforation in the chicken breast is indicated by the black arrow. The release of steam from the perforation is also depicted by the dashed circle.

The rate of heat generation inside tissue during microwave ablation, $\dot{q}_{\text{mwa}}$ (W m^{-3}) can be estimated from (Hall *et al* 2014):

$$\dot{q}_{\text{mwa}} = \frac{1}{2}\sigma_{\text{eff}}\mathbf{E}^2, \tag{4.34}$$

where σ_{eff} (S m^{-1}) is the effective electrical conductivity of tissue and E (V m^{-1}) is the electric field, which can be obtained by solving (Hall *et al* 2014):

$$\nabla \times \left[\left(\varepsilon_{\text{r}} - j\frac{\sigma_{\text{eff}}}{\omega\varepsilon_0} \right)^{-1} \nabla \times \mathbf{H} \right] - \mu_{\text{r}}k_0^2\mathbf{H} = 0, \tag{4.35}$$

where H (A m^{-1}) is the magnetic field, ε_{r} (dimensionless) is the relative permittivity, ε_0 (dimensionless) is the permittivity of free space, ω (rad s^{-1}) is the angular frequency, μ_{r} (H m^{-1}) is the relative permeability, and $k_0 = \omega\sqrt{\varepsilon_0\mu_0}$, with μ_0 (H m^{-1}) the free space permeability. The tissue dielectric properties (ε_{r} and σ_{eff}) play an important role during microwave ablation as they determine the solution of equations (4.34) and (4.35). These properties are not only temperature dependent, but also frequency and water content dependent (Hall *et al* 2014). As such, accurate representations of these properties are crucial to the modelling of microwave ablation.

4.5.2.3 Laser ablation

Laser ablation employs light as the energy source to generate heat inside the tissue. Heating is achieved from the conversion of optical energy into heat. Laser ablation is usually carried out using lasers emitted in the wavelength of 750–1400 nm, i.e., in the near infrared region. This is because light in the near infrared region has the highest penetration depth in biological tissues (Smith *et al* 2009), which allows photons to reach deeper parts of the tissue to be absorbed and converted into heat. Laser ablation is typically used in prostate cancer treatment (Zhou *et al* 2020), although some studies have also found it to be effective in liver cancer treatment (Sartori *et al* 2017).

Two modes of laser delivery are available, namely continuous and pulse mode. In continuous mode, the laser power typically ranges from 2 to 30 W, and ablation is carried out usually over a long period. Pulse mode refers to the intermittent laser irradiation into the target tissue and is usually carried out using laser power that is higher than in continuous mode. During operation, laser is transmitted via a fibre optic cable and into the target tissue. For superficial lesion such as skin cancer, the tip of the fibre optic cable can be placed directly or at a distance from the skin surface. For tissues located inside the body, a guiding needle is usually used to guide

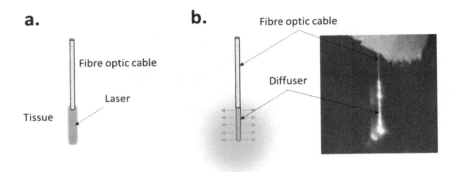

Figure 4.18. Laser emission from (a) bare tip fibre optic cable and (b) cylindrical diffuser.

the fibre optic tip to the target lesion. When in position, light can be emitted either through a bare tip or through a cylindrical diffuser, such as shown in figure 4.18. The latter emits laser radially into the tissue and over a larger area, which allows a larger coverage of ablation.

The rate of volumetric heat generation inside the tissue during laser ablation, $\dot{q}_{\text{laser}}$ (W m^{-3}) can be quantified through the following mathematical expression:

$$\dot{q}_{\text{laser}} = \mu_a P_{\text{laser}} \Phi_{\text{laser}}, \tag{4.36}$$

where μ_a (m^{-1}) is the optical absorption coefficient of the tissue, P_{laser} (W) is the laser power, and Φ_{laser} (m^{-2}) is the light fluence distribution per unit laser power. To obtain Φ_{laser}, one must first solve for the propagation of light inside the tissue. This can be done through several means, although the most reliable approach is to use the Monte Carlo method; a numerical technique widely regarded as the gold standard for modelling light propagation (Jacques 2011). Briefly, in a Monte Carlo algorithm, photons or packets of photons are launched into the tissue. Probability distributions are used to describe the physical events such as absorption, scattering, transmission, and reflection of the photons at the boundaries and interfaces. The superposition of these events provides an accurate description of the light propagation inside the tissue, from where the fluence distribution can be obtained. For more details on the Monte Carlo method, readers may refer to the seminal paper by Jacques and Wang (1995).

4.5.2.4 High intensity focused ultrasound (HIFU)
HIFU is a thermal ablation technique that converts acoustic energy into heat to raise the tissue temperature. Unlike RFA, microwave ablation and laser ablation, HIFU does not require the insertion of needles or probes into the tissue, which makes the treatment completely non-invasive. High intensity ultrasound waves are focused onto the targeted tissue from a transducer that is positioned at a distance away from the human body. This is illustrated in figure 4.19. Because of the high level of focusing, HIFU is very effective at treating very small tumours that are surrounded by critical structures.

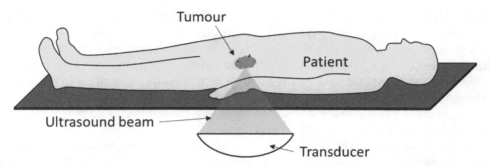

Figure 4.19. Typical set up of a HIFU treatment. The transducer has a shape resembling that of a paraboloid, which plays a significant role in focusing high intensity acoustic radiation to the target tumour.

The rate of volumetric heat generation during HIFU, $\dot{q}_{us}$ (W m^{-3}) is mathematically given by:

$$\dot{q}_{us} = 2\alpha I, \tag{4.37}$$

where α (m^{-1}) is the acoustic absorption coefficient of tissues and I (W m^{-2}) is the magnitude of the acoustic intensity, which can be estimated based on the acoustic pressure distribution inside the tissue. The acoustic pressure inside the tissue can be obtained by solving the acoustic wave equation. Since the ultrasound waves propagate significantly faster than heat, one may solve the acoustic wave equation in the frequency domain, which is given by:

$$\nabla^2 p + \frac{\omega^2}{c^2} p = 0, \tag{4.38}$$

where p (Pa) is the acoustic pressure, ω (rad s^{-1}) is the angular frequency of the acoustic wave and c (m s^{-1}) is the speed of sound in tissue.

4.5.2.5 Cryoablation

Although cryoablation is not a hyperthermic treatment, it is a form of thermal ablation technique and analysis of the temperature distribution during the treatment can be carried out using the bioheat transfer models presented in section 4.3. Hence, it is fitting to also discuss and introduce cryoablation to readers here. Unlike hyperthermic treatments, cryoablation is hypothermic, which utilises extreme cold to destroy tissues. During cryoablation, tissue temperature is lowered to freezing conditions (usually <-10 °C) to induce cell death through intracellular ice formation and dehydration (Mazur 1984). The temperatures reached during cryoablation varies depending on the type of tissues (He and Bischoff 2003).

In a typical cryoablation treatment, a needle-like probe, also known as a cryoprobe, is inserted into the target tissue. Just like an internally-cooled RF electrode, cryoprobes contain an inner and an outer lumen where working fluid circulates. When cryoablation was first introduced, liquid nitrogen circulates within the lumen of the cryoprobe, where the very cold temperature helps to freeze the surrounding tissue (Nomori *et al* 2017). A modern cryoablation system uses the

Joule–Thomson effect; a phenomenon where a drastic drop in tissue temperature to sub-zero levels is achieved by the sudden expansion of gas (Song 2016). This process is also known as throttling. In this case, argon gas at high pressure flows through the inner lumen of the cryoprobe. At the tip, the sudden change in cross sectional area causes the gas to expand, thus causing a drop in temperature according to the Joule–Thomson effect. This is illustrated in figure 4.20.

To describe tissue cooling due to the Joule–Thomson effect, one may choose to model the throttling process inside the cryoprobe as part of the heat transfer process. However, this step is very complicated and requires large computational resources since throttling occurs inside the tip of the cryoprobe, which is orders of magnitude smaller than the scale of the ablation zone. Instead, researchers commonly employ a convective boundary condition to simulate the cooling effect induced around the surface of the cryoprobe, such that (Chan and Ooi 2016):

$$-k_t\frac{\partial T_t}{\partial n} = h_{\text{cryo}}\big(T - T_{\text{cryo}}\big), \qquad (4.39)$$

where h_{cryo} (W (m^2·K)$^{-1}$) is the convection heat transfer coefficient that can be estimated from experimental conditions and T_{cryo} (K) is the temperature of the argon gas following its expansion at the tip.

An important point to consider when performing thermal analysis of cryoablation is the freezing process, which involves phase change. During freezing, heat is released by the tissue in the form of latent heat, which can affect the heat transfer analysis if they are not taken into consideration. Modelling of the freezing process can be accomplished using one of three methods, namely the front tracking method,

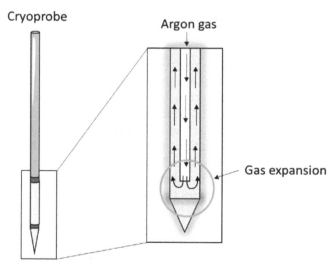

Figure 4.20. The Joule–Thomson effect inside a cryoprobe, which involves the expansion of argon gas inside the cryoprobe.

enthalpy method and the effective heat capacity method (He and Bischoff 2003). In this section, only the effective heat capacity method will be presented.

The effective heat capacity assumes the freezing process in biological tissue to occur over a range of temperature, $T_f \leqslant T \leqslant T_u$, where T_f (K) and T_u (K) are respectively the frozen and unfrozen temperature thresholds. In other words, they represent the lower and upper phase transition temperatures of the tissue, respectively. Water in tissue is assumed to be completely liquid at $T > T_u$ and completely solid at $T < T_f$. Between T_u and T_f, tissue exists as both liquid and solid states, and is commonly referred to as the mushy zone (He and Bischoff 2003). The existence of a mushy zone is due to biological tissues being non-ideal materials, where freezing occurs over a range of tissue rather than at a fixed temperature. Using the effective heat capacity method, tissue thermal properties, specifically the density, thermal conductivity and specific heat are expressed according to the state the tissue is in, such that:

$$\rho_{t,\,eff} = \begin{cases} \rho_f, & T < T_f \\ \rho_f(1 - \theta) + \theta\rho_u, & T_f \leqslant T \leqslant T_u, \\ \rho_u, & T > T_u \end{cases} \tag{4.40}$$

$$k_{t,\,eff} = \begin{cases} k_f, & T < T_f \\ k_f(1 - \theta) + \theta k_u, & T_f \leqslant T \leqslant T_u, \\ k_u, & T > T_u \end{cases} \tag{4.41}$$

$$c_{t,\,eff} = \begin{cases} c_f, & T < T_f \\ c_f(1 - \theta) + \theta c_u + \dfrac{h_{fg}}{\rho_w(T_u - T_f)}, & T_f \leqslant T \leqslant T_u, \\ c_u, & T > T_u \end{cases} \tag{4.42}$$

where the subscripts 'u' and 'f' represent unfrozen and frozen states, respectively, ρ_w (kg m^{-3}) is the density of water, h_{fg} (J kg^{-1}) is the latent heat of solidification and θ (dimensionless) is a parameter that quantifies the fraction of liquid in the mushy region, and is given by (Chan and Ooi 2016):

$$\theta = \frac{T - T_f}{T_u - T_f}. \tag{4.43}$$

When performing bioheat transfer analysis on cryoablation treatment, equations (4.40)–(4.42) are substituted into the relevant terms of the bioheat transfer model.

4.5.3 Summary

Four thermal ablation techniques based on hyperthermia (RFA, microwave ablation, laser ablation and HIFU) and their basic concepts have been presented in this section. Each technique differs in the mechanism used to generate heat inside the tissue. However, all of them involve the conversion of some form of energy to heat. Other forms of thermal ablation techniques that are derivatives of these four exist. For instance, several researchers have explored the use of gold nanorods as photo-enhancers to increase the amount of energy absorption inside the tissue during laser ablation (Cheong *et al* 2021, Vines *et al* 2019). Similarly, some studies that explored methods to overcome the limiting factor in RFA have resulted in the use of nanofluids and cationic polymer solutions to augment the physical properties of tissues to intensify Joule heating (Wu *et al* 2015, Zheng *et al* 2020).

The choice of which technique to use to treat a patient depends on a variety of factors such as the size of the cancerous tissue, the type of cancer and the location of the tumours. Furthermore, each technique has its pros and cons that make one technique a better choice over the others for the treatment of a particular patient. A non-exhaustive list of the pros and cons is presented in table 4.4.

The planning of a thermal ablation treatment protocol is a complicated process. Under most circumstances, the success of the planned protocol is determined by the experience of the doctors. Computational modelling can play a huge part in assisting with the planning of the treatment protocol. Models that are based on the medical images of the patient can be developed and simulation based on a bioheat transfer analysis can be carried out to inform the doctors on the predicted outcome of a planned protocol. This approach is known as patient-specific modelling and is an area of study that is growing in popularity. One of the main advantages of patient-specific modelling is the ability to optimise and customise clinical treatments of various therapies and surgical interventions based on the computational prediction of the treatment outcome (Voglreiter *et al* 2018).

Table 4.4. Summary of the different thermal ablation techniques and their limitations.

	RFA	Microwave	Laser	HIFU
Energy Delivery	Electric Minimally invasive	Microwaves Minimally invasive	Optic Minimally invasive/ non-invasive	Acoustic Non-invasive
Limitations	• Small ablation zone. • Risk of under-ablation. • Susceptible to heat sink effect due to presence of blood vessel.	• Energy delivery into tissue is more complex. • Steam pop is common and dangerous. • Over-ablation is a concern. • Larger probe compared to RFA.	• Limited by laser penetration depth. • Effects of some laser treatment may not last long. • Requires strict precautionary measures.	• Adverse effects from US reflection in bone. • Tumours must be in the range of the ultrasound focal depth. • Lengthy treatment time due to small ablation zone (require multiple overlapping application).

4.5.3.1 Case study 4.2: bioheat transfer analysis during radiofrequency ablation
This case study[4] examines the rise in tissue temperature during RFA treatment of liver cancer and demonstrates the use of bioheat transfer analysis to facilitate treatment planning of RFA. Consider a patient with liver cancer who is scheduled for an RFA treatment. A CT scan revealed that the tumour is spherical with a diameter of 1.5 cm and is located at the centre of the liver. The tumour is not in the vicinity of large blood vessels. The RF probe that is available for treatment is internally cooled, 1 mm in diameter and has an active length[5] of 1 cm. A constant voltage RF generator that produces an output electric potential of 40 V was used. To assist interventional radiologist in planning the RFA treatment, it is of interest to determine the ablation time required for the temperature of the entire tumour to rise above 50 °C.

To solve this problem, the model of the tumour and the surrounding liver tissue was developed. Since the ablation zone is smaller than the size of the liver, it suffices to model the liver as a sphere that surrounds the tumour. This is shown in figure 4.21(a). Note that the size of the sphere must be sufficiently large to negate any boundary effects. Typically, a domain convergence study must be carried out, where simulations are repeated for increasingly large domain until the difference in the numerical solution becomes negligible. The geometry of the tumour was modelled in 2D axisymmetry to further reduce the requirement for computational resources. This is shown in figure 4.21(b). The bioheat transfer analysis is carried out using the Pennes model, which is reproduced here as:

$$\rho_t c_t \frac{\partial T_t}{\partial t} = \nabla \cdot (k_t \nabla T_t) + \rho_b c_b \omega_b (T_{body} - T_t) + \dot{q}_{met} + \dot{q}_{ext}. \tag{4.44}$$

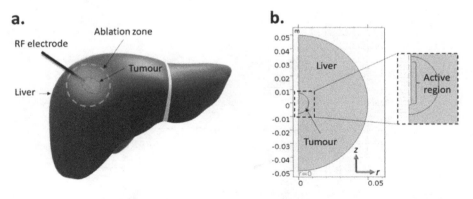

a.

b.

Figure 4.21. (a) Truncation of the liver domain to a sphere around the tumour and (b) the model of the tumour and surrounding liver in 2D axisymmetry.

---

[4] Source files for case study 4.2 are available at https://doi.org/10.1088/978-0-7503-4016-8.
[5] Active length of an RF electrode is the region of the electrode where electric current flows and is the region where direct heating occurs.

Values of the thermal properties of liver and tumour are summarised in table 4.5. Metabolic heat generation, $\dot{q}_{met}$ was assumed to be zero since its contribution is negligible under the presence of Joule heating (Hall *et al* 2015). The external heat source, $\dot{q}_{ext}$ was evaluated by solving equations (4.32) and (4.33). Values of the electrical conductivity for both the liver and tumour are listed in table 4.5.

The boundary conditions prescribed to the model are presented in figure 4.22. Across the active tip of the electrode, a constant electric potential of 40 V was applied. Internal cooling of the electrode was simulated by assuming convective heat transfer at the boundary of the active electrode, such that:

$$-k_t \frac{\partial T_t}{\partial n} = h_{cool}(T - T_{cool}),\qquad (4.45)$$

where h_{cool} (W $(m^2 \cdot K)^{-1}$) is the convection heat transfer coefficient between the coolant and tissue and T_{cool} (K) is the temperature of the coolant. The value of h_{cool} can be estimated based on the dimension of the electrode and the flow rate of the

Table 4.5. Thermal and electrical properties used in case study 4.2.

Parameter	Liver	Tumour
Electrical conductivity, σ_t (S m^{-1})	0.12	0.2
Thermal conductivity, k_t (W (m·K)$^{-1}$)	0.56	0.58
Density, ρ_t (kg m^{-3})	1040	1060
Specific heat, c_t (J (kg·K)$^{-1}$)	4180	4180
Blood perfusion rate, ω_b (s^{-1})	0.0016	0.002
Blood density, ρ_b (kg m^{-3})	1060	
Blood specific heat, c_b (J (kg·K)$^{-1}$)	3300	

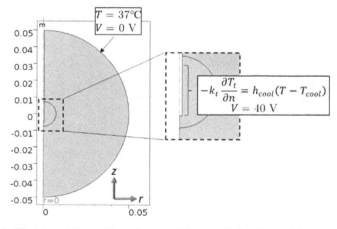

Figure 4.22. Electric and thermal boundary conditions applied to the model in case study 4.2.

internally circulating coolant (Burdío *et al* 2009). Here, we assume that $h_{cool} = 4000$ W $(m^2 \cdot K)^{-1}$ and set $T_{cool} = 10$ °C. Across the outer boundary of the liver tissue, a zero electric potential and a constant temperature of 37 °C were applied. The former simulates ground condition, while the latter assumes the outer boundary to be sufficiently far from the ablation zone around the electrode, such that thermo-regulation of the surrounding tissue can maintain the temperature here at constant body temperature. All other boundaries were electrically and thermally insulated. The initial temperature of the tumour and liver was set to $T = T_{body} = 37$ °C.

Simulations were carried out for a treatment duration of 900 s (15 min) and temperature contours at different times were plotted to identify the time when the temperature of the entire tumour increased beyond 50 °C. Results indicate that 240 s or 4 min of ablation is sufficient to achieve this. This is shown in figure 4.23, where the 50 °C isotherm (thick white curve) has completely encapsulated the tumour. If 50 °C is taken as the threshold at which thermal damage occurs, then the results from the model suggest that a minimum of 4 min treatment time is required for the entire tumour to be thermally destroyed.

It is acknowledged that the analysis carried out in this case study is highly simplified. The actual planning of the treatment protocol is in fact much more complicated and involves the consideration of many other factors. For example, some of the tissue electrical and thermal properties are unlikely to remain constant during treatment. Studies have shown that tissue electrical and thermal conduc-tivity changes with temperature and RFA models will have to account for these behaviours to obtain an accurate representation of the treatment outcome (Hall *et al* 2015). Some studies carried out on animal tissues have also reported on an increase in blood perfusion rate when tissue temperature increases to 45 °C; as the tissue responds to heat through vasodilation. Beyond 45 °C, the blood vessels lose their capacity to response and vascular stasis begin to occur that leads

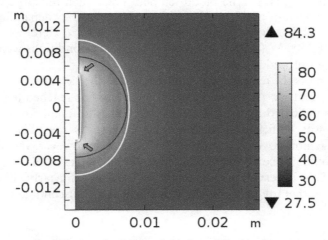

Figure 4.23. Contours of temperature after 4 min of ablation, with white line representing the isotherm at 50 °C. Red arrows point to the region of peak temperatures.

to a decrease in blood perfusion rate. Blood perfusion ceases when complete thermal damage occurs (He *et al* 2004, Schutt and Haemmerich 2008). Changes in the blood flow during RFA are expected to influence the tissue thermal response (Hall *et al* 2015). These factors must be taken into consideration when developing computational models to predict the treatment outcome of RFA.

4.5.3.2 Case study 4.3: heat sink effect from a nearby blood vessel during radiofrequency ablation

One of the limitations of RFA, as shown in table 4.4, is its susceptibility to heat sink effect when there is the presence of a large blood vessels. Large blood vessels carry enough blood at a large enough flow rate to become a significant heat sink that draws heat away from the tumour. This will be investigated in this case study[6]. Consider a spherical tumour of diameter 1.5 cm that is surrounded by homogeneous liver tissue, similar to that in case study 4.2. An infinitely long and straight blood vessel of diameter 5 mm is located at a distance of 5 mm from the tumour boundary. To investigate the effects of the blood vessel, a 3D model must be developed since the presence of blood vessel disrupts the conditions for axisymmetry modelling. The 3D model is shown in figure 4.24. Note that the surrounding liver tissue is approximated as a cuboid instead of a sphere. Nevertheless, this assumption does not affect the numerical predictions for the truncated model approach considered here.

Across the surface of the blood vessel, the convection heat transfer condition can be used to describe the heat exchange between tissue and blood (see table 4.5), such that (Payne *et al* 2011):

$$-k_t\frac{\partial T_t}{\partial n} = h_{\text{blood}}(T - T_{\text{blood}}),\tag{4.46}$$

where h_{blood} (W $(\text{m}^2 \cdot \text{K})^{-1}$) is the convection heat transfer coefficient between tissue and blood, and T_{blood} (K) is the blood temperature, which for large vessels, can be assumed to be constant at 37 °C. The value of h_{blood} varies depending on the flow rate. Naturally, higher flow rates will result in larger h_{blood}. Here, we set h_{blood} to an ad hoc value of 2500 W $(\text{m}^2 \cdot \text{K})^{-1}$. All other boundary conditions were set to be the same as those employed in case study 4.2.

Figure 4.25 plots the temperature contours across the xy plane at $z = 0$ after 4, 10 and 15 min of ablation. At 4 min, not all the tumour has reached temperature of at least 50 °C, as indicated by the yellow arrow. This is different from case study 4.2, where 4 min was sufficient to achieve this target. As the ablation duration is extended, the region covered by the 50 °C increases; however, the side facing the blood vessel could not be extended due to the cooling effect from the blood flow (see red arrows). This observation demonstrates the role of nearby blood vessels in thermal ablation therapy and how RFA is particularly susceptible to this heat sink effect.

---

[6] Source files for case study 4.3 are available at https://doi.org/10.1088/978-0-7503-4016-8.

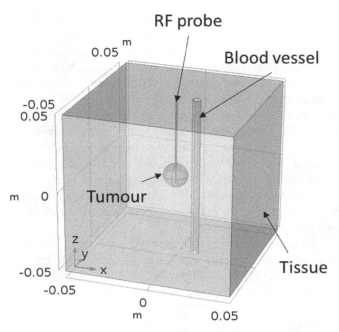

Figure 4.24. 3D model developed for case study 4.3. Blood vessel is located 5 mm next to the tumour domain.

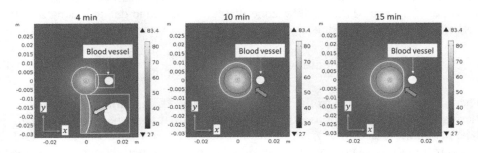

Figure 4.25. Contours of the temperature across the *xy* plane at *z*=0 at 4, 10 and 15 min after RFA treatment.

4.6 Thermal damage

The case studies in section 4.5 demonstrate the potential of using bioheat transfer analysis to predict the rise in tissue temperatures during thermal ablation treatments. Knowledge of the tissue temperature rise provides an indication of the effectiveness of the treatment procedure; however, it does not correctly measure the level of thermal damage sustained by the tissue. This may be better quantified by accounting for the physical processes that occur inside the tissue during heat exposure.

Two mechanisms are involved in the formation of thermal damage inside the tissue, namely direct (primary) and delayed (secondary) injury. Direct thermal injury occurs due to the physical interaction between heat and the cellular structures of the tissues, including proteins, lipoproteins, and water (Thomsen 2005). Direct injury occurs during the heating event, which can be detected visually and instantaneously after a certain heating threshold (temperature and duration) is reached. The process is known to disrupt normal cellular structure and function. Thermal denaturation or coagulation is an example of direct thermal damage.

Unlike direct thermal injury, delayed thermal injury does not occur instantaneously. Instead, it can happen several seconds, hours, days and even weeks after the heating event. The process by which delayed thermal injury occurs is pathophysiological. An example of delayed thermal injury is cell death due to apoptosis (also known as programmable cell death); a cellular response to biochemical events that lead to cellular changes and eventually death. Since delayed thermal injury is a pathophysiological response, experimental studies on this mechanism can only be carried out on living cells and tissues.

Quantifying the amount of thermal damage inside the tissue after exposure to heat is an important part of bioheat transfer analysis. Some of the methods available to quantify thermal damage will be presented in this section. However, focus will be given only to methods related to direct thermal injury.

4.6.1 Critical isotherm

Critical isotherm represents the simplest method to represent thermal damage. In fact, case studies 4.2 and 4.3 demonstrate how an isotherm can be used to represent the zone of thermal damage. The zone of thermal damage defined using a critical isotherm can be expressed as:

$$\text{Tissue condition} = \begin{cases} \text{no damage,} & \text{if } T < T_c \\ \text{damage,} & \text{if } T \geqslant T_c \end{cases}, \tag{4.47}$$

where T_c (K) is the critical isotherm that when exceeded, will induce the formation of thermal damage. It is obvious from equation (4.47) that the zone of thermal damage depends on the selection of T_c. A value of T_c that is too low or too high will result in an overestimation or underestimation of the zone of thermal damage, respectively. This is demonstrated in figure 4.26, where a 50 °C (black) isotherm clearly predicts a larger zone of thermal damage than a 60 °C (orange) and 70 °C (blue) isotherm. Several studies have shown that a value of T_c = 60 °C is a good indicator of immediate thermal damage during thermal ablation treatment (Heisterkamp et al 1999).

Although critical isotherms provide a fast and easy way to quantify thermal damage, they do not fully capture the physical processes that are involved. This is because the formation of thermal damage depends not only on the tissue temperature, but also the duration of heat exposure. In other words, heating the tissue at 50 °C for a longer duration may induce similar thermal damage as heating the tissue at 60 °C for a shorter duration. Unfortunately, the effects of exposure duration on the formation of thermal damage cannot be accounted for using the critical isotherm method.

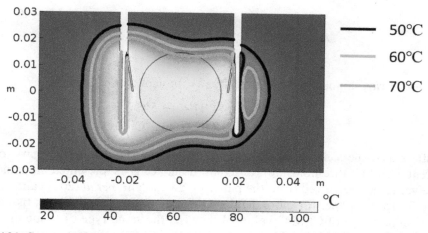

Figure 4.26. Contrast in the thermal damage zone represented by critical isotherms of 50 °C, 60 °C and 70 °C. Temperature contours obtained from a saline-infused bipolar RFA study.

4.6.2 Cumulative equivalent minutes

Cumulative equivalent minutes (CEM) is a simple concept of quantifying thermal damage by combining the temperature history of the heating event into a single number. In essence, CEM measures the exposure of tissue to heat in terms of the number of minutes of heating at a particular temperature that is needed to obtain equivalent thermal effects. The most prominent CEM is the one that is measured at 43 °C or CEM43 due to tissue hyperthermic response occurring at 43 °C.

CEM43 can be evaluated from the expression (Yarmolenko *et al* 2011):

$$\text{CEM43} = \int_{t_0}^{t_f} R^{43-T(t)}dt, \tag{4.48}$$

where t is time (in minutes) and $T(t)$ is a smooth function describing the transient temperature changes during heating (in °C). During experiments, tissue temperature is typically measured at discrete time points. In this case, CEM43 can be evaluated using:

$$\text{CEM43} = \sum_{i=1}^{N} t_i R^{43-T_i}, \tag{4.49}$$

where t_i (in min) and T_i (°C) are the discrete time and temperature points, and N is the number of time points at which temperature is measured. The parameter R in equations (4.48) and (4.49) is a constant whose value can be obtained experimentally. Different cells give rise to different values of R. For instance, the R value of Chinese hamster ovary cells is given by (Yarmolenko *et al* 2011):

$$R = \begin{cases} 0, & \text{for } T(t) < 39°C \\ 0.25, & 39°C \leqslant T(t) < 43°C, \\ 0.5, & T \geqslant 43°C \end{cases} \qquad (4.50)$$

while for *in vitro* human cells, is given by (Yarmolenko *et al* 2011):

$$R = \begin{cases} 0.233, & \text{for } T(t) < 43.5°C \\ 0.428, & \text{for } T(t) \geqslant 43.5°C \end{cases} \qquad (4.51)$$

Different tissues/cells have different CEM43 thresholds. A summary of the different CEM43 thresholds for different tissues/cells is presented in table 4.6. These values are retrieved from the paper of Yarmolenko *et al* (2011) and readers may refer to this paper for more details. One may notice that different tissues can have similar range of CEM43 values. Likewise, the same type of tissue may also lead to different CEM43 values, where higher CEM43 values are often accompanied by significant histological and gross tissue changes. The values in table 4.6

Table 4.6. CEM43 thresholds of some tissues/cells retrieved from Yarmolenko *et al* (2011).

| CEM43 (min) | Tissue type | *Type of tissue change | | | | Animal |
| | | Acute | | Chronic | | |
		Minor	Significant	Minor	Significant	
0–20	Blood brain barrier		H/F			Rat, rabbit, dog
	Bone marrow	F/H	H			Mouse, rat
	Kidney	H	F			Rabbit
	Testis	F/H	H/F/G			Mouse
21–40	Blood brain barrier		H/F			Rabbit, dog
	Cornea	G		F/H	F	Rabbit
	Mammary gland		H			Goat
	Skin	F				Mouse
41–80	Bladder		F			Rat
	Bone				G	Rabbit
	Kidney		H			Pig
	Liver	F/H				Dog/rabbit
80–240	Bladder		F		G	Rat, dog
	Bone				G	Rabbit
	Muscle		H		G/H	Rat, pig
	Brain		H		H	Monkey
> 240	Kidney		H			Pig, dog
	Liver		H			Rabbit, pig
	Muscle		H/G			Rabbit, pig
	Brain		H/G		H	Rabbit, pig, monkey

*F: functional; H: histological; G: gross.

provide the threshold in terms of the heating duration that is required to induce thermal damage. For example, if kidney tissue is heated such that the CEM43 values estimated from equation (4.51) are between 41 and 80 min, then one should expect the formation of thermal damage that is characterised by significant histological changes to the tissue.

The use of CEM to quantify thermal damage is an improvement over the use of critical isotherm since it accounts for the effects of both temperature and time. This is valid across a wide range of temperature and accounts for functional, histological, and gross changes to the tissue (see table 4.6), thus making it highly applicable to a variety of different thermal and physical effects. Nevertheless, CEM also has its limitation. Primarily, this approach does not account for the physical and physiological changes in tissue during hyperthermia, such as changes to the blood perfusion rate in response to tissue temperature elevation.

4.6.3 The Arrhenius thermal damage model

Just like the bioheat transfer model, there exists numerous thermal damage models in the literature, each with their pros and cons. For a complete review, one may refer to the paper of Pearce (2013). Among the different thermal damage models available, the one that is most frequently used is the thermal damage model of Henriques Jr and Moritz (1947). According to this model, the formation of thermal damage in tissues is similar to thermal denaturation or thermal coagulation, where its rate of formation follows the first order Arrhenius reaction, such that:

$$k = Ae^{-\frac{\Delta E}{RT}}, \tag{4.52}$$

where k (s^{-1}) is the reaction rate, A (s^{-1}) is the frequency factor, ΔE (J mol^{-1}) is the activation energy, R (J (mol·K)$^{-1}$) is the universal gas constant and T (K) is temperature. From equation (4.52), one may observe that the rate of thermal damage formation depends on temperature. The activation energy represents the energy threshold that must be overcome by the supplied heat in order for the reaction to occur. This is represented by the schematic in figure 4.27. Thermal coagulation described by the Arrhenius process is irreversible, meaning that coagulated tissues cannot be 'uncoagulated' by cooling them.

Taking Ω as the dimensionless parameter that quantifies thermal damage, one may set the rate of change of Ω, i.e., the rate of thermal damage formation, to be equivalent to k, such that:

$$\frac{d\Omega}{dt} = k = Ae^{-\frac{\Delta E}{RT(t)}}, \tag{4.53}$$

or

$$\Omega(t) = \int_0^{\tau} Ae^{-\frac{\Delta E}{RT(t)}}dt. \tag{4.54}$$

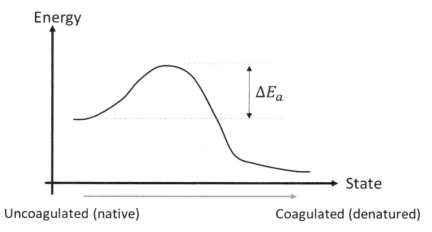

Figure 4.27. The Arrhenius process describing how tissues change from an uncoagulated (native) to coagulated (denatured) state after overcoming the activation energy ΔE.

Equation (4.54) is known as the Arrhenius thermal damage integral and is one of the most frequently used thermal damage models alongside bioheat transfer analysis.

To use equations (4.53) or (4.54) to predict thermal damage, knowledge of the frequency factor A and activation energy ΔE_a must be known. These values are determined experimentally, and they vary depending on the type of cells/tissues. Fortunately, numerous studies have measured and quantified them for a variety of different cells and tissues. Table 4.7 presents the values of A and ΔE_a for some cells retrieved from the review paper of Pearce (2013).

The dimensionless thermal damage parameter can be expressed as:

$$\Omega(t) = \ln\left[\frac{C(0)}{C(\tau)}\right], \tag{4.55}$$

where $C(0)$ is the initial concentration (mol m^{-3}) of the uncoagulated tissue and $C(\tau)$ is the concentration (mol m^{-3}) of uncoagulated tissue after exposure to heat for a duration defined by τ (s). The logarithmic term in equation (4.55) suggests that below a critical temperature, the formation of thermal damage is slow. Beyond that, the rate of thermal damage formation increases rapidly. It is helpful to define this critical temperature T_{crit} at which thermal damage increases rapidly. If we assume this event to occur when $d\Omega/dt = 1$, using equation (4.53), we have:

$$Ae^{-\frac{\Delta E}{RT_{crit}}} = 1, \tag{4.56}$$

where the critical temperature depends on the parameters A and ΔE_a. If we select[7] $A = 1.3 \times 10^{95}$ s^{-1} and $\Delta E_a = 6.05 \times 10^5$ J mol^{-1}, then T_{crit} can be estimated from equation (4.56) to be 331.8 K or 58.5 °C. Figure 4.28 plots the variation in $d\Omega/dt$ for the aforementioned values of A and ΔE_a for a range of temperature values. As expected, below the critical temperature of 58.5 °C, there is negligible change

Table 4.7. Summary of the values of A, ΔE_a and T_{crit} for different cell type.

Damage process	A (s^{-1})	ΔE_a (J mol^{-1})	T_{crit} (°C)	Remarks
Cell death				
Sapareto *et al* (1978)	1.67×10^{280}	1.71×10^6	45.6	CHO cells $\leqslant$ 43 °C
	2.84×10^{99}	6.19×10^5	51.4	CHO cells $\geqslant$ 43 °C
Diller and Klutke (1993)	1.3×10^{95}	6.04×10^5	58.5	Skin cells $T \leqslant$ 50 °C
Weaver and Stoll (1967)	2.2×10^{124}	7.82×10^5	55.4	$T \leqslant$ 50 °C
	1.82×10^{51}	3.27×10^5	60.1	$T >$ 50 °C
Retinal damage				
Welch and Polhamus (1984)	3.1×10^{99}	6.28×10^5	57.6	Damage
Muscle				
Jacques and Gaeeni (1989)	2.94×10^{39}	2.6×10^5	70.4	Myocardium whitening
Liver				
Jacques *et al* (1991)	5.51×10^{41}	2.77×10^5	73.4	Whitening, pig liver
Erythrocytes				
Flock *et al* (1993)	1×10^{31}	2.12×10^5	84	Membrane denaturation

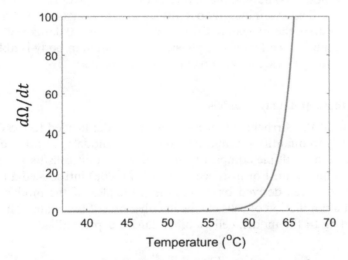

Figure 4.28. Plot of the rate of thermal damage formation against temperature for $A = 1.3 \times 10^{95}$ s^{-1} and $\Delta E_a = 6.05 \times 10^5$ J mol^{-1}.

to $d\Omega/dt$. Beyond that, the rate of thermal damage formation increased rapidly. The critical temperatures obtained for other cells and tissues are summarised in table 4.7. In general, a larger ΔE_a leads to a higher critical temperature, since greater amount of heat must be supplied to overcome the activation energy (see figure 4.27).

---

[7] These values are selected for matter of convenience and demonstration purposes.

The dimensionless thermal damage parameter Ω does not provide any meaningful information to our understanding of the physical effects of thermal damage. From equation (4.55), one may notice that as the concentration of the uncoagulated state approaches zero $C(\tau) \to 0$, i.e., complete thermal coagulation, the value of Ω will approach infinity. A more intuitive way to quantify thermal damage is to use the probability of thermal damage, which is defined as:

$$P(\Omega) = 100\% \times (1 - e^{-\Omega}). \qquad (4.57)$$

It is easy to show that a value of $\Omega = 4.6$ will lead to $P(\Omega) = 99\%$, or a probability of 99% thermal coagulation, a threshold that has been used by many researchers in thermal ablation studies as an indication that the tissue has undergone complete thermal damage (Cheong *et al* 2021, Ooi and Ooi 2021, Kho *et al* 2020). A less conservative threshold of $\Omega = 1$ has also been adopted by other researchers (Singh and Repaka 2016), which works out to a thermal damage probability of 63%.

The Arrhenius thermal damage model accounts for the effects of both temperature and exposure duration, thus making it versatile in thermal ablation studies. Furthermore, the parameter Ω can be incorporated into bioheat transfer models to account for the dependence of blood perfusion with the state of the tissue (Ooi *et al* 2019). Despite these advantages, the nature of the model gives rise to a limitation. As the model is described by an integral over time (see equation (4.54)), a small increase in temperature can in theory lead to the formation of thermal damage if the exposure is sufficiently long. This effect is not physical, as the human body is able to recover from exposure to moderate elevations in temperature.

4.6.4 Other thermal damage models

The limitation of the Arrhenius thermal damage model has led to the development of other models to quantify thermal damage. These models are often characterised by the existence of multiple compartments and states that cells/tissues may assume during the heating event. For instance, Feng *et al* (2008) introduced a two-state cell death model that was derived based on the principles of thermodynamics. They assumed that a population of cells can be in either one of two states, alive (viable) or dead. According to the model, cell viability can be expressed as:

$$C(t, T) = \frac{e^{-\frac{f(t,T)}{kT}}}{1 + e^{-\frac{f(t,T)}{kT}}}, \qquad (4.58)$$

where k is a constant and $f(t,T)$ is a function that is fitted based on experimental results.

In theory, the higher the number of compartment/states in the model, the better the model is at predicting the thermal damage phenomenon. O'Neill *et al* (2011) proposed a three-state cell death model, where at any given time, cells can be in either the alive (A_1), vulnerable (V_n) or dead (D_d) state. The process by which cells transition from alive to dead follows:

$$A_l \overset{k_f}{\underset{k_b}{\rightleftarrows}} V_n \overset{k_f}{\rightarrow} D_d, \tag{4.59}$$

where k_f (s^{-1}) and k_b (s^{-1}) are the forward and backward reaction rates, respectively. According to equation (4.59), cells in the alive state must transition to the vulnerable state when exposed to heat. At this point, if heat is removed, the vulnerable cells will recover and return to the alive state. However, if heating continues, vulnerable cells will transition to the dead state. Cells in the dead state cannot return to the vulnerable or alive states, i.e., the process is irreversible. Assuming that $A_l + V_n + D_d = 1$, the equations describing the transition of cell states are given by:

$$\frac{dA_l}{dt} = -k_f A_l + k_b (1 - A_l - D_d), \tag{4.60}$$

$$\frac{dD_d}{dt} = k_f (1 - A_l - D_d). \tag{4.61}$$

Although the multiple state cell death models have been shown to describe better the thermal damage response of cells, their usage is limited due to need to perform parameter fitting to obtain the values of the parameters of the model. Although this is also true for the Arrhenius thermal damage model, an extensive database of the values of A and ΔE_a for different types of cells and tissues already exists from years of research. The same cannot be said of the other models, where values for only a few cells, usually those from the authors who developed the model, are available.

4.6.4.1 Case study 4.4: thermal damage formation during RFA

In this case study[8], the formation of thermal damage during RFA will be quantified using the Arrhenius thermal damage model. The results will be compared against the thermal damage estimated using critical isotherm of 50 °C. Let us consider the problem defined in case study 4.2. The values of the frequency factor and the activation energy used for the liver and the tumour tissues are presented in table 4.8. To account for the loss in blood perfusion when tissue is completely damaged, we set the blood perfusion to depend on the state of the tissue. For simplicity, we assume a stepwise behaviour, such that:

$$\omega_b(\Omega) = \begin{cases} \omega_{b,o}, & \text{for } \Omega < 4.6 \\ 0, & \text{for } \Omega \geqslant 4.6' \end{cases} \tag{4.62}$$

where $\omega_{b,o}$ is the blood perfusion rate of the tissue at basal level. Equation (4.62) states that blood perfusion is zero when complete thermal damage has formed.

Figures 4.29(a) and (b) plot the contours of the thermal damage Ω and the region of complete thermal damage ($\Omega \geqslant 4.6$), respectively after 4 min of RFA treatment. The 50 °C isotherm, which we have assumed to define the thermal damage region in

---

[8] Source files for case study 4.4 are available at https://doi.org/10.1088/978-0-7503-4016-8.

Table 4.8. Values of the frequency factor and the activation energy used for the liver and the tumour tissues (Kim *et al* 1996, Reddy *et al* 2013).

Parameter	Tissue	
	Liver	Tumour
Frequency factor, A (s^{-1})	7.39×10^{39}	3.25×10^{43}
Activation energy, ΔE_a (J mol^{-1})	2.56×10^5	2.81×10^5

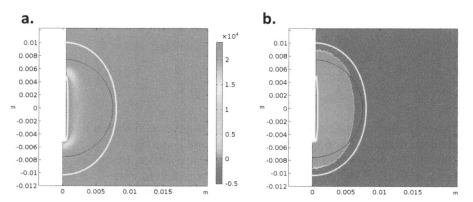

Figure 4.29. Contours of the (a) thermal damage parameter (Ω) and (b) thermal damage zone ($\Omega \geqslant 4.6$) obtained after 4 min of RFA treatment. The yellow curve indicates the isotherm at 50 °C.

case study 4.2, is depicted by the thick yellow curve. The plot of the thermal damage parameter Ω provided no indication on the region of thermal damage (figure 4.29(a)). On the other hand, the condition $\Omega \geqslant 4.6$, which is illustrated by the red region in figure 4.29(b), clearly shows the zone where there is at least a 99% probability of thermal damage. It is evident that the use of the 50 °C isotherm overestimates the region of thermal coagulation, as it does not account for the duration of heat exposure of the tissue.

4.6.4.2 Case study 4.5: analysis of skin burn injury
Burn injury is commonly associated with heat, although other factors may also cause burns, including chemical, electrical, radiation, friction and even cold. The degree of burn injury varies from first degree (minor) to third degree (severe) burns. Severe cases of burn injury may result in death. Patient survival after burn injury depends on the seriousness of the injury. In that aspect, bioheat transfer and thermal damage analyses play important roles in helping doctors understand better the temperature rise inside the skin tissue and correlate them with the degree of burn injury, see figure 4.30. The pioneering study on thermal damage formation using the Arrhenius model by Henriques Jr and Moritz (1947) was in fact carried out on skin burns.

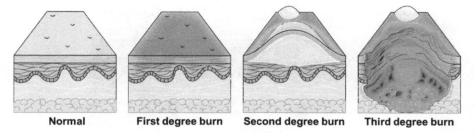

Normal **First degree burn** **Second degree burn** **Third degree burn**

Figure 4.30. Different degrees of burn of the skin tissue due to exposure to heat. Copyright © smart.servier. com. The figure was partly generated using Servier Medical Art, provided by Servier, licensed under a Creative Commons Attribution 3.0 unported license.

In this case study[9], we will demonstrate how the Pennes model can be coupled with the Arrhenius thermal damage model to predict the formation of thermal damage in skin due to exposure to heat. In this case, skin is assumed to be in contact with a hot surface at constant temperature. The skin consists of three domains, i.e., the epidermis (0.05 mm), dermis (1.5 mm) and subcutaneous fat (2.5 mm). For simplicity, the skin tissue is assumed to be cylindrical with a radius of 2 cm and is modelled in 2D axisymmetry. This is shown in figure 4.31. A circular disk of radius 1 cm, which acts as the hot surface, is placed on top of the epidermis with the disk axis aligned with the cylinder axis to preserve the axisymmetry assumption. Across the surface of the epidermis that is in contact with the disk, natural convection to the ambient was assumed, such that:

$$-k_t\frac{\partial T_t}{\partial n} = h_{\mathrm{amb}}(T_t - T_{\mathrm{amb}}),\qquad(4.63)$$

where $h_{\mathrm{amb}} = 10$ W $(\mathrm{m^2 \cdot K})^{-1}$ is the ambient convection coefficient and $T_{\mathrm{amb}} = 25\ ^\circ$C is the ambient temperature. The temperature at the bottom surface of the skin tissue was set to a constant temperature of 37 °C. Three temperatures of the hot disk were investigated, i.e., 70 °C, 80 °C and 90 °C.

Heat transfer inside the skin is described using the Pennes model. Values of the thermal properties for the epidermis, dermis and subcutaneous fat are summarised in table 4.9. Blood perfusion was assumed to be damage dependent according to equation (4.62). The initial temperature of the skin was obtained by solving the steady state Pennes equation without exposure to the heat source.

Figure 4.32 illustrates the temperature contours obtained due to the exposure of the skin to the constant temperature heat source after 60 and 300 s exposure. The white iso-contour represents the threshold of $\Omega = 4.6$, which is indicative of the thermal damage region. A higher disk temperature and longer exposure duration contribute to greater formation of thermal damage across the skin. Contact with a 90 °C surface for 60 s is sufficient to cause thermal damage that is far greater than a 300 s exposure to a 70 °C surface.

---

[9] Source files for case study 4.5 are available at https://doi.org/10.1088/978-0-7503-4016-8.

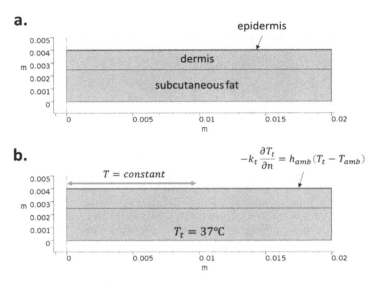

Figure 4.31. (a) Geometry of the skin model and (b) the boundary conditions applied.

Table 4.9. Thermal and cell damage properties of the epidermis, dermis and subcutaneous fat.

Parameter	Epidermis	Dermis	Subcutaneous fat
Thermal conductivity (W $(m \cdot K)^{-1}$)	0.24	0.45	0.69
Density (kg m^{-3})	1200	1200	2000
Specific heat (J $(kg \cdot K)^{-1}$)	3590	3300	6500
Blood perfusion rate (s^{-1})	—	0.001 25	0.0025
Frequency factor (s^{-1})	3.1×10^{98}	2.86×10^{69}	2.86×10^{69}
Activation energy (J mol^{-1})	6.27×10^5	4.60×10^5	4.60×10^5

4.7 General summary

Heat transfer in biological tissues plays an important role in our understanding of the different physical and physiological conditions inside the human body. In this chapter, we have presented the different models that can be used to investigate human body heat transfer. This was demonstrated through various case studies involving thermoregulation and the role of blood flow, and thermal therapy. Except for case study 4.1, all other case studies have adopted the Pennes model as the equation that governs heat transfer inside tissues. It is important to note that the selection of the Pennes model in these case studies was based on its simplicity and availability of parameters to carry out the required analysis. As mentioned in section 4.3.8, the complexity of biological tissues and the variability among different organs and individuals have led to failed attempts at deriving a universal bioheat transfer that can account for all types of tissues. This remains an unfulfilled challenge. Hence, the selection of the bioheat transfer model to use in each analysis should be

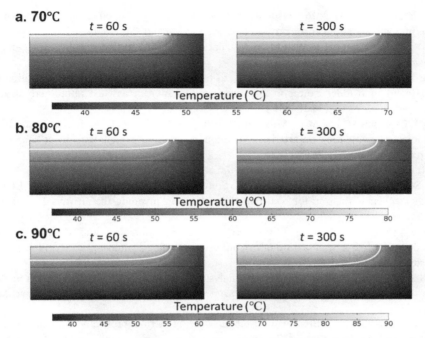

Figure 4.32. Contours of temperature obtained at $t = 60$ and 300 s for skin tissue in contact with a hot surface at (a) 70 °C, (b) 80 °C and (c) 90 °C. White iso-contour depict the interface where $\Omega = 4.6$.

based on the circumstances of the problem and driven by appropriate judgement and justifications.

References

Andreozzi A, Brunese L, Iasiello M, Tucci C and Vanoli G P 2019 Bioheat transfer in a spherical biological tissue: a comparison among various models *J. Phys. Conf. Ser.* **1224** 012001

Andreuccetti D and Zoppetti N 2006 Quasi-static electromagnetic dosimetry: from basic principles to examples of applications *Int. J. Occup. Saf. Ergonom.* **12** 201–15

Arens E A and Zhang H 2006 *The Skin's Role in Human Thermoregulation and Comfort* (UC Berkeley: Center for the Built Environment) https://escholarship.org/uc/item/3f4599hx

Astani S A, Brown M L and Steusloff K 2014 Comparison of procedure costs of various percutaneous tumor ablation modalities *Radiol. Manage* **36** 12–17

Aydin A M *et al* 2020 Focal bipolar radiofrequency ablation for localised prostate cancer: safety and feasibility *Int. J. Urol.* **27** 882–9

Bagavathiappan S, Saravanan T, Philip J, Jayakumar T, Raj B, Karunanithi R, Panicker T M R, Korath M P and Jagadeesan K 2009 Infrared thermal imaging for detection of peripheral vascular disorders *J. Med. Phys.* **34** 43–7

Brace C L 2009 Radiofrequency and microwave ablation of the liver, lung, kidney and bone: what are the differences? *Curr. Probl. Diagn. Radiol.* **38** 135–43

Burdío F *et al* 2009 Research and development of a new RF-assisted device for bloodless rapid transection of the liver: computational modeling and in vivo experiments *Biomed. Eng. Online* **8** 6

Chan J Y and Ooi E H 2016 Sensitivity of thermophysiological models of cryoablation to the thermal and biophysical properties of tissues *Cryobiology* **73** 304–15

Chen M M and Holmes K R 1980 Microvascular contributions in tissue heat transfer *Ann. N. Y. Acad. Sci.* **335** 137–50

Cheong J K K *et al* 2021 A numerical study to investigate the effects of tumour position on the treatment of bladder cancer in mice using gold nanorods assisted photothermal ablation *Comput. Biol. Med.* **138** 104881

Chiang J, Cristescu M, Lee M H, Moreland A, Hinshaw J L, Lee F T and Brace C L 2016 Effects of microwave ablation on arterial and venous vasculature after treatment of hepatocellular carcinoma *Radiology* **281** 617–24

Choudhuri S K R 2007 On a thermoelastic three-phase-lag model *J. Therm. Stresses* **30** 231–8

Chung S R, Baek J H, Choi Y J, Sung T Y, Song D E, Kim T Y and Lee J H 2021 Efficacy of radiofrequency ablation for recurrent thyroid cancer invading the airways *Eur. Radiol.* **31** 2153–60

Costanzo A, Sandri A, Regis D, Trivellin G, Pierantoni S, Samaila E and Magnan B 2017 CT-guided radiofrequency ablation of osteoid osteoma using a multi-tined expandable electrode system *Acta Biomed.* **88** 31–7

Diller K R and Klutke G A 1993 Accuracy analysis of the Henriques model for predicting thermal burn injury ed R B Roemer *Advances in Bioheat and Mass Transfer* (New York: ASME) pp 117–23

Ekici S and Jawzal H 2020 Breast cancer diagnosis using thermography and convolutional neural networks *Med. Hypotheses* **137** 109542

Febbraio M A 2003 Alterations in energy metabolism during exercise and heat stress *Sports Med.* **31** 47–59

Feng Y, Oden J T and Rylander M N 2008 A two-state cell damage model under hyperthermic conditions: theory and in vitro experiments *J. Biomech. Eng.* **130** 041016

Flock S T, Smith L and Warner M D 1993 Quantifying the effects on blood of irradiation with four different vascular-lesion lasers *Proc. SPIE* **1882** 237–72

Gao J, Wang S H, Ding X M, Sun W B, Li X L, Xin Z H, Ning C M and Guo S G 2015 Radiofrequency ablation for single hepatocellular carcinoma 3 cm or less as first-line treatment *World J. Gastroenterol.* **21** 5287–94

Gatt A, Mercieca C, Borg A, Grech A, Camilleri L, Gatt C, Chockalingam N and Formosa C 2019 A comparison of thermographic characteristic of the hands and wrists of rheumatoid arthritis patients and healthy controls *Sci. Rep.* **9** 17204

Gordon C J 2012 Thermal physiology of laboratory mice: defining thermoneutrality *J. Thermal Biol.* **37** 654–85

Hall S K, Ooi E H and Payne S J 2014 A mathematical framework for minimally invasive tumor ablation therapies *Crit. Rev. Biomed. Eng.* **42** 383–417

Hall S K, Ooi E H and Payne S J 2015 Cell death, perfusion and electrical parameters are critical in models of hepatic radiofrequency ablation *Int. J. Hyperth.* **31** 538–50

He X and Bischoff J C 2003 Quantification of temperature and injury response in thermal therapy and cryosurgery *Crit. Rev. Biomed. Eng.* **34** 355–421

He X, McGee S, Coad J E, Schmidlin F, Iaizzo P A, Swanlund D J, Kluge S, Rudie E and Bischoff J C 2004 Investigation of the thermal and tissue injury behaviour in microwave thermal therapy using a porcine kidney model *Int. J. Hyperth.* **2** 567–93

Heisterkamp J, van hillegersberg R and Ijzermans J 1999 Critical temperature and heating time for coagulation damage: implications for interstitial laser coagulation (ILC) of tumors *Lasers Surf. Med.* **25** 257–62

Henriques F Jr and Moritz A 1947 Studies of thermal injury: I. The conduction of heat to and through skin and the temperatures attained therein. A theoretical and an experimental investigation *Am. J. Pathol.* **23** 530–49

Ilo A, Romsi P and Mäkelä J 2020 Infrared thermography and vascular disorders in diabetic feet *J. Diabetes Sci. Tech.* **14** 28–36

Ito T *et al* 2018 Radiofrequency ablation of breast cancer: a retrospective study *Clin. Breast Cancer* **18** e495–500

Jacques S L and Wang L 1995 Monte Carlo modeling of light transport in tissues ed A J Welch and M J C van Gemert *Optical-Thermal Response of Laser-Irradiated Tissue* (Boston, MA: Springer)

Jacques S L and Gaeeni M O 1989 Thermally induced changes in optical properties of heart *IEEE Eng. Med. Biol. Mag.* **11** 1199–200

Jacques S L, Newman C and He X Y 1991 Thermal coagulation of tissues: liver studies indicate a distribution of rate parameters not a single rate parameter describes the coagulation process Proc. Winter Annu. Meeting Am. Soc. Mech. Eng. *(Atlanta, GA)* pp 71–3

Jacques S L 2011 Monte Carlo modeling of light transport in tissues *Optical Thermal Response of Laser* (New York: Springer) pp 109–44

Keener J and Sneyd J 2009 *Mathematical Physiology—Systems Physiology.* 2nd edn (New York: Springer)

Keller K H and Seiler L 1971 An analysis of peripheral heat transfer in man *J. Appl. Physiol.* **30** 779–89

Kho A S K, Foo J J, Ooi E T and Ooi E H 2020 Shape-shifting thermal coagulation zone during saline-infused radiofrequency ablation: a computational study on the effects of different infusion location *Comput. Methods Programs Biomed.* **184** 105289

Kho A S K, Foo J J, Ooi E T and Ooi E H 2022 Saline-infused radiofrequency ablation: a review on the key factors for a safe and reliable tumour treatment *IEEE Rev. Biomed. Eng.* https://doi.org/10.1109/RBME.2022.3179742

Kim B M, Jacques S, Rastegar S, Thomsen S and Motamedi M 1996 Nonlinear finite element analysis of the role of dynamic changes in blood perfusion and optical properties in laser coagulation of tissue *IEEE J. Sel. Top Quant. Electron* **2** 922–33

Klinger H G 1974 Heat transfer in perfused biological tissue—I: general theory *Bull. Math. Biol.* **36** 403–15

Kok H P, Wust P, Stauffer P R, Bardati F, van Rhoon G C and Crezee J 2015 Current state of the art of regional hyperthermia treatment planning: a review *Radiat. Oncol.* **10** 196

Kwiecien S Y and McHugh M P 2021 The cold truth: the role of cryotherapy in the treatment of injury and recovery from exercise *Eur. J. Appl. Physiol.* **121** 2126–42

Lee D H, Lee J M, Lee J Y, Kim S H, Yoon J H, Kim Y J, Han J K and Choi B I 2014 Radiofrequency ablation of hepatocellular carcinoma as first-line treatment: long-term results and prognostic factors in 162 patients with cirrhosis *Radiology* **270** 900–9

Lim C L 2020 Fundamental concepts of human thermoregulation and adaptation to heat: a review in the context of global warming *Int. J. Environ. Res. Public Health* **17** 7795

Lim C L, Byrne C and Lee J K 2008 Human thermoregulation and measurement of body temperature in exercise and clinical settings *Ann. Acad. Med. Singap.* **37** 347–53

Lorentzen T 1996 A cooled needle electrode for radiofrequency tissue ablation: thermodynamic aspects of improved performance compared with conventional needle design *Acad. Radiol.* **3** 556–63

Mazur P 1984 Freezing of living cells: mechanisms and implications *Am. J. Physiol.* **247** C125–42

McDermott S and Gervais D A 2013 Radiofrequency ablation of liver tumors *Semin. Intervent. Radiol.* **30** 49–55

Mitchell J W and Myers G E 1968 An analytical model of the counter-current heat exchange phenomena *Biophys. J.* **8** 897–911

Nakayama A and Kuwahara F 2008 A general bioheat transfer model based on the theory of porous media *Int. J. Heat Mass Transf.* **51** 3190–9

Ni Y, Mulier S, Miao Y, Michel L and Marchal G 2005 A review of the general aspects of radiofrequency ablation *Abdom. Imaging* **30** 381–400

Nomori H, Yamazaki I, Kondo T and Kanno M 2017 The cryoablation of lung tissue using liquid nitrogen in gel and the ex vivo pig lung *Surg. Today* **47** 259–64

O'Neill D P, Peng T, Stiegler P, Mayrhauser U, Koestenbauer S, Tscheilienssnigg K and Payne S J 2011 A three-state mathematical model of hyperthermic cell death *Ann. Biomed. Eng.* **39** 570–9

Ooi E H and Ooi E T 2021 Unidirectional ablation minimizes unwanted thermal damage and promotes better thermal ablation efficacy in time-based switching bipolar radiofrequency ablation *Comput. Biol. Med.* **137** 104832

Ooi E H, Lee K W, Yap S, Khattab M, Liao I Y, Ooi E T, Foo J J, Nair S R and Mohd Ali A F 2019 The effects of electrical and thermal boundary condition on the simulation of radio-frequency ablation of liver cancer for tumours located near to the liver boundary *Comput. Biol. Med.* **106** 12–23

Payne S J, Flanagan R, Pollari M, Alhonnoro T, Bost T, O'Neill D, Peng T and Stiegler P 2011 Image-based multi-scale modelling and validation of radio-frequency ablation in liver tumours *Phil. Trans. Roy. Soc.* A **369** 4233–54

Pearce J A 2013 Comparative analysis of mathematical models of cell death and thermal damage processes *Int. J. Hyperth.* **29** 262–80

Peng T, O'Neill D P and Payne S J 2011 A two-equation coupled system for determination of liver tissue temperature during thermal ablation *Int. J. Heat Mass Transf.* **54** 2100–9

Pennes H H 1948 Analysis of tissue and arterial blood temperatures in the resting human forearm *J. Appl. Physiol.* **1** 93–122

Qian P C, Barry M A, Tran V T, Lu J, McEwan A, Thiagalingam A and Thomas S P 2020 Irrigated microwave catheter ablation can create deep ventricular lesions through epicardial fat with relative sparing of adjacent coronary arteries *Circ. Arrhythm. Electrophysiol.* **13** e008251

Ramos G V, Pinheiro C M, Messa S P, Delfino G B, Marquetti R, Salvini T and Durigan J L Q 2016 Cryotherapy reduces inflammatory response without altering muscle regeneration process and extracellular matrix remodeling of rat muscle *Sci. Rep.* **6** 18525

Reddy G, Dreher M R, Rossmann C, Wood B J and Haemmerich D 2013 Cytotoxicity of hepatocellular carcinoma cells to hyperthermic and ablative temperature exposures: *in viro* studies and mathematical modelling *Int. J. Hyperth.* **20** 318–23

Roetzel W and Xuan Y 1998 Transient response of the human limb to an external stimulus *Int. J. Heat Mass Transf.* **41** 229–39

Sapareto S A, Hopwood L E, Dewey W C, Raju M R and Gray J W 1978 Effects of hyperthermia on survival and progression of Chinese hamster ovary cells *Cancer Res.* **38** 393–400

Sartori S, Vece F, Ermili F and Tombesi P 2017 Laser ablation of liver tumors: an ancillary technique, or an alternative to radiofrequency and microwave? *World J. Radiol.* **28** 91–6

Schramm W, Yang D, Wood B J, Rattay F and Haemmerich D 2007 Contribution of direct heating, thermal conduction and perfusion during radiofrequency and microwave ablation *Open Biomed. Eng. J.* **1** 47–52

Schutt D J and Haemmerich D 2008 Effects of variation in perfusion rates and of perfusion models in computational models of radio frequency tumor ablation *Med. Phys.* **35** 3462–70

Singh S and Repaka R 2016 Temperature-controlled radiofrequency ablation of different tissues using two-compartment models *Int. J. Hyperth.* **33** 122–34

Singh D and Singh A K 2020 Role of image thermography in early breast cancer *Comput. Methods Programs Biomed.* **183** 105074

Smith A M, Mancini M C and Nie S 2009 Second window for in vivo imaging *Nat. Nanotechnol.* **4** 710–1

Song K D 2016 Percutaneous cryoablation for hepatocellular carcinoma *Clin. Mol. Hepatol.* **22** 509–15

Su T Y, Chiang H K, Hwa C K, Liu P H, Wu M H, Chang D O, Su P F and Chang W S 2011 Noncontact detection of dry eye using a custom designed infrared thermal image system *J. Biomed. Opt.* **16** 046009

Tan L L, Sanjay S and Morgan P B 2016 Screening for dry eye disease using infrared ocular thermography *Cont. Lens Anterior Eye* **39** 442–9

Tan Y K, Hong C, Li H, Allen J C Jr and Thumboo J 2020 Thermography in rheumatoid arthritis: a comparison with ultrasonography and clinical joint assessment *Clin. Radiology* **75** 963.e17–22

Thomsen S 2005 Non-thermal effects in thermal treatment applications of non-ionizing irradiation *Proc. SPIE* **5698** 1–14

Tucci C, Trujillo M, Berjano E, Iasiello M, Andreozzi A and Vanoli G P 2021 Pennes bioheat equation vs. porous medial approach in computer modeling *Sci. Rep.* **11** 5272

Vines J B, Yoon J-H, Ryu N-E, Lim D-J and Park H 2019 Gold nanoparticles for photothermal cancer therapy *Front. Chem.* **7** 167

Voglreiter P, Mariappan P, Pollari M, Flanagan R, Sequeiros R B, Portugaller R H, Fütterer J, Schmalstieg D, Kolesnik M and Moche M 2018 RFA guardian: comprehensive simulation of radiofrequency ablation treatment of liver tumors *Sci. Rep.* **8** 787

Weaver J A and Stoll A M 1967 Mathematical model of skin exposed to thermal radiation *Aerosp. Med.* **40** 24–30

Welch A J and Polhamus G D 1984 Measurement and prediction of thermal injury in the retina of Rhesus monkey *IEEE Trans. Biomed. Eng.* **31** 631–44

Weinbaum S, Jiji L M and Lemons D E 1984a Theory and experiment for the effect of vascular microstructure on surface tissue heat transfer—part I: anatomical foundation and model conceptualization *J. Biomech. Eng.* **106** 321–30

Weinbaum S, Jiji L M and Lemons D E 1984b Theory and experiment for the effect of vascular microstructure on surface tissue heat transfer—part II: model formulation and solution *J. Biomech. Eng.* **106** 331–41

Wu Q, Zhang H, Chen M, Zhang Y, Huang J, Xu Z and Wang W 2015 Preparation of carbon-coated iron nanofluid and its application in radiofrequency ablation *J. Biomed. Mater. Res.* B **103** 908–14

Wulff W 1974 The energy conservation equation for living tissue *IEEE Trans. Biomed. Eng.* **21** 494–5

Xia L Y, Hu Q L and Xu W Y 2021 Efficacy and safety of radiofrequency ablation for breast cancer smaller than 2 cm: a systematic review and meta-analysis *Front. Oncol.* **11** 651646

Xu F, Lu T and Seffen K A 2008 Dual-phase-lag model of skin bioheat transfer 2008 *Int. Conf. Biomed. Eng. Inform. (Sanya China) vol 1 pp 505–11*

Xuan Y and Roetzel W 1997 Bioheat equation of the human thermal system *Chem. Eng. Technol.* **20** 268–76

Yarmolenko P S, Moon E J, Landon C, Manzoor A, Hochman D W, Viglianti B L and Dewhirst M W 2011 Thresholds for thermal damage to normal tissues: an update *Int. J. Hyperth.* **27** 320–43

Yu F C, Lu K C, Lin S H, Chen G S, Chu P, Gao G W and Lin Y F 1997 Energy metabolism in exertional heat stroke with acute renal failure *Nephrol. Dial. Transplant.* **12** 2087–92

Zheng F, Moser M A J, Zhang E M, Zhang W and Zhang 2020 A novel method to increase tumor ablation zones with RFA by injecting the cationic polymer solution to tissues: *in vivo* and computational studies *IEEE Trans. Biomed. Eng.* **67** 1787–96

Zhou X, Jin K, Qiu S, Jin D, Liao X, Tu X, Zheng Z, Li J, Yang L and Wei Q 2020 Comparative effectiveness of radiotherapy versus focal laser ablation in patients with low and intermediate risk localized prostate cancer *Sci. Rep.* **10** 9112

Zhu L 2009 Heat transfer applications in biological systems ed M Kutz *Biomedical Engineering and Design Handbook, Volume 1: Fundamentals* (New York: McGraw Hill) ch 2

Chapter 5

Haemodynamics

5.1 Introduction

Haemodynamics is the study of blood flow, which is integral to human body functions. In chapter 4, we have shown how blood flow in tissues play an important role in human body thermoregulation. Other than that, blood flow is crucial for the transport of oxygen and carbon dioxide to and from cells at different parts of the body, respectively. It also functions as a medium that delivers nutrients to cells and collects waste products to be discharged. Blood flows in the circulatory system of the human body, which consists of the systemic and the pulmonary circulation, both of which are connected to the heart. The systemic circulation, which accounts for 84% blood volume within the circulatory system, delivers oxygenated blood from the left ventricle of the heart to the rest of the body through the arteries and capillaries. Deoxygenated blood is transported through the veins and back to the right atrium. The pulmonary system carries deoxygenated blood from the right atrium to the lungs and returns oxygenated blood to the heart through the left atrium where it then enters the systemic circulation. The pathways of blood through the systemic and pulmonary system are illustrated in figure 5.1.

5.2 Arteries, veins, and capillaries

The circulatory system is made up of three types of blood vessels, i.e., arteries, veins, and capillaries. Arteries typically branch off into smaller arterioles before forming the capillary bed. Likewise, capillaries converge into larger venules before they merge to form veins. This is shown in figure 5.2. These blood vessels are differentiated primarily by their size and functions. Table 5.1 summarises the typical radius of arteries, veins, and capillaries. The exact radius of each vessel varies depending on the organs and location within the organs. Blood flow in the arteries, veins and capillaries are different due to their different sizes and anatomical features, such as the presence of valves and bifurcations. Consequently, different fluid dynamic analysis is required to elucidate the blood flow phenomena inside different blood vessels.

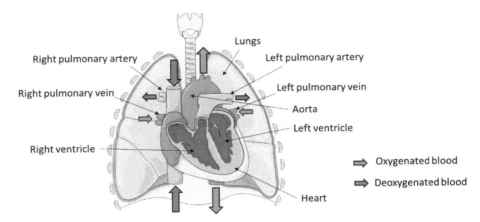

Figure 5.1. The systemic and pulmonary circulatory system of the human body. Copyright © smart.servier. com. The figure was partly generated using Servier Medical Art, provided by Servier, licensed under a Creative Commons Attribution 3.0 unported license.

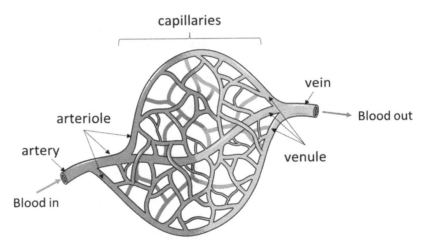

Figure 5.2. Blood flow through the arteries, capillaries, and veins. Arteries branch into arterioles before separating into capillaries. Capillaries converge into venules before merging to the vein. Copyright © smart. servier.com. The figure was partly generated using Servier Medical Art, provided by Servier, licensed under a Creative Commons Attribution 3.0 unported license.

5.2.1 Arteries

Arteries carry oxygen-rich blood from the heart to other organs and tissues of the body. Artery walls are thicker than veins and capillaries since they must be structurally strong to withstand the high blood flow pressure from the heart. The walls of the arteries consist of three layers known as the intima (innermost layer), media (middle layer) and adventitia (outermost layer). These are illustrated in figure 5.3(a). The media is the thickest of the three layers and provides the required structural support to the vessel to withstand the high pressures from the heart.

Table 5.1. Typical values of radius in arteries, veins, and capillaries (Chen and Holmes 1980).

Blood vessel type	Radius (mm)
Large arteries	1.5
Arterial branches	0.5
Terminal arterial branches	0.3
Arterioles	0.01
Capillaries	0.004
Venules	0.015
Terminal veins	0.75
Venous branches	1.2
Large veins	3

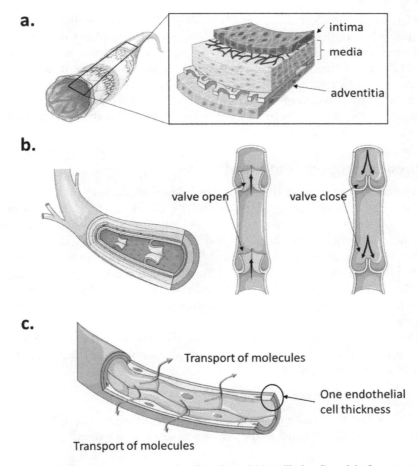

Figure 5.3. Anatomical features of the (a) arteries, (b) veins and (c) capillaries. Copyright © smart.servier.com. The figure was partly generated using Servier Medical Art, provided by Servier, licensed under a Creative Commons Attribution 3.0 unported license.

5.2.2 Veins

Veins carry deoxygenated blood from the tissue back to the heart, where it then enters the pulmonary system for oxygenation. Since pressure in the veins is significantly lower than in the artery, the walls of veins are typically thinner than arteries. One of the main features of veins is the presence of valves to prevent backflow of blood. This is shown in figure 5.3(b). Prevention of backflow is necessary to avoid blood accumulation inside the veins, which can potentially cause damage. Valves are not present in arteries since the high pressure from the heart is sufficient to prevent backflow from occurring. Two types of veins exist in the human body, namely deep and superficial veins. The former is situated deep inside the muscle tissue and has a corresponding artery nearby. The latter is located beneath the skin surface and do not have corresponding arteries.

5.2.3 Capillaries

Capillaries are the smallest blood vessels inside the body. The capillary bed functions as a platform for solutes and nutrients to transport between blood and tissue. Unlike arteries and veins, capillaries exist as a complex and tortuous[1] network. Pressure inside capillaries is significantly lower than in arteries and veins; as such, the radii and thicknesses of capillaries are several orders of magnitude smaller than arteries and veins. Capillary walls consist of a single layer of endothelial cells. The walls are fenestrated[2] to allow transport of molecules from blood to the surrounding tissue. This is shown in figure 5.3(c).

5.3 Physical properties of blood

To carry out a proper fluid dynamics analysis of blood flow, it is important to understand the relevant physical properties of blood, as they can influence the behaviour of blood flow in arteries, veins, and capillaries. Blood comprises plasma and cellular contents such as red blood cells (erythrocytes), white blood cells (leukocytes) and platelets (thrombocytes); all of which contribute to some extent in determining the physical properties of blood. Blood rheology plays an important role in the fluid dynamics analysis of blood flow. However, blood rheology is not constant and its behaviour, either as a Newtonian or a non-Newtonian fluid, varies depending on the vessels.

A Newtonian fluid is one where its viscosity is independent of the viscous stress. In a Newtonian fluid, the flow-induced viscous stress is a linear function of the shear rate, such that (Panton 2013):

$$\tau = -\mu\dot{\gamma}, \tag{5.1}$$

where τ (N m^{-2} or Pa) is the viscous stress, μ (Pa·s) is dynamic viscosity and $\dot{\gamma}$ (s^{-1}) is the strain rate, which is defined as the velocity gradient in the direction parallel to the

---

[1] Full of twists and turns.
[2] Having tiny holes or perforations.

direction of shear. The linear dependence of shear stress on strain rate is typically observed in blood flowing inside large arteries. Hence, when performing fluid dynamics analysis in these cases, blood may be assumed to behave as a Newtonian fluid.

A non-Newtonian fluid is one where the viscosity varies depending on the shear stress. The shear stress in this case exhibits a nonlinear dependence on the shear rate and typically follows a power law (Bird *et al* 1987):

$$\tau = -\mu' \dot{\gamma}^n, \tag{5.2}$$

where μ' (Pa·s^n) is the flow consistency index and $n > 0$ is a constant. Non-Newtonian behaviour is typically observed in blood that is flowing inside very small vessels such as the capillaries. One of the most common models that describe non-Newtonian blood viscosity is the Carreau model (Carreau 1972):

$$\mu = \mu_\infty + (\mu_0 - \mu_\infty)[1 + (\lambda\dot{\gamma})^2]^{(n-1)/2}, \tag{5.3}$$

where μ_0 (Pa·s) is the dynamic viscosity at zero shear rate, μ_∞ (Pa·s) is the viscosity at infinite shear rate and λ (s) is the relaxation time.

5.4 Haemodynamics of a single blood vessel

5.4.1 Poiseuille's law in blood flow analysis

A simple analysis of flow in blood vessels can be carried out using Poiseuille's law. Let us assume a blood vessel that is straight with a constant radius of r_b (m) and length ℓ_b (m). This is illustrated in figure 5.4. Two factors determine the blood flow rate Q (m^3 s^{-1}) through the vessel:

(i) the pressure difference Δp (Pa) between the two ends of the vessel, and
(ii) the flow resistance R (kg·s m^{-4}) of blood flow through the vessel.

The blood flow rate, pressure difference and flow resistance are related to one another through the relation:

$$Q = \frac{\Delta p}{R} \text{ or } R = \frac{\Delta p}{Q}. \tag{5.4}$$

Equation (5.4) is also known as the Darcy's law or Ohm's law; the latter because it shares similarities with Ohm's law for electric current flow. In this case, the blood flow rate is analogous to the electric current (I), pressure difference is analogous

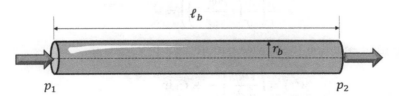

Figure 5.4. Poiseuille's law analysis of blood flow through a straight vessel with uniform radius.

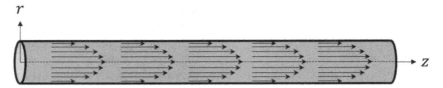

r

z

Figure 5.5. Parabolic velocity profile under the fully developed assumption. Velocity in the radial direction is zero ($u = 0$), while velocity in the axial direction is independent of z ($w(r, z) = w(r)$).

to the electric potential difference (ΔV), and the flow resistance is analogous to electrical resistance (R_i).

To determine the blood flow rate, first, we assume the flow inside the blood vessel to be fully developed, such that the velocity profile inside the vessel is parabolic (more details in section 5.5.2) and is independent of the position along the vessel. This is shown in figure 5.5. Next, the Navier–Stokes equations in the absence of body force (more details in section 5.5.1) is expressed in 2D axisymmetry, which is made possible by the assumption of fully developed flow. These are given by:

$$\frac{\partial u}{\partial r} + \frac{u}{r} + \frac{\partial w}{\partial z} = 0, \tag{5.5}$$

$$\frac{\partial u}{\partial t} + u\frac{\partial u}{\partial r} + \frac{u}{r} + w\frac{\partial u}{\partial z} = -\frac{1}{\rho}\frac{\partial p}{\partial r} + \frac{\mu}{\rho}\left(\frac{\partial^2 u}{\partial r^2} + \frac{1}{r}\frac{\partial u}{\partial r} - \frac{u}{r^2} + \frac{\partial^2 u}{\partial z^2}\right), \tag{5.6}$$

$$\frac{\partial w}{\partial t} + u\frac{\partial w}{\partial r} + w\frac{\partial w}{\partial z} = -\frac{1}{\rho}\frac{\partial p}{\partial z} + \frac{\mu}{\rho}\left(\frac{\partial^2 w}{\partial r^2} + \frac{1}{r}\frac{\partial w}{\partial r} + \frac{\partial^2 w}{\partial z^2}\right), \tag{5.7}$$

where $u = (u,w)$ (m s^{-1}) is the velocity vector, t (s) is time, (r, z) is the coordinate in 2D axisymmetry, ρ (kg m^{-3}) is fluid density and p (Pa) is pressure.

Under the fully developed flow assumption, velocity in the radial direction is zero, such that $u = 0$. Velocity in the axial direction becomes independent of z such that $w(r, z) = w(r)$. Using these assumptions and further assuming the flow to be in steady state ($\partial u/\partial t = \partial w/\partial t = 0$), equations (5.5)–(5.7) can be simplified to:

$$\mu\left(\frac{d^2 w}{dr^2} + \frac{1}{r}\frac{dw}{dr}\right) = \frac{dp}{dz}, \tag{5.8}$$

or

$$\frac{\mu}{r}\left(\frac{d}{dr}\left(r\frac{dw(r)}{dr}\right)\right) = \frac{dp}{dz}. \tag{5.9}$$

Integrating equation (5.9) twice with respect to r leads to:

$$w(r) = \left(\frac{1}{\mu}\frac{dp}{dz}\right)\frac{r^2}{4} + C_1 \ln r + C_2, \tag{5.10}$$

where C_1 and C_2 are integration constants. Using the conditions $w(r_b) = 0$ (velocity at the vessel wall is zero) and $dw(0)/dr = 0$ (velocity gradient is zero at point of maximum w), one obtains the expressions of C_1 and C_2, which upon substituting into equation (5.10), yields:

$$w(r) = -\frac{1}{4\mu}\left(\frac{dp}{dz}\right)r_b^2\left[1 - \left(\frac{r}{r_b}\right)^2\right].$$

(5.11)

Equation (5.11) describes the velocity profile of blood flow inside a vessel that is cylindrical and straight. Note that the pressure gradient in the axial direction dp/dz is negative due to the direction of blood flow from points of high to low pressure. For a uniform pressure drop along the vessel, one may express the pressure gradient as $dp/dz = \Delta p/\ell_b$. Substituting this into equation (5.11) and performing some mathematical rearrangements, one obtains:

$$w(r) = -\left(\frac{\Delta p}{4\mu\ell_b}\right)[r_b^2 - r^2],$$

(5.12)

which describes the velocity in the z-direction as a function of r. The parabolic flow profile as a result from the fully developed flow assumption is evident from the term r^2.

Knowledge of the velocity profile allows us to obtain an expression for the blood flow rate inside the vessel, which is attainable by performing a double integral of equation (5.12) across the circular cross section of the vessel:

$$Q = \iint_A w(r)dA = \int_0^{2\pi}\int_0^{r_b} w(r)rdrd\theta = -2\pi\int_0^{r_b}\left(\frac{\Delta p}{4\mu\ell_b}\right)[r_b^2 - r^2]rdr,$$

(5.13)

where the $dA = rdrd\theta$ denotes the area of an infinitesimal portion of the region A expressed in polar coordinates. Integrating equation (5.13) results in:

$$Q = -\frac{\pi\Delta pr_b^4}{8\mu\ell_b},$$

(5.14)

which describes the flow rate inside the blood vessel.

Equation (5.14) is also known as the Poiseuille's law, which relates flow rate to the pressure drop for a fully developed flow in a cylindrical tube. Note that the negative term from $\Delta p = p_2 - p_1$ cancels off the negative term on the right-hand side of equation (5.14). Substituting equation (5.14) into (5.4) leads to the expression for the flow resistance:

$$R = \frac{8\mu\ell_b}{\pi r_b^4}.$$

(5.15)

According to equation (5.15), the resistance to flow in blood vessel is proportional to the dynamic viscosity of blood and vessel length, but inversely proportional to the fourth power of the vessel radius. Blood viscosity depends on the concentration of various constituents of plasma and the amount of red blood cells (haematocrit), as well as size, shape, and deformability. In healthy individuals, blood viscosity is typically a constant. Under some pathological conditions such as anaemia, the low haematocrit count can lead to a decrease in blood viscosity (Connes *et al* 2013). Vessel length is also typically constant within a section of blood flow and does not change considerably in the human body. Hence, the main factor that governs the flow resistance of blood according to equation (5.15) is the vessel radius. The inverse dependence of the flow resistance on the fourth power of the vessel radius suggests that a small change in the vessel radius can result in a significant increase in flow resistance, which can have severe consequences to the blood flow rate.

Equation (5.15), and by that extension, equation (5.14), allows one to understand the regulation of blood flow in response to some external stimuli, such as the enlargement and the narrowing of blood vessel through vasodilation and vaso-constriction, respectively, in response to a thermal stimulus (see chapter 4). This can be further demonstrated through the simple example below:

> A climate change scientist working in the Arctic Circle steps out of his tent and into the frozen tundra. His blood vessels begin to constrict to prevent heat loss to the environment. If there is vasoconstriction of 25% in the vessel radius, determine the change in the blood flow along the constricted blood vessel. Assume the vessel pressure, vessel length and blood viscosity remain unchanged.

To determine the change in the blood flow due to vasoconstriction, we may use the Poiseuille's law defined by equation (5.14). Since the vessel pressure remains constant, we have:

$$\Delta p_1 = \Delta p_2, \tag{5.16}$$

where '1' and '2' refer to the state of the vessel before and after vasoconstriction, respectively. Rearranging equation (5.14) in terms of Δp:

$$\Delta p = \frac{8 Q \mu \ell_b}{\pi r_b^4} \tag{5.17}$$

and substituting it into equation (5.16), we obtain:

$$\frac{8 \mu Q_1 \ell_{b,1}}{\pi r_{b,1}^4} = \frac{8 \mu Q_2 \ell_{b,2}}{\pi r_{b,2}^4}. \tag{5.18}$$

A vasoconstriction that leads to 25% change in vessel radius implies that $r_{b,2} = 0.75 r_{b,1}$. Substituting this into equation (5.18) and eliminating identical terms, one obtains:

$$Q_2 = \frac{(0.75 r_{b,1})^4}{r_{b,1}^4} Q_1 = 0.316 Q_1, \tag{5.19}$$

where blood flow rate after vasoconstriction is reduced to 0.316 times its value before vasoconstriction. The decrease in blood flow rate minimises the amount of heat loss from the body to the ambient through the skin, which helps to conserve body heat under freezing conditions.

5.4.2 Application of Poiseuille's law in atherosclerosis

Atherosclerosis is a cardiovascular disease defined by the accumulation and formation of plaque (fatty deposits) around the blood vessel wall that if left untreated, will cause blockage or occlusion (Rafieian-Kopaei *et al* 2014). Figure 5.6 illustrates the formation of atherosclerosis, where an increase in occlusion results in a more severe atherosclerosis. As the occlusion increases, the area available for blood flow decreases, which according to equation (5.15), can increase the flow resistance significantly. Poiseuille's law provides a simple yet effective approach to understand how the different levels of occlusion can affect the dynamics of blood flow.

For simplicity, let us assume that the level of occlusion is directly correlated with the radius of the vessels. In other words, a 10% occlusion results in a 10% decrease in vessel radius. Hence, for 30%, 65% and 90% occlusions, as illustrated in figure 5.6, we have $r_{b,2} = 0.7r_{b,1}$, $r_{b,2} = 0.35r_{b,1}$ and $r_{b,2} = 0.1r_{b,1}$, respectively. Assuming blood viscosity and vessel length to remain constant, and blood pressure before and after the event of occlusion to be the same, we obtain:

$$\Delta p_1 = \Delta p_2,$$

which upon substituting for the expressions in equation (5.17) and eliminating identical terms on the left- and right-hand side, yields:

$$\frac{Q_1}{r_{b,1}^4} = \frac{Q_2}{r_{b,2}^4}, \tag{5.20}$$

where '1' and '2' represent the pre-occluded and occluded states, respectively.

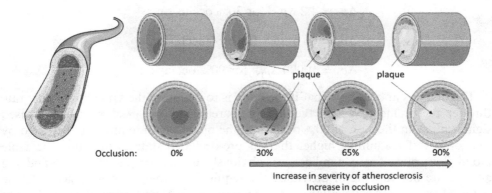

Figure 5.6. Atherosclerosis at various degrees of occlusion. Copyright © smart.servier.com. The figure was partly generated using Servier Medical Art, provided by Servier, licensed under a Creative Commons Attribution 3.0 unported license.

Substituting the expressions for $r_{b,2}$ in terms of $r_{b,1}$ for the different degrees of occlusion into equation (5.20), yields:

$$Q_2 = 0.24Q_1, \text{ for 30\% occlusion,}$$

$$Q_2 = 0.015Q_1, \text{ for 65\% occlusion,}$$

$$Q_2 = 0.0001Q_1, \text{ for 90\% occlusion.}$$

At 30% occlusion, the decrease in the vessel radius results in 0.24 times decrease in blood flow rate. At 65% occlusion, the flow rate decreases to 0.015 times its basal value. At the severe case of 90% occlusion, flow rate decreases by four orders of magnitude. At this point, blood flow through the vessel becomes almost negligible. If the occlusion occurs in the internal carotid artery, i.e., the major artery supplying blood to the head, the decrease in blood flow will result in insufficient blood supply to the brain that can eventually lead to a stroke (Madulanda-Londoño and Chaturvedi 2016).

In the example above, we have considered changes to the blood flow rate in occluded vessels under the condition that the blood pressure remains unchanged. It is also possible to use Poiseuille's law to investigate the pressure that is required to maintain the same blood flow rate through the occluded vessels. Under the condition of equal blood flow rate, we have:

$$Q_1 = Q_2,$$

which upon substituting equation (5.14) and after some mathematical operations and rearrangements, yields:

$$\Delta p_2 = \left(\frac{r_{b,1}}{r_{b,2}}\right)^4 \Delta p_1. \tag{5.21}$$

Substituting $r_{b,2} = 0.7r_{b,1}$, $r_{b,2} = 0.35r_{b,1}$ and $r_{b,2} = 0.1r_{b,1}$ into equation (5.21) results in:

$$\Delta p_2 = 4.2 \, \Delta p_1, \text{ for 30\% occlusion,}$$

$$\Delta p_2 = 66.6 \, \Delta p_1, \text{ for 65\% occlusion,}$$

$$\Delta p_2 = 10000 \, \Delta p_1, \text{ for 90\% occlusion.}$$

The findings above show that if the body is to maintain the same blood flow rate through the occluded vessels, then the pressure inside the vessel must be increased significantly. In the case of 90% occlusion, the blood pressure must be increased by four orders of magnitude higher than its pre-occluded state to maintain the same blood flow rate. These numbers are obviously unrealistic, as the heart and the arteries are not capable of providing the required pumping power to generate the required pressure. An elevation in the pressure causes hypertension that can lead to various cardiovascular disorders (Fuchs and Whelton 2020).

5.4.3 Limitations of the Poiseuille's law in blood flow analysis

Poiseuille's law presents a simple approach for understanding blood flow dynamics. However, its application is limited to cases that satisfy the following conditions:
1. Blood vessel is long and straight.
2. Flow inside the vessel is laminar, fully developed and in steady state.
3. Blood behaves as a Newtonian fluid.

Unfortunately, these conditions are not always satisfied.

Not all blood vessels inside the body are long and straight. Except for certain sections of some major arteries, most blood vessels will bifurcate and branch off into smaller vessels, thus negating the first assumption above. Moreover, as pointed out in section 5.2.2, some vessels like veins have valves that can cause variation in the blood flow profile. Blood flow inside the human body is also not in steady state. The heart pumps blood in a cyclic pattern, which gives rise to pulsatile blood flow through the vessels. This causes unsteady flow that can disrupt the fully developed flow profile. Several anatomical characteristics and vascular disorders can cause blood flow to be turbulent. Some examples include flow through venous valves and flow through constricted vessels due to occlusion; both of which cause blood flow to be turbulent. As pointed out in section 5.3, whether blood behaves as a Newtonian or non-Newtonian fluid depends on the blood vessel. While flow in large arteries demonstrate Newtonian-like flow behaviour, the same cannot be said for flow in small vessels such as the capillaries.

Despite these limitations, the Poiseuille's law provides a simple yet important understanding of various vascular conditions and how they are influenced by the blood vessel radius. Other than vasoconstriction and atherosclerosis as discussed above, Poiseuille's law can be used to describe changes in the blood flow dynamics due to vascular toning, a condition defined by the degree of vessel constriction relative to its state at maximum dilation (Fernández-Alfonso 2004), and vascular stenosis, a pathological condition defined by the abnormal narrowing of blood vessels (Thiriet *et al* 2015).

5.5 Computational fluid dynamics in blood flow analysis

Computational fluid dynamics (CFD) is a sub discipline of fluid mechanics study that employs numerical modelling and digital computers to predict fluid flow phenomena based on solutions of conservation laws, such as the mass, momentum, and energy conservations (Hu 2012). CFD plays a huge role in the study of haemodynamics as it can provide solutions to problems that cannot be described using Poiseuille's law (see section 5.4). They allow complicated blood vessel geometries to be developed and complex flow analysis (for e.g. turbulent and non-Newtonian flows) to be carried out. CFD is a very broad topic and understanding its principles and concept requires some background knowledge on numerical modelling, which is beyond the scope of this book. Nevertheless, we will present some of the important elements of CFD in the subsequent sections that should be given due consideration when carrying out haemodynamics analysis.

5.5.1 Navier–Stokes equations

Navier–Stokes equations are a set of partial differential equations that describe viscous fluid in motion. It consists of two equations, namely the mass conservation (also known as the continuity equation) and the momentum conservation equations. Their expressions in 2D axisymmetry have been presented in section 5.4.1 (see equations (5.5)–(5.7)), but are reproduced here in 3D vector form as:

$$\nabla \cdot \mathbf{v} = 0, \tag{5.22}$$

$$\frac{\partial \mathbf{v}}{\partial t} + (\mathbf{v} \cdot \nabla)\mathbf{v} = -\frac{\nabla p}{\rho} + \frac{\mu}{\rho}\nabla^2\mathbf{v} + \mathbf{F}, \tag{5.23}$$

where $\mathbf{v} = (u, v, w)$ (m s^{-1}) is the velocity vector, u, v and w are the velocity components in the x-, y- and z-directions, respectively, and $\mathbf{F}$ (N m^{-3}) is the body force vector that accounts for external forces acting on the flow, such as gravity and buoyancy. Equations (5.22) and (5.23) are respectively the continuity and momentum conservation equations and are valid when the flow is incompressible.

To solve equations (5.22) and (5.23), initial and boundary conditions must be prescribed to the model. For the initial conditions, the initial velocity and pressure associated to the given problem can be applied. For a fluid domain at rest, i.e., stationary fluid (no flow), one may set:

$$\mathbf{v} = 0 \text{ and } p = 0, \tag{5.24}$$

as the initial velocity and pressure. The type of boundary conditions that can be applied are summarised in table 5.2. In the case of prescribed inlet velocity, one may choose to apply a constant velocity with a uniform velocity profile across the inlet boundary or an inlet velocity profile that is fully developed. Depending on the problem, the latter can facilitate convergence of the numerical model.

5.5.2 Boundary layer

The boundary layer is an important concept in fluid mechanics. When fluid flows across a flat surface, a layer of fluid known as the boundary layer forms above it. This is shown in figure 5.7, where U_∞ is the free stream velocity. The effects of viscosity are significant inside this layer. As the flow hits the leading edge, a laminar boundary layer forms across the surface. Within the laminar region, fluid flows uniformly and in regular patterns, effectively demonstrating layer-by-layer flow paths. The velocity in this layer follows a parabolic profile that increases from zero on the surface to the free stream velocity outside of the boundary layer.

The thickness of the boundary layer increases at points further from the leading edge, which causes the flow to transition from laminar to turbulent. Turbulent flow is characterised by a disordered flow pattern, with fluctuations in both the velocity and pressure, such that the magnitude and direction (for velocity only) undergo changes throughout the flow regime. Turbulence creates higher resistance to flow and results in the loss of mechanical energy due to the chaotic motion of fluid particles.

Table 5.2. Summary of some of the boundary conditions that can be used to represent the physical conditions in haemodynamics analysis.

Condition	Expression	Remarks
Prescribed inlet velocity	$\mathbf{v} \cdot \mathbf{n} = -U_0$	• Sets the velocity in the normal direction to a given value. • U_0 in this case can represent the uniform inlet velocity magnitude or the average inlet velocity derived from a fully developed flow profile. • The negative sign is introduced since the normal vector points outward of the boundary.
Prescribed inlet pressure	$p = p_0$	• Sets the inlet pressure to a given value p_0. • This condition is usually accompanied with the condition $\mathbf{v} \cdot \mathbf{t} = 0$, where $\mathbf{t}$ is the unit tangential vector. This condition states that the tangential velocity is zero such that the inlet pressure induces only inflow in the normal direction.
Prescribed outlet velocity	$\mathbf{v} \cdot \mathbf{n} = U_0$	• Sets the velocity in the normal direction to a given value. • U_0 in this case can represent the uniform inlet velocity magnitude or the average outlet velocity derived from a fully developed flow profile.
Prescribed outlet pressure	$p = p_0$	• Sets the outlet pressure to a given value p_0. • This condition is usually accompanied with the condition $\mathbf{v} \cdot \mathbf{t} = 0$, where $\mathbf{t}$ is the unit tangential vector. This condition states that the tangential velocity is zero such that the outlet pressure induces only outflow in the normal direction.
Wall condition (stationary, no slip)	$\mathbf{v} \cdot \mathbf{n} = 0$	• This is used to describe conditions at stationary walls with no slip, where velocity is zero.

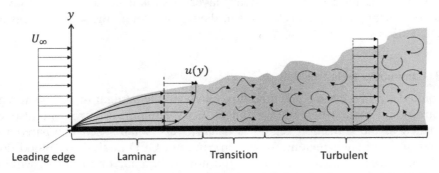

Figure 5.7. The laminar, transitional, and turbulent boundary layer for flow across a flat surface.

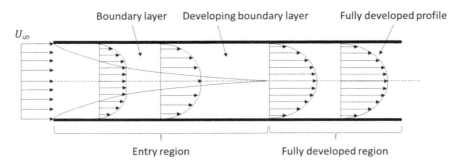

Figure 5.8. Formation of the boundary layer and the development of fully developed profile for flow in a cylindrical tube.

A similar phenomenon occurs when fluid flows through a cylindrical tube. This is shown in figure 5.8. In this case, the boundary layer forms around the surface of the cylinder. Flow in a cylinder is defined by an entry region, where the boundary layer grows from the leading edge, and a fully developed region, where the boundary layers growing from the surface of the tube merges. Here, the flow becomes fully developed and the velocity follows a paraboloid profile (parabolic in 2D).

The boundary layer and the fully developed region plays an important role in the CFD analysis of haemodynamics. Assumption of a fully developed flow at the entrance of a blood vessel model is crucial to facilitate convergence in the numerical algorithm. Without the fully developed flow assumption, flow entering the blood vessel must undergo boundary layer development, where the velocity transitions from a uniform to a parabolic profile such as shown in figure 5.8. Describing such phenomenon numerically is complex and usually requires sufficiently refined meshes around the surfaces of the vessel where the boundary layer forms. Even when flow at the vessel entrance is assumed to be fully developed, it is critical for meshes in the regions near the surface to be sufficiently refined to capture accurately the large velocity gradients here.

Many computational modelling software today comes with meshing functionality that refines the mesh around solid surfaces for CFD simulations. For instance, COMSOL provides an option for users to assign boundary layer mesh to solid surfaces in CFD models. The boundary layer mesh is defined by several layers of prismatic (rectangular in 2D) elements in the region around the solid surfaces of the model. This is shown in figure 5.9.

5.5.3 Laminar vs turbulent flow

As pointed out in section 5.5.2, fluid flow can be in the laminar or turbulent regime. A transitional state where flow changes from laminar to turbulent also exist. Nevertheless, the transition region is usually very small when compared to the laminar and turbulent regions. When carrying out CFD analysis on blood flow in vessels, it is important to ascertain if the flow is laminar or turbulent within the region of analysis. This can be determined by evaluating the Reynolds number, Re:

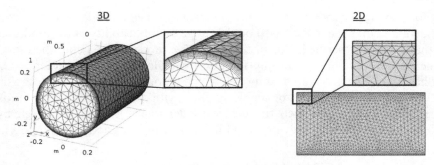

Figure 5.9. Boundary layer mesh in 3D and 2D in COMSOL.

$$\mathrm{Re} = \frac{\rho U d_{\mathrm{h}}}{\mu}, \qquad (5.25)$$

where d_{h} is the hydraulic diameter, which for a blood vessel with a circular cross section, is given by the inner diameter of the vessel. Using equation (5.25), blood flow is laminar if $\mathrm{Re} < 2300$, in the transitional region if $2300 \leqslant \mathrm{Re} \leqslant 4000$ and turbulent if $\mathrm{Re} > 4000$.

While blood flow in the laminar regime can be predicted by numerically solving equations (5.22) and (5.23) without much difficulty, the same cannot be said for turbulent blood flow. This is because of the large computational resources that is needed to discretise the computational domain to numerically resolve the length and time scale of both large and small eddies (Jeyapaul *et al* 2015). To overcome this, it is possible to combine equations (5.22) and (5.23) with turbulence models that simulate the mean flow characteristics for turbulent flow conditions.

Several turbulence models are available including but not limited to the k-epsilon (k-ε) model (Launder and Spalding 1974), the k-omega (k-ω) model (Wilcox 2008), the shear stress transport (SST) model (Menter 1994), and the Spalart–Allmaras model (Spalart and Allmaras 1994). Among these models, the k-ε model is the most used turbulence model for CFD studies of turbulent flow due to numerous studies that have validated its accuracy against experimental and industrial problems (Papageorgakis and Assanis 1999, Avva *et al* 1990). It is a two-equation system that describes turbulence by the transport of two turbulence parameters, i.e., the turbulent kinetic energy, k (J kg^{-1}) and the turbulent energy dissipation rate, ε (m^2 s^{-3}). The k-ω is also a two-equation system that describes the transport of the turbulent kinetic energy and the dissipation of turbulent energy into heat, also known as the specific dissipation rate, ω (s^{-1}). The SST model combines both the k-ε and the k-ω model such that the former is used to describe flow in the inner region of the boundary layer, while the latter is used for flow outside of the boundary layer. Unlike the k-ε, k-ω and SST models, the Spalart–Allmaras model comprises only one equation that describes the transport of the eddy turbulent kinematic viscosity, ν (m^2 s^{-1}).

Most of the commercial software that can perform CFD analysis, such as Ansys Fluent and COMSOL, are equipped with several turbulence models that users can select for their applications. The choice of which turbulence model to use is problem-dependent and must be made based on the range of applicability of the models to the flow that is to be described. For instance, the k-ε model while being the most used turbulence model, is accurate only for flows with low pressure gradients. On the other hand, the Spalart–Allmaras model, which is computationally cheaper as it has only one equation, is only applicable in flow with very high-pressure gradients. Hence, the selection of which turbulence model to use should be driven by the problem. For problems involving blood flow, the k-ε is a good starting point.

5.5.4 Applications of CFD in blood flow analysis

The approach in carrying out a CFD analysis on blood flow depends on the type of blood vessel. For large blood vessels, the geometry of the blood vessel can be explicitly constructed and flow simulations inside the blood vessel can be carried out. These vessel geometries can be constructed based on images obtained from medical imaging systems such as computerised tomography (CT), magnetic resonance imaging (MRI) and ultrasounds scans, or medical procedures such as angiography. These methods allow an accurate representation of the geometry of the vessel and form the foundation behind patient-specific modelling (Neal and Kerckhoffs 2010). An example of the liver vasculature reconstructed from segmentation of the vascular boundary of multiple slices of CT images and stacking them is shown figure 5.10(a).

Alternatively, the geometry of the blood vessel can be approximated as the union of several primitive shapes, such as cylinders, that are constructed based on the dimensions measured from the blood vessel. Figure 5.10(b) shows an idealisation of a vessel bifurcation for CFD analysis.

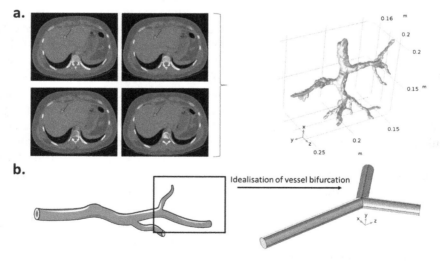

Figure 5.10. Construction of the blood vessel model. (a) Reconstruction of the liver vasculature based on images obtained from CT scans. (b) Idealisation of vessel bifurcation. (a) Adapted from Almotairi *et al* (2020) © 2020 MDPI, (b) Copyright © smart.servier.com. The figure was partly generated using Servier Medical Art, provided by Servier, licensed under a Creative Commons Attribution 3.0 unported license.

5.5.4.1 Case study 5.1: blood flow through a vessel bifurcation

Blood flow through a vessel bifurcation is an important study in haemodynamics due to the changes in the blood flow pattern that can lead to conditions that accelerate the occurrence of several vascular disorders, such as atherosclerosis. A good comprehension of the flow profile in such conditions can assist doctors to better understand the hydrodynamic contribution to these diseases. Essentially, shear stresses that are laminar and physiologic are critical to maintain normal vascular function, while regions of the blood vessel with low wall shear stress or highly oscillatory wall shear stress are at most risk of developing atherosclerosis. This will be demonstrated in this case study[3].

A 3D model representing vessel bifurcation is shown in figure 5.11. The parent vessel, which has a radius of 3 mm, branches into two daughter vessels at an angle of 45° from its central axis. Both daughter vessels have the same radius as the parent vessel. The parent vessel has a length of 30 mm, while each daughter vessel has a length of 7.5 mm. At the vessel inlet, a fully developed inlet velocity that follows a pulsatile profile was prescribed (Peattie *et al* 2004):

$$U(t) = \begin{cases} U_0\sin(4\pi[t + 0.016]), & t \leqslant 0.218 \\ 0.2U_0, & 0.218 < t \leqslant 0.3 \end{cases} \quad (5.26)$$

where U_0 is the amplitude of the parabolic velocity profile assumed here to be 0.2 m s^{-1}. At the vessel outlet, the pressure was set to zero. All other surfaces were prescribed with the no slip wall condition:

$$\mathbf{v} = 0. \quad (5.27)$$

The properties of blood used in this case study are presented in table 5.3. Blood was assumed to be Newtonian and flow inside the vessel was assumed to be laminar.

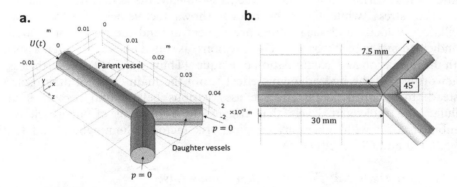

Figure 5.11. Model of the bifurcated vessel (a) in 3D and (b) viewed from the *xz* plane.

---

[3] Source files for case study 5.1 are available at https://doi.org/10.1088/978-0-7503-4016-8.

Table 5.3. Physical properties of blood.

Property	Value
Dynamic viscosity, μ (Pa · s)	0.001
Density, ρ (kg m^{-3})	1050

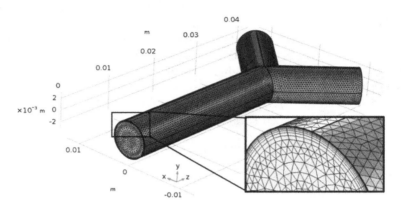

Figure 5.12. Model of the bifurcated vessel discretised into tetrahedral elements. The presence of boundary layer mesh is clearly depicted.

Figure 5.12 shows the model of the bifurcated vessel following discretisation into finite elements. The use of boundary layer mesh is clearly illustrated.

Figure 5.13 plots the contours of shear stress and velocity around the region of bifurcation at various time frames. Due to symmetry, the left branch is used to plot the shear stress, while the right branch shows the velocity profile. Low and oscillatory velocity and shear stress are evident around the region of bifurcation, as indicated by the black arrows. These regions, as stated above, are often associated with the formation and accumulation of plaques (Thim *et al* 2012). Nevertheless, it is noteworthy that the hydrodynamic effect is not the main cause of atherosclerosis. Instead, the hydrodynamic effect causes various behavioural responses at the cellular and molecular levels that trigger the formation of atherosclerosis in combined effect with other physiological risk factors (Cunningham and Gotlieb 2005, Chiu and Chien 2011).

5.5.4.2 Case study 5.2: flow through a venous valve
Just like vessel bifurcation, blood flow through venous valves creates hydrodynamic events that can potentially lead to several pathological conditions. An example is deep vein thrombosis (DVT), a vascular disorder that is characterised by the formation of blood clot (Stone *et al* 2017). DVT has a pathological origin, however, blood flow through the veins creates a region of low pressure behind the valve, such

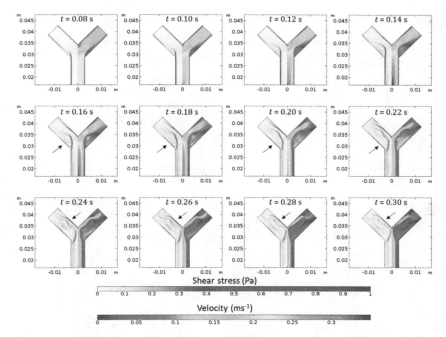

Figure 5.13. Shear stress (left branch) and velocity (right branch) contours at various time levels. Arrows point to the oscillatory flow behaviour that promotes the accumulation of plaque and the formation of atherosclerosis.

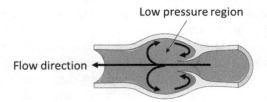

Figure 5.14. Low pressure region generated behind the valve promotes thrombus formation. Copyright © smart.servier.com. The figure was partly generated using Servier Medical Art, provided by Servier, licensed under a Creative Commons Attribution 3.0 unported license.

as shown in figure 5.14, that promotes thrombus formation (Ibrahim *et al* 2017). This phenomenon will be demonstrated in this case study[4].

A 3D model of the vein and its valve was developed. For simplicity, the shape of the vein was idealised into a smooth straight cylinder. This is shown in figure 5.15(a). To reduce the requirement for computational resources, only half of the model was constructed by making use of symmetry. The vein has a radius and length of 5 and 100 mm, respectively. The valve is positioned 20 mm from the inlet. Four different

---

[4] Source files for case study 5.2 are available at https://doi.org/10.1088/978-0-7503-4016-8.

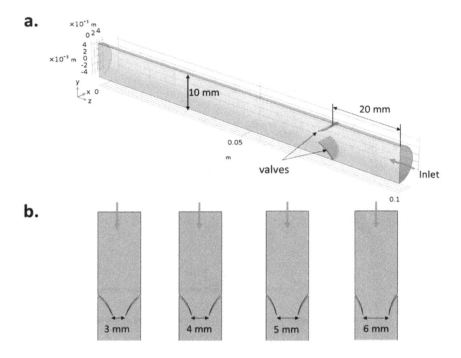

Figure 5.15. (a) 3D model of the venous valve, (b) models with the four different valve openings.

valve openings, namely 3, 4, 5 and 6 mm, to replicate different stages of blood flow through the valve will be considered. These are shown in figure 5.15(b).

A pulsatile velocity profile identical to equation (5.26) was prescribed at the inlet boundary, while zero pressure was prescribed at the outlet. No slip wall condition was applied to the walls of the vessel and valve. The symmetry condition, which describes zero flow penetration and vanishing shear stress, was applied at the symmetry plane. Blood was assumed to be Newtonian with values of density and dynamic viscosity identical to those presented in table 5.3. Since blood flow past the valve is turbulent, the models were solved using the k-ε turbulence model[5].

Figure 5.16 illustrates the iso-surfaces of the velocity magnitude obtained for the different valve openings at 0.05, 0.1, 0.15, 0.2 and 0.25 s. A smaller valve opening results in a higher velocity magnitude. A vortex can be seen to form behind the valve (see red arrows), with a larger vortex developing in the models with smaller valve openings. These vortices induce a region of low pressure just behind the valve, thus creating conditions that are favourable for thrombus formation.

Note that the simulation of blood flow through the venous valve presented above is a simplified representation of the actual flow phenomenon. In the actual vein, the

---

[5] Turbulence models are available in versions of COMSOL where the CFD module is present. Users without the CFD module can reduce the value of U_0 in equation (5.26) and perform the simulations using the Laminar Flow model.

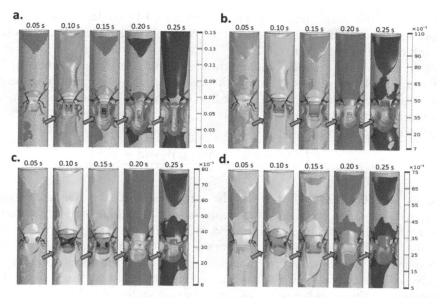

Figure 5.16. Iso-surfaces depicting the velocity magnitude (m s^{-1}) at 0.05, 0.1, 0.15, 0.2 and 0.25 s obtained for the model with valve opening of (a) 3, (b) 4, (c) 5 and (d) 6 mm. Red arrows indicate the formation of vortex behind the valve.

valve will open and close in response to the pulsatile blood flow, thus creating a highly dynamic flow through the valve. To properly investigate this, one must adopt a fluid–structure interaction study, whereby the force exerted by the blood flow causes the structure of the valve to deform (Hajati *et al* 2020, Liu *et al* 2020). Fluid–structure interaction simulations are more complicated to execute and require very high computational resources, especially in 3D, to accurately solve them. This is beyond the scope of this book; however, interested readers may refer to other resources available in the literature, such as by Bodnár *et al* (2014).

5.5.4.3 Case study 5.3: vascular models in bioheat transfer

CFD analysis can be coupled with bioheat transfer models from chapter 4 to understand the heat sink effect of blood flow during thermal ablation treatment. One may recall from chapter 4 that the thermal effects of blood flow are accounted for mathematically either by introducing a perfusion term (the Pennes model), a velocity term (the Wulff and Klinger models) or by using a separate differential equation to describe their distribution (the Chen and Holmes model, the porous medium models). In cases where large blood vessels are present, the use of these bioheat transfer models may not be appropriate since these models assume a distributed vasculature within the tissue domain. Instead, the large vessel can be explicitly modelled such that blood flow inside the vessel can be solved and coupled to the bioheat transfer model. This in fact, has been addressed in case study 4.3. However, in that case study, blood flow inside the vessel was not modelled and the heat sink effect was accounted for by imposing a Robin type boundary condition across the vessel wall. In this case study[6], we will couple the CFD model of blood flow in a large vessel with the bioheat transfer model to demonstrate the role of blood as a heat sink during heating of tissues.

Consider a spherical tissue domain of radius 50 mm. A straight cylindrical blood vessel of radius 1.5 mm passes through the tissue with its axis 5 mm from the tissue centre. This is shown in figure 5.17. Note that only half of the model was developed by assuming symmetry across the midplane. The tissue is subjected to an external Gaussian heat source given by:

$$\dot{q}_{\text{ext}} = \dot{q}_0 \exp\left(-\frac{(x - x_0)^2 + (y - y_0)^2 + (z - z_0)^2}{s^2}\right), \tag{5.28}$$

where $\dot{q}_0 = 500\ 000$ W m^{-3} is the amplitude of the Gaussian profile, $(x_0, y_0, z_0) = (0, 0, 0)$ represents the coordinate of the Gaussian peak and $s = 5$ mm is the width of the Gaussian profile.

At the inlet boundary, a fully developed velocity profile was assumed. Blood enters the vessel at a constant flow rate of 25 ml min^{-1}. At the outlet boundary, zero pressure was prescribed. The walls of the vessel were set to no slip wall condition. Temperature at the outer boundary of the tissue was set to normal body temperature of 37 °C. The same value was prescribed as the temperature of blood entering the vessel. Hydrodynamic and thermal properties of blood and tissue adopted in this case study are presented in table 5.4.

Simulations were carried out in steady state and the temperature distributions across the symmetrical plane for the cases with and without blood flow inside the

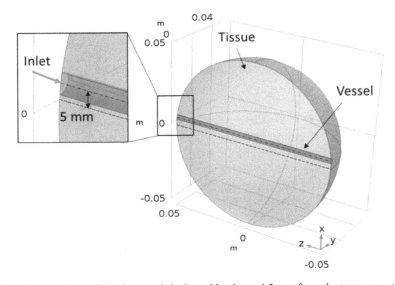

Figure 5.17. Model of the tissue and the large blood vessel 5 mm from the tumour centre.

---

[6] Source files for case study 5.3 are available at https://doi.org/10.1088/978-0-7503-4016-8.

Table 5.4. Thermal properties of tissue and blood.

Property	Tissue	Blood
Thermal conductivity $(W (m K)^{-1})$	0.58	0.60
Specific heat $(J (kg K)^{-1})$	4180	3300
Density $(kg m^{-3})$	1060	1050
Blood perfusion rate (s^{-1})	—	0.0065
Blood dynamic viscosity $(Pa \cdot s)$	—	0.001

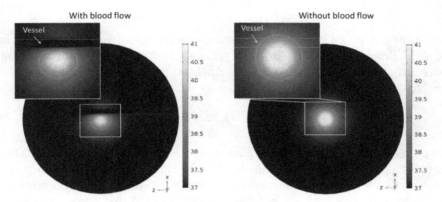

Figure 5.18. Comparison of the temperature distribution across the symmetrical plane with and without the presence of blood flow inside the vessel.

vessel are presented in figure 5.18. In the presence of blood flow, the regions of high temperature are confined only within the tissue domain, while the temperature of blood inside the vessel remains largely unaffected by the Gaussian heat source. This is because any heat that is generated inside the vessel is constantly transferred away by the blood flow. The maximum temperature attained by the tissue in this case is 41.3 °C. Without blood flow, temperature inside the blood vessel increased due to the Gaussian heat source. The maximum temperature attained by the tissue in this case is 41.9 °C, which is higher than in the case with blood flow. This is not surprising as the absence of blood flow removes the heat sink effect from the tissue, which results in an increase in tissue temperature.

5.6 Blood flow in capillaries

Capillaries exist as a complex and tortuous network of vessels inside the body (see figure 5.1). As such, constructing individual capillary vessel for blood flow simulation and analysis becomes impractical. A different kind of analysis is thus required to understand blood flow in capillaries. One way is to treat the entire capillary network as a porous medium, where the pores represent the network of vessels where blood flows and the solid matrix represents the surrounding tissue.

By assuming the capillary network to mimic the pores of a porous medium, it is then possible to describe blood flow inside the capillaries using Darcy's law (Darcy 1856).

5.6.1 Darcy's law

Darcy's law is an equation that governs the flow through porous medium. According to Darcy's law, the fluid flux, q'' (m s^{-1}) (flow per unit area) through a porous medium is proportional to the pressure difference, Δp (Pa) and inversely proportional to the length, L (m) of the porous medium, such that:

$$q'' \propto -\frac{\Delta p}{L}, \tag{5.29}$$

where the negative sign is introduced to overcome the negative value arising from Δp since fluid flows from points of high pressure to low pressure. Introducing the constant of proportionality and writing $\Delta p/L$ in differential form, equation (5.29) can be rewritten as:

$$q''_x = -K\frac{dp}{dx}, \tag{5.30}$$

where dp/dx (Pa m^{-1}) is the pressure gradient in the flow direction, and K (m^2 (Pa·s)$^{-1}$) is the hydraulic conductivity; a parameter that determines the ease of which fluid flows through a porous medium. The value of the hydraulic conductivity depends not only on the type of porous medium, but also the type of fluid that flows through it. The hydraulic conductivity is related to the fluid dynamic viscosity through:

$$K = \frac{\kappa}{\mu}, \tag{5.31}$$

where κ (m^2) is the porous medium permeability and μ (Pa·s) is the dynamic viscosity of the fluid. For flow in 3D, the fluid flux can be expressed as:

$$\mathbf{q}'' = \left(q''_x, q''_y, q''_z\right) = \nabla p, \tag{5.32}$$

where $\nabla p = \{\partial p/\partial x, \partial p/\partial y, \partial p/\partial z\}$ is the pressure gradient and (q''_x, q''_y, q''_z) represent each component of the fluid flux vector in the x-, y- and z-directions, respectively, such that:

$$q''_x = -\frac{\kappa}{\mu}\frac{\partial p}{\partial x}, \ q''_y = -\frac{\kappa}{\mu}\frac{\partial p}{\partial y}, \ q''_z = -\frac{\kappa}{\mu}\frac{\partial p}{\partial z}, \tag{5.33}$$

where $\nabla p = \{\partial p/\partial x, \partial p/\partial y, \partial p/\partial z\}$ is the pressure gradient.

Flow in a porous medium must satisfy mass conversation or the continuity equation. Applying equation (5.22) to equation (5.32) yields:

$$\nabla \cdot \mathbf{q}'' = 0, \ \text{or} \ \nabla \cdot \left(-\frac{\kappa}{\mu}\nabla p\right) = 0, \tag{5.34}$$

which can be solved to obtain the pressure distribution inside the porous medium. Once this is obtained, the flow distribution inside the porous medium can be estimated from equation (5.33).

It is important to note that the fluid flux $\mathbf{q}''$ is not the same as the actual flow velocity inside the porous medium. This is because fluid can only flow through the pores of the porous medium (see figure 5.19). The actual velocity $\mathbf{v}$ is related to the fluid flux through:

$$\mathbf{v} = \frac{\mathbf{q}''}{\varphi}, \tag{5.35}$$

where φ is the porosity of the porous medium, which is a measure of the ratio of the pore volume (V_{pore}) to that of the porous medium (V_{total}):

$$\varphi = \frac{V_{\text{pore}}}{V_{\text{total}}}. \tag{5.36}$$

5.6.2 Permeability

An important parameter in the Darcy equation that governs the flow through the porous medium is the medium permeability. Permeability is a material property that quantifies the ability for fluid to flow through the porous medium. A medium with higher permeability allows greater flow through the porous medium. Permeability can be isotropic or anisotropic. An isotropic permeability indicates that the permeability is independent of direction, which leads to uniform flow in all directions. An anisotropic porous medium has permeability that varies according to the flow direction. Consequently, flow in one direction can be either larger or smaller than in the other directions. These are illustrated in figure 5.20.

It is possible to estimate the permeability of a porous medium by using the Carman–Kozeny equation (Kozeny 1927, Carman 1937), an empirical formula that relates permeability with the parameters that characterise the porous medium. Different types of porous medium yield different empirical relations. For a porous medium defined by a packed bed of solid spheres, the formula to calculate the pressure drop across the porous medium is given by (Carman 1937):

$$\frac{\Delta p}{L} = -\frac{180\mu}{\Phi_s^2 D_p^2} \frac{(1 - \varphi)^2}{\varphi^3} q'', \tag{5.37}$$

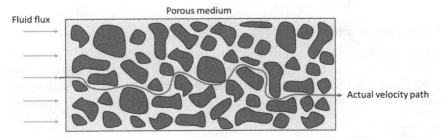

Figure 5.19. Difference between fluid flux and the actual velocity path.

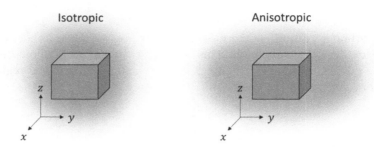

Figure 5.20. Example of fluid flow in an isotropic and anisotropic porous medium. In the anisotropic case, permeability is the largest in the y-direction; hence, the greater flow in this direction.

where D_p (m) is the hydraulic diameter of the spherical particle and Φ_s (dimensionless) is the sphericity of the particles. For a packed bed of spherical particles, D_p is given by the diameter of each sphere, while $\Phi_s = 1$. From Darcy's law, we have:

$$\frac{\Delta p}{L} = -\frac{\mu}{\kappa}q'', \qquad (5.38)$$

which upon substituting into equation (5.37), gives the expression for permeability:

$$\kappa = \Phi_s^2 \frac{\varphi^3 D_p^2}{180(1 - \varphi)^2}, \qquad (5.39)$$

which be used to estimate the permeability of a porous medium.

Obviously, neither biological tissues nor the capillary network resembles a packed bed of spherical particles. Hence, slight variation in the Carman–Kozeny formula is needed to estimate the permeability. For instance, Overby *et al* (2001) suggested the following expression to estimate the permeability of the trabecular meshwork[7]:

$$\kappa = \frac{\varphi D_p^2}{80}, \qquad (5.40)$$

where φ and D_p can be estimated based on images obtained from scanning electron microscopy (SEM) or transmission electron microscopy (TEM).

5.6.3 Capillary as a porous medium

The anatomy of the capillary bed and the low velocity in capillary blood flow allow the use Darcy's law to describe its flow dynamics. To do so, biological tissues are assumed to be a porous medium, where the solid matrix is represented by the cells, connective tissues and extracellular matrix that constitute the tissue, while the pores

---

[7] A small ring-like domain that has structure that can be characterised as a porous medium.

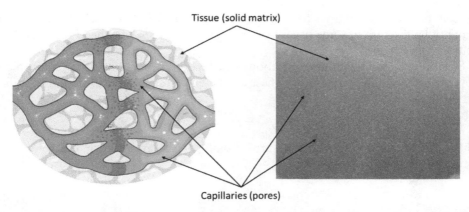

Figure 5.21. Blood capillaries inside tissues represented as a porous medium, where solid matrix represents the tissues, while pores represent the capillary network. A sponge (right) is used as an illustration of a porous medium. Copyright © smart.servier.com. The figure was partly generated using Servier Medical Art, provided by Servier, licensed under a Creative Commons Attribution 3.0 unported license.

are represented by the capillary network where blood flows. This is illustrated in figure 5.21, where the analogy of a sponge is used to describe the tissue-blood architecture.

Under the porous medium assumption, the velocity of blood flow through the capillaries, $\mathbf{v}_b$ (m s^{-1}) is given by:

$$\mathbf{v}_b = -\frac{\kappa_b}{\mu_b}\nabla p_b, \qquad (5.41)$$

where κ_b (m^2) is the permeability of the capillary network, μ_b (Pa·s) is blood dynamic viscosity and p_b (Pa) is pressure inside the capillaries. Applying the continuity equation to equation (5.41) yields:

$$\nabla \cdot \left(-\frac{\kappa_b}{\mu_b}\nabla p_b\right) = 0. \qquad (5.42)$$

Equation (5.42) can be solved to obtain the pressure distribution across the capillary network once boundary conditions relevant to the problem have been prescribed. With knowledge of the pressure distribution, the velocity distribution inside the capillaries can be obtained by evaluating equation (5.41).

There are several points to note regarding the use of Darcy's law to describe blood flow in capillaries. Firstly, equation (5.42), which describes the pressure distribution inside the capillary bed, is in steady state. This means that any change in the pressure gradient induces an instantaneous blood flow across the entire capillary bed. Secondly, the equation assumes the capillaries to be rigid and do not have the capacity to expand. This is a reasonable assumption under normal physiologic conditions but may not be the case in pathologic cases or circumstances that may cause the capillaries to expand, such as vasodilation. Thirdly, by approximating the capillary network as a porous medium and using Darcy's law to describe its flow, we have assumed the capillaries to be homogeneously distributed inside the tissue. This may not be the case in some organs of the human body such as the kidney (Molema and Aird 2012).

Several types of boundary conditions can be prescribed to solve capillary blood flow problems using Darcy's law. These can be in the form of the Dirichlet boundary condition:

$$p_b = p_0, \tag{5.43}$$

where p_0 (Pa) is the applied pressure (usually of the arteriole or the venule), or Neumann boundary condition:

$$-\frac{\kappa_b}{\mu_b} \frac{\partial p_b}{\partial n} = q_0, \tag{5.44}$$

where $\partial p_b / \partial n$ is the rate of change of the vascular pressure in the outward direction normal to the surface, and q_0 (m s^{-1}) is the magnitude of the fluid flux. The Neumann condition in equation (5.44) may be viewed as the velocity prescribed in the normal direction across the boundary of the porous medium. This follows from equation (5.41), where:

$$-\frac{\kappa_b}{\mu_b} \frac{\partial p_b}{\partial n} = -\frac{\kappa_b}{\mu_b} \nabla p_b \cdot \mathbf{n} = \mathbf{v}_b \cdot \mathbf{n} = q_0. \tag{5.45}$$

If the boundary is impermeable to flow, then:

$$\mathbf{v}_b \cdot \mathbf{n} = 0. \tag{5.46}$$

5.6.3.1 Case study 5.4: analysis of blood flow in capillaries using Darcy's law
This case study[8] demonstrates the use of Darcy's law to describe blood flow in capillaries. Consider the domain shown in figure 5.22(a), which consists of the tissue and an embedded capillary bed. Blood enters the capillary from a single artery and exits through a single vein. The capillary network is assumed to be complex and tortuous such that it approximates the pores inside a porous medium. This is shown in figure 5.22(b).

Consider a 2D porous tissue domain represented by a square of sides 5 cm such as shown in figure 5.23(a). The boundaries representing the artery and the vein where blood enters and leaves the capillary network, respectively, are 3 mm in length. At the inlet, a constant pressure of 15 mmHg was prescribed. At the outlet, zero pressure was prescribed. The remaining boundaries were set to be impermeable to blood flow. These conditions are illustrated in figure 5.23(a). Properties of blood are identical to those summarised in table 5.3. Permeability of the capillary network was set to 1.5×10^{-14} m^2, while porosity was set to 0.15.

Figure 5.23(b) illustrates the pressure contours across the capillary bed. The arrows represent the velocity vector of blood flow through the capillaries. The higher

[8] Source files for case study 5.4 are available at https://doi.org/10.1088/978-0-7503-4016-8.

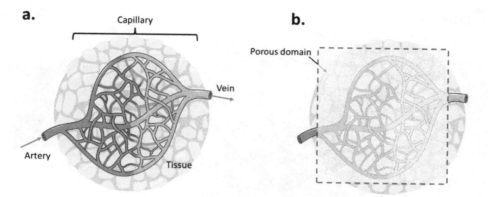

Figure 5.22. (a) The tissue-capillary structure considered in case study 5.4 and (b) the porous domain assumption. Copyright © smart.servier.com. The figure was partly generated using Servier Medical Art, provided by Servier, licensed under a Creative Commons Attribution 3.0 unported license.

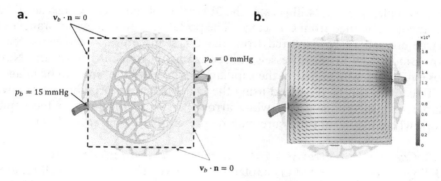

Figure 5.23. (a) Model geometry and boundary conditions applied in case study 5.4, (b) contours of pressure (Pa) and velocity vector of blood flow inside the capillaries. Copyright © smart.servier.com. The figure was partly generated using Servier Medical Art, provided by Servier, licensed under a Creative Commons Attribution 3.0 unported license.

pressure at the artery drives blood flow through the capillaries and into the vein. Case study 5.4 demonstrates a simplified approach to modelling blood flow in capillaries, where only one artery and one vein supplies and drains blood to and from a 2D capillary bed, respectively. A more complex analysis based on the Darcy's law can be carried out with the aid of medical imaging systems through the visualisation of the intricate capillary network inside biological tissues.

MRI and CT scanners can assist with identifying regions of tissues where large blood vessels reside. In these regions, the blood vessels can be segmented and reconstructed where CFD analysis similar to that in section 5.5.4 can be carried out. Vessels that are smaller than the resolution of the medical imaging system cannot be imaged and blood flow in these regions can be modelled using Darcy's law.

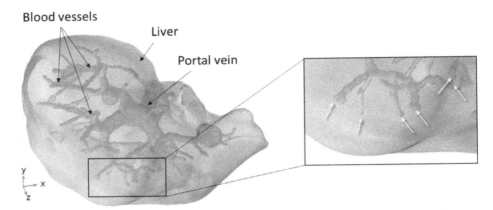

Figure 5.24. Model reconstruction of the liver and portal vein. White arrows indicate the termination of the large vessels. A constant pressure condition can be applied here to drive the flow through the capillaries that are smaller than the resolution of the imaging system.

For example, figure 5.24 illustrates the 3D model of the liver reconstructed based on the images obtained from CT scans[9]. The portal vein and its major branches that are large enough to be captured from the CT scans are also reconstructed and shown. Blood flow in these vessels can be explicitly modelled using the Navier–Stokes equations, while those in the capillaries, which are too small to be imaged by the CT scanner, can be described using the Darcy equation. The boundaries where the large vessels terminate (see white arrows) serve as the inlet to the capillary network where a constant pressure may be prescribed (Payne *et al* 2011).

5.6.3.2 Case study 5.5: revisiting the Klinger bioheat transfer model
The Klinger model presented in chapter 4 was derived to overcome the limitation of the global perfusion term assumed by the Pennes model. For convenience, the Klinger model is reproduced here:

$$\rho_t c_t \frac{\partial T_t}{\partial t} + \rho_b c_b (\mathbf{v}_b \cdot \nabla T_t) = \nabla \cdot (k_t \nabla T_t) + \dot{q}_{\text{ext}}. \tag{5.47}$$

Solving equation (5.47) requires the knowledge of the velocity vector $\mathbf{v}_b$, which is usually not known. Nevertheless, the ability to describe blood flow in capillaries using Darcy's law makes it possible for the Klinger model to be solved. This will be demonstrated in this case study[10].

Consider a 2D circular tissue of radius 5 mm with embedded capillaries such as shown in figure 5.25. Blood enters the capillaries from a single artery of radius 0.5 mm located at $(x, y) = (-0.004, 0)$ and exits the network from a single vein of radius 0.5 mm located at $(x, y) = (0.004, 0)$. The tissue experiences a Gaussian heat source that can be expressed mathematically as:

---

[9] Publicly available from 3D-IRCADb 01, https://www.ircad.fr/research/3d-ircadb-01/.
[10] Source files for case study 5.5 are available at https://doi.org/10.1088/978-0-7503-4016-8.

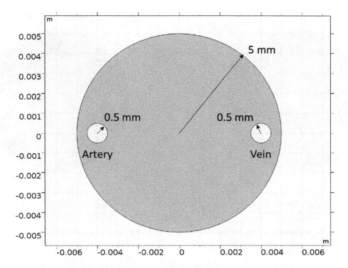

Figure 5.25. Model of the 2D tissue with embedded capillaries in case study 5.5.

Table 5.5. Properties of blood and tissue used in case study 5.5.

Parameter	Value
Permeability of capillary, κ_b (m^2)	1×10^{-12}
Tissue porosity, φ	0.2
Blood dynamic viscosity, μ_b (Pa·s)	0.001
Blood density, ρ_b (kg m^{-3})	1050
Blood specific heat, c_b (J (kg K)$^{-1}$)	3600
Tissue thermal conductivity, k_t (W (m K)$^{-1}$)	0.58

$$\dot{q}_{ext} = \dot{q}_0 \exp\left(-\frac{(x-x_0)^2 + (y-y_0)^2}{s^2}\right), \tag{5.48}$$

where $\dot{q}_0 = 10$ W cm^{-3} is the amplitude of the Gaussian heat source, $(x_0, y_0) = (0, 0)$ is the coordinate where the Gaussian heat source peaks and s=0.5 mm is the width of Gaussian heat source. We are interested in the steady state temperature distribution inside the tissue obtained using the Klinger model. For comparison purposes, a second model that was solved using the Pennes model was also developed. Hydraulic properties of the capillaries and thermal properties of the tissues are summarised in table 5.5.

The following boundary conditions were applied:
1. Blood pressure across the boundary of the artery was 15 mmHg.
2. Blood pressure across the boundary of the vein was 0 mmHg.

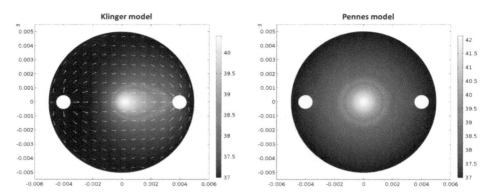

Figure 5.26. Contours of the steady state temperature obtained using the Klinger and the Pennes models. Arrows in the Klinger model results represent the velocity vector. The direction of blood flow influences the heat transfer process and the temperature distribution inside the tissue.

3. Outer boundary of the tissue was impermeable to flow, i.e., $\mathbf{v}_b \cdot \mathbf{n} = 0$.
4. Temperature at the outer boundary was constant at 37 °C.
5. All other boundaries were thermally insulated.

Figure 5.26 plots the contours of the steady state temperature obtained using the Klinger and the Pennes models. For the latter, a blood perfusion rate of $\omega_b = 0.0065\ \text{s}^{-1}$ was assumed. The temperature distribution obtained using the Klinger model is asymmetrical and skewed to the right-hand side due to blood flow in the capillaries from the artery in the left to the vein in the right. With the Pennes model, the temperature distribution is symmetrical since the thermal effects of blood flow is homogeneous across the tissue domain. The results clearly contrast the predictions made between the Klinger and the Pennes models, where the direction of blood flow influences heat transfer and resulting temperature distribution inside the tissue.

5.7 General summary

We have presented some of the modelling approaches to investigate blood flow in the vasculature. A simple analysis based on the Poiseuille's law is helpful in elucidating how flow resistance changes with the blood vessel parameters, especially the vessel radius. However, its application is limited by the assumptions that bound the Poiseuille's law. More complex flow analysis can be carried out using CFD, which were demonstrated in this chapter through several relevant case studies. This includes flow through vessel bifurcation and flow past a venous valve. For blood flow in capillaries, the intricacy and tortuosity of the capillary network prevents the construction of each individual vessel within the network. A more practical approach is to approximate the capillary bed as a porous medium and the flow described using Darcy's law.

It is important to note that the approaches to performing haemodynamic analysis presented in this chapter are limited to the fluid dynamics aspect. Several aspects of the vessel-blood flow interaction have not been considered. For instance, the walls of arteries are elastic and the pumping pressure from the heart can cause these arteries to expand, thus storing some blood instead of directing flow through them. There are simple approaches to investigate this. For instance, the ability of the arteries to expand and 'store' blood can be thought of as simple capacitance where the storage capacity is simply the ratio of the volume difference to the pressure difference (Eilad and Einav 2009). Incorporating such expansion of the arteries into CFD becomes technically more complicated.

Finally, blood flow analysis extends beyond the considerations of a single vessel and flow in the capillary bed. The analysis could be carried out on a larger scale such as for the entire cardiovascular system. A physiological modelling approach that accounts for the entire cardiovascular system is better suited in this case. The use of the lumped modelling approach, such as the three-chamber model to describe blood flow in the cardiovascular system is presented in chapter 10.

References

Almotairi S, Kareem G, Aouf M, Almutairi B and Salem M A-M 2020 Liver tumor segmentation in CT scans using modified SegNet *Sensors* **20** 1516

Avva R, Smith C and Singhal A 1990 Comparative study of high and low Reynolds number versions of *k*-epsilon models *28th Aerospace Sciences Meeting (January 8–11) (Reno Nevada) vol 90-0246 (Reston, VA: AIAA), pp 1–9*

Bird R B, Armstrong R C and Hassager O 1987 *Dynamics of Polymeric Liquids, Vol. 1: Fluid Mechanics* 2nd edn (New York: Wiley-Interscience)

Bodnár T, Galdi G P and Nečasová S 2014 *Fluid–Structure Interaction and Biomedical Applications* (Basel: Springer)

Carman P C 1937 Fluid flow through granular beds *Trans. Inst. Chem. Engrs.* **15** 150–66

Carreau P J 1972 Rheological equations from molecular network theories *Trans. Soc. Rheol.* **116** 99–127

Chen M M and Holmes K R 1980 Microvascular contributions in tissue heat transfer *Ann. N. Y. Acad. Sci.* **335** 137–50

Chiu J-J and Chien S 2011 Effects of disturbed flow on vascular endothelium: pathophysiological basis and clinical perspectives *Physiol. Rev.* **91** 327–81

Connes P *et al* 2013 Decreased hematocrit-to-viscosity ratio and increased lactate dehydrogenase level in patients with sickle anemia and recurrent leg ulcers *PLoS One* **8** e79680

Cunningham K and Gotlieb A I 2005 The role of shear stress in the pathogenesis of atherosclerosis *Lab Invest.* **85** 9–23

Darcy H 1856 *Les fontaines publiques de la ville de Dijon* (Paris: Dalmont)

Eilad D and Einav S 2009 Physical and flow properties of blood ed M Kutz *Biomedical Engineering and Design Handbook. Vol. 1: Fundamentals* (New York: McGraw Hill) ch 3

Fernández-Alfonso M 2004 Regulation of vascular tone: the fat connection *Hypertension* **44** 255–56

Frank O 1990 The basic shape of the arterial pulse. First treatise: mathematical analysis *J. Mol. Cell. Cardiol.* **22** 255–77

Fuchs F D and Whelton P K 2020 High blood pressure and cardiovascular disease *Hypertension* **75** 285–92

Hajati Z, Moghanlou F S, Vajdi M, Razavi S E and Matin S 2020 Fluid–structure interation of blood flow around a vein valve *Bioimpacts* **10** 169–75

Hu H 2012 Computational fluid dynamics ed P K Kundu, I M Cohen and D R Dowling *Fluid Mechanics* (Amsterdam: Academic) ch 10

Jeyapaul E, Coleman G N and Rumsey C L 2015 Higher-order and length-scale statistics from DNS of a decelerated planar wall-bounded turbulent flow *Int. J. Heat Fluid Flow* **54** 14–27

Kozeny J 1927 Ueber kapillare Leitung des Wassers im Boden *Sitzungsber Akad. Wiss.* **136** 271–306

Launder N E and Spalding D B 1974 The numerical computation of turbulent flows *Comput. Methods Appl. Mech. Eng.* **3** 269–89

Liu X, Sun L, Wang M, Li B and Liu L 2020 Modeling and simulation of valve cycle in vein using an immersed finite element method *Comput. Model. Eng. Sci.* **123** 153–83

Madulanda-Londoño E and Chaturvedi S 2016 Stroke due to large vessel atherosclerosis *Neurol. Clin. Pract.* **6** 252–8

Menter F 1994 Two-equation eddy-viscosity turbulence models for engineering applications *AIAA J.* **32** 1589–605

Ibrahim N, Aziz N S A and Manap A N A 2017 Vein mechanism simulation study for deep vein thrombosis early diagnosis using CFD *J. Phys. Conf. Ser.* **822** 012040

Molema G and Aird W C 2012 Vascular heterogeneity in the kidney *Semin. Nephrol.* **32** 145–55

Neal M L and Kerckhoffs R 2010 Current progress in patient-specific modelling *Brief Bioinform.* **11** 111–26

Overby D, Ruberti J, Gong H, Freddo T F and Johnson M 2001 Specific hydraulic conductivity of corneal stroma as seen by quick-freeze/deep-etch *J. Biomech. Eng.* **123** 154–61

Panton R L 2013 *Incompressible Flow* 4th edn (Hoboken, NJ: Wiley), p 114

Papageorgakis G C and Assanis D N 1999 Comparison of linear and nonlinear RNG-based k-epsilon models for incompressible turbulent flow *Numer. Heat Transf.* B **35** 1–22

Payne S J, Flanagan R, Pollari M, Alhonnoro T, Bost T, O'Neill D, Peng T and Stiegler P 2011 Image-based multi-scale modelling and validation of radio-frequency ablation in liver tumours *Phil. Trans. Roy. Soc.* A **369** 4233–54

Peattie R A, Riehle T J and Bluth E I 2004 Pulsatile flow in fusiform models of abdominal aortic aneurysms: flow fields, velocity patterns and flow-induced wall shear stress *J. Biomech. Eng.* **126** 438–46

Rafieian-Kopaei M, Setorki M, Doudi M, Baradaran A and Nasri H 2014 Atherosclerosis: process, indicators, risk factors and new hopes *Int. J. Prev. Med.* **5** 927–46

Spalart P R and Allmaras S R 1994 A one-equation turbulence model for aerodynamic flows *AIAA Pap.* **1** 5–21

Stone J, Hangge P, Albadawi H, Wallace A, Shamoun F, Knuttien M G, Naidu S and Oklu R 2017 Deep vein thrombosis: pathogenesis, diagnosis, and medical management *Cardiovasc. Diagn. Ther.* **7** S276–84

Thim T, Hagensen M K, Hørlyck A, Kim W Y, Niemann A K, Thrysøe S A, Drouet L, Paaske W P, Bøtker H E and Falk E 2012 Wall shear stress and local plaque development in stenosed carotid arteries of hypercholesterolemic mappings *J. Cardiovasc. Dis. Res.* **3** 76–83

Thiriet M, Delfour M and Garon A 2015 Vascular stenosis: an introduction ed P Lanzer *PanVascular Medicine* (Berlin: Springer)

Wilcox D C 2008 Formulation of the k-ω turbulence model revisited *AIAA J.* **46** 2823–38

IOP Publishing

Model-Based Approaches in Biomedical Engineering

Ean Hin Ooi and Yeong Shiong Chiew

Chapter 6

Mass transport in biological tissues

6.1 Introduction

Mass transport is the process where mass or matter is transferred from one point to another via diffusion or/and convection. Mass transport in biological tissues plays an important role in the human body, especially in understanding the effectiveness of drug delivery systems. Upon entering the body, drugs are carried along the blood stream and through the circulatory system. Understanding the transport mechanism involved is important in healthcare as it can help with the design and development of new and improved drug delivery systems. In this chapter, some of the theories involved in describing the mass transport inside biological tissues, such as the convection–diffusion equation and the dual porosity model will be presented. Central to these are Fick's law of diffusion, which governs the transport of matter (mass) in a medium, and Starling's law, which describes transvascular fluid exchange.

6.2 Fick's law of diffusion

Mass transport can occur via diffusion or convection. Diffusion is described using Fick's law (Fick 1855), which states that mass in a medium move from points of higher concentration to points of lower concentration. The term 'mass' in this case can refer to either matter, solutes, or particles, and is usually measured in terms of the number of moles, χ (mol). For a medium contained in a domain of length L (m) and cross-sectional area A (m^2), such as shown in figure 6.1, Fick's law states that the rate of mass transfer J (mol s^{-1}) is proportional to the concentration difference, Δc (mol m^{-3}) and the cross-sectional area, and inversely proportional to the length of the domain:

$$J \propto -A\frac{\Delta c}{L},$$

(6.1)

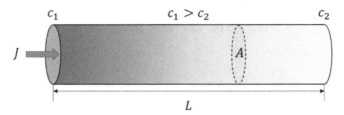

Figure 6.1. Diffusion flux in a domain of length L and cross-sectional area A.

Table 6.1. Similarity between Fick's law of diffusion and Fourier's law of heat conduction.

Fick's law	Fourier's law
• Mass diffusion flux is driven by concentration gradient.	• Heat flux is driven by temperature gradient.
• $\mathbf{j} = -D\nabla c$	• $\mathbf{q} = -k\nabla T$
• Proportionality constant is defined by the mass diffusion, D.	• Proportionality constant is defined by the thermal conductivity, k.

where the negative sign on the right-hand side is introduced to eliminate the negative resulting from Δc being smaller than zero, since $c_2 < c_1$ and $\Delta c = c_2 - c_1$.

Introducing the constant of proportionality, equation (6.1) becomes:

$$J = -DA\frac{\Delta c}{L}, \tag{6.2}$$

where the proportionality constant D $(\mathrm{m}^2\ \mathrm{s}^{-1})$ is known as the mass diffusion coefficient. It is also convenient to express the mass transfer as the rate over unit area, such that:

$$j = \frac{J}{A} = -D\frac{\Delta c}{L}, \tag{6.3}$$

where j $(\mathrm{mol}\ (\mathrm{m}^2{\cdot}\mathrm{s})^{-1})$ is the mass diffusion flux. In differential form, the mass diffusion flux is a vector, whose components are given by:

$$j_x = -D\frac{\partial c}{\partial x},\ j_y = -D\frac{\partial c}{\partial y},\ j_z = -D\frac{\partial c}{\partial z}, \tag{6.4}$$

or

$$\mathbf{j} = -D\nabla c. \tag{6.5}$$

There are similarities between Fick's law of diffusion and Fourier's law of heat conduction (see appendix A). These are summarised in table 6.1.

The diffusion coefficient in equations (6.2)–(6.5) measures the ability of the mass (solute, substance, etc) to diffuse inside a medium. Different substances diffusing in different media give rise to different mass diffusion coefficient values. The temperature and dynamic viscosity of the medium through which diffusion occurs also affect the diffusion coefficient. For diffusion in solids, the temperature dependence of the diffusion coefficient can be describe reasonably well using the Arrhenius equation:

$$D = D_0 \exp\left(-\frac{\Delta E}{RT}\right), \tag{6.6}$$

where D_0 (m^2 s^{-1}) is the diffusion coefficient at a reference temperature, ΔE (J mol^{-1}) is the activation energy, R (J (mol·K)$^{-1}$) is the universal gas constant and T (K) is temperature.

In liquids, the equation describing the dependence of the diffusion coefficient on temperature is given by the Stokes–Einstein equation:

$$D = \frac{kT}{6\pi\mu a}, \tag{6.7}$$

where k (kg·m^2 (s^2·K)$^{-1}$) is the Boltzmann constant, μ (Pa·s) is the medium dynamic viscosity and a (m) is the radius of the molecule. The Stokes–Einstein equation above also describes the dependence of the diffusion coefficient on the dynamic viscosity of the medium. From equation (6.7), an increase in temperature results in a larger diffusion coefficient. On the other hand, a more viscous medium decreases the diffusion coefficient.

Other than temperature and dynamic viscosity, the diffusion coefficient is dependent on the size of the molecules of the diffusing substance. Substances with larger molecules have smaller diffusion coefficient. For biological molecules diffusing in biological tissues, the diffusion coefficient is very small and is typically in the range from 10^{-12} to 10^{-11} m^2 s^{-1}. This explains why diffusion is ineffective for drug transport in the human body.

6.3 Convection–diffusion equation

The convection–diffusion equation, also known as Fick's second law of diffusion, is a partial differential equation that describes mass transfer in the 3D space and is given by (Incropera *et al* 2006):

$$\frac{\partial c}{\partial t} + \left(u\frac{\partial c}{\partial x} + v\frac{\partial c}{\partial y} + w\frac{\partial c}{\partial z}\right) = D\left(\frac{\partial^2 c}{\partial x^2} + \frac{\partial^2 c}{\partial y^2} + \frac{\partial^2 c}{\partial z^2}\right) + \dot{R}, \tag{6.8}$$

or in a more concise form:

$$\frac{\partial c}{\partial t} + \mathbf{v} \cdot \nabla c = D\nabla^2 c + \dot{R}, \tag{6.9}$$

where c (mol m^{-3}) is the concentration of the substance, $\mathbf{v} = (u,v,w)$ (m s^{-1}) are the velocity components in the (x,y,z) directions, and $\dot{R}$ (mol (m^3·s)$^{-1}$) is a reaction term that can be either a source or a sink. In the case of the latter, $\dot{R}$ is negative. In drug

Table 6.2. Boundary conditions to complement the convection–diffusion equation.

Condition	Expression	Remarks
Prescribed concentration (Dirichlet)	$c = c_0$	• Sets the concentration at the boundary to the value c_0. • Typically used for modelling inflow conditions where concentration is known.
Prescribed mass flux (Neumann)	$\mathbf{j} \cdot \mathbf{n} = N_0$ $\mathbf{j} = \mathbf{u}c - D\nabla c$	• Sets the mass flux at the boundary to the value N_0. • $\mathbf{j}$ is the mass flux, which includes contribution from both convection ($\mathbf{u}c$) and diffusion ($D\nabla c$).
No flux	$\mathbf{j} \cdot \mathbf{n} = 0$ $\mathbf{j} = \mathbf{u}c - D\nabla c$	• Sets the flux at the boundary to zero. • Typically used to describe boundaries that are impermeable to flow and mass transfer.
Outflow	$(-D\nabla c) \cdot \mathbf{n} = 0$	• Sets the diffusive flux at the boundary to zero. • Typically used to describe conditions at the far-end boundary where mass is transported out of the solution domain by fluid.

transport inside biological tissues, the metabolisation of drugs by the cells and the clearance of drugs from the systemic circulation are examples of processes that can contribute to the presence of the sink term.

The terms inside the bracket on the left-hand side of equation (6.8) represents mass transfer via convection, while those inside the bracket on the right-hand side represent contributions due to diffusion. In biological tissues, the contribution from diffusion is usually smaller than convection due to the small diffusion coefficient. It is possible to determine if the transport process in a medium is diffusion- or convection-dominated by evaluating the dimensionless Peclet number, Pe:

$$\text{Pe} = \frac{UL}{D}, \tag{6.10}$$

where U is the velocity magnitude of the flow inside the domain and L is the characteristic length. A large Pe implies that mass transfer is convection-dominated, while a small Pe implies that mass transfer is diffusion-dominated. As pointed out in section 6.2, the diffusion coefficient in biological tissues can be of the order of $10^{-12}\,\text{m}^2\,\text{s}^{-1}$. Taking U to be on the order of $10^{-3}\,\text{m}\,\text{s}^{-1}$ for flow in capillaries (see table 4.2) and a characteristic length of 0.01 m, Pe is estimated to be 10^7. The large value of Pe indicates that convection is the primary contributor to mass transfer in biological tissues even at the capillary level.

The solution of equations (6.8) or (6.9) subject to appropriate initial-boundary conditions yields the spatio-temporal concentration distribution across the solution domain. The three types of boundary conditions that are commonly employed in mass transport problems are summarised in table 6.2.

6.4 Transvascular fluid exchange

The circulatory system is responsible for the exchange of oxygen, nutrients and waste products between blood and the surrounding tissue. This exchange occurs at the capillary level, where the fenestrated capillary walls allow fluid to filter out into the surrounding tissue, carrying with it the solutes (oxygen, nutrients, and drugs) mentioned above. Hence, studies of mass transfer in biological tissues are typically focused on transvascular fluid exchange, i.e., the exchange that occurs between the capillaries and the surrounding tissue rather than the transport through the vasculature. In general, fluid flows from the capillaries into the surrounding tissue at the arteriole end, while waste products are transported from the surrounding tissue to the capillaries at the venule end. This is shown in figure 6.2. The outflow of fluid from the capillaries and inflow of fluid into the capillaries are determined by the local pressure difference across the capillary wall.

6.4.1 Starling law

Fluid exchange across the capillary wall can be described using Starling's law (Starling 1896), which states that the rate of fluid flow across the capillary wall is governed by two forces (also known as Starling forces), namely the hydrostatic pressure and the osmotic pressure. Mathematically, Starling's law is given by:

$$J_v = L_p S \left[p_v - p_i - \sigma_s(\pi_v - \pi_i) \right], \tag{6.11}$$

where J_v (m^3 s^{-1}) is the volumetric flow rate through the capillary wall, L_p (m (Pa·s)$^{-1}$) is the hydraulic conductivity of the capillary wall, S (m^2) is the surface area of the capillary wall from where fluid exchange occurs, p_v (Pa) and p_i (Pa) are the

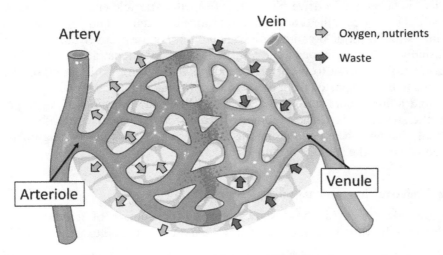

Figure 6.2. Fluid outflow (green arrows) at the arteriole end, and fluid inflow (grey arrows) at the venule end driven by the local pressure difference (hydrostatic and osmotic) between the capillary wall and the surrounding tissue. Copyright © smart.servier.com. The figure was partly generated using Servier Medical Art, provided by Servier, licensed under a Creative Commons Attribution 3.0.

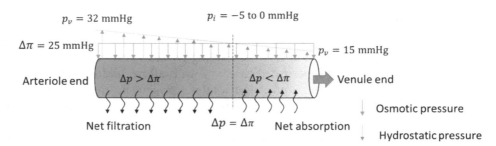

Figure 6.3. Single capillary with hydrostatic and osmotic pressures.

vascular and interstitial pressures, respectively, π_v (Pa) and π_i (Pa) are the vascular and interstitial osmotic pressures[1] (Pa), respectively, and σ_s (dimensionless) is the osmotic reflection coefficient, which determines the effectiveness of the osmotic driving force. A value of $\sigma_s = 0$ suggests that the boundary is infinitely permeable, while $\sigma_s = 1$ indicates an impermeable boundary.

According to equation (6.11), whether fluid flows out of or into the capillary depends on the balance between the hydrostatic pressure difference ($\Delta p = p_v - p_i$) and the osmotic pressure difference ($\Delta \pi = \sigma_s(\pi_v - \pi_i)$). If $\Delta p > \Delta \pi$, then $J_v > 0$; implying a net outflow of fluid from the capillary. This is termed as fluid efflux. On the other hand, if $\Delta p < \Delta \pi$, then $J_v < 0$; implying a net inflow of fluid into the capillary, or fluid influx.

To better understand Starling's law, consider the simplest case of one capillary vessel such as shown in figure 6.3. At the arteriole end, the pressure is around 32 mmHg, while at the venule end, the pressure is around 15 mmHg. This pressure gradient is necessary to drive blood flow from the arteriole end to the venule end. Interstitial pressure on the other hand, can range between −5 and 0 mmHg. Vascular and interstitial osmotic pressures are 25 and 0 mmHg, respectively, and these values are usually constants. From these values, it can be demonstrated that fluid efflux occurs at regions closer to the arteriole end where $\Delta p > \Delta \pi$. This allows solutes and nutrients to be transported from blood to the surrounding tissue. Towards the venule end, fluid influx occurs since $\Delta p < \Delta \pi$. This allows the transport of waste product from the surrounding tissue to blood. Because of the negative vascular pressure gradient, there will be a point along the capillary where $\Delta p = \Delta \pi$ (see figure 6.3). At this point no fluid exchange occurs.

6.4.2 Understanding oedema through Starling's law

The example presented above shows how the production of interstitial fluid is regulated by Starling forces. Under normal conditions, the efflux is balanced by the

---

[1] Osmotic pressure is defined as the minimum pressure required to prevent fluid transport across a semi-permeable membrane.

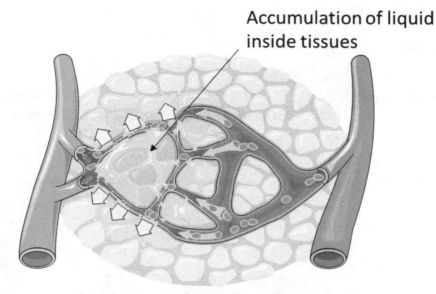

Figure 6.4. Oedema formation due to the leakage of excess fluid (white arrows) to the surrounding tissue. Copyright © smart.servier.com. The figure was partly generated using Servier Medical Art, provided by Servier, licensed under a Creative Commons Attribution 3.0.

influx to maintain homeostasis. An imbalance in the Starling forces can cause excess fluid to leak from the capillary and into the surrounding tissue. This is shown in figure 6.4. The failure to drain the excess fluid will cause the fluid to accumulate inside the tissue, which gives rise to a pathological condition known as oedema (also spelled edema); a medical condition that is characterised by tissue swelling caused by the accumulation of fluid (Reed *et al* 2010). Several factors can lead to an imbalance in Starling forces. These include: (i) increase in hydrostatic pressure, (ii) changes in osmotic pressure and (iii) increase in vessel wall hydraulic conductivity, while other factors such as obstructed lymphatic drainage and water retention in tissues present conditions that encourage oedema formation.

6.4.2.1 Increase in hydrostatic pressure
Elevation of hydrostatic pressure can be caused by various factors such as an elevation in venous pressure by gravitational forces (Hinghofer-Szalkay 2011), volume expanded states in heart failure (Watkins Jr *et al* 1976) and venous obstruction (Levick and Michel 2010). From equation (6.11), an increase in hydrostatic pressure such that Δp is always greater than $\Delta \pi$ will lead to a net transfer of fluid from the capillary to the surrounding tissue throughout the capillary bed. This is represented by figure 6.5. Since the hydrostatic pressure across the entire capillary is now greater than the osmotic pressure, there will be no influx of fluid. As a result, fluid retention inside the tissue occurs, which subsequently leads to swelling and build-up of pressure inside the tissue.

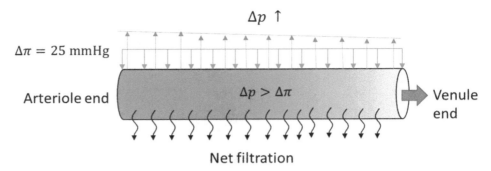

Figure 6.5. Net filtration of fluid out of the capillary due to elevation in the hydrostatic pressure.

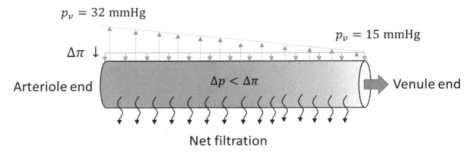

Figure 6.6. Net filtration of fluid out of the capillary due to decrease in vascular osmotic pressure.

6.4.2.2 Changes in osmotic pressure

Changes in osmotic pressure can occur due to changes in the protein content in either blood or interstitial fluid inside the tissue (Michel *et al* 2020). Using equation (6.11), it is possible to demonstrate that a decrease in the vascular osmotic pressure ($\pi_v\downarrow$) leads to a larger positive value of J_v, implying a net filtration of fluid out of the capillary. This is shown in figure 6.6. Similarly, an increase in interstitial osmotic pressure ($\pi_i\uparrow$) will result in greater efflux of fluid due to the increase in J_v. The increase in fluid efflux without the compensating fluid influx results in greater fluid retention inside the tissue and subsequently oedema.

6.4.2.3 Increase in vessel wall hydraulic conductivity

Several pathological conditions, such as vascular injury and pneumonia can result in an increase in vessel wall permeability, L_p (Duan *et al* 2017, Ong *et al* 2003). Capillaries with elevated wall hydraulic conductivity are known as leaky vessels and they are characterised by excessive fluid efflux from the capillaries to the tissue. If all other conditions remain the same, then one can easily show from equation (6.11) that an increase in L_p will result in larger fluid efflux than influx. The net outflow of fluid from the capillaries causes excess fluid inside the tissue, which leads to oedema if left untreated.

6.5 Interstitial fluid flow

6.5.1 Tissue as a porous medium

The fluid that filters out from the capillary walls mixes with the interstitial fluid and flows through the tissue interstitial space. Understanding the flow through the interstitial space is an important part of understanding the efficacy of drug delivery inside the human body. To describe the interstitial fluid flow, one may adopt a similar assumption as when describing blood flow in capillaries. By neglecting the presence of vasculature, the structure of tissue can be assumed to be porous, where the solid matrix is represented by cells, connective tissues, and extracellular matrix, while the pores are represented by the interstitial space that is filled with interstitial fluid. This is shown in figure 6.7.

With the porous medium assumption, fluid flow inside the interstitial space can be described using Darcy's equation, such that:

$$\mathbf{v}_i = -\frac{\kappa_i}{\mu}\nabla p_i, \tag{6.12}$$

where $\mathbf{v}_i$ (m s^{-1}) is the velocity of the interstitial fluid, κ_i (m^2) is the permeability of the interstitial space, μ (Pa·s) is the dynamic viscosity of the interstitial fluid and p_i (Pa) is the interstitial fluid pressure. Flow inside the interstitial space must satisfy the continuity equation. Applying mass conservation to equation (6.12), one obtains:

$$\nabla \cdot \left(-\frac{\kappa_i}{\mu}\nabla p_i \right) = 0, \tag{6.13}$$

which can be solved for the interstitial fluid pressure distribution subject to appropriate boundary conditions.

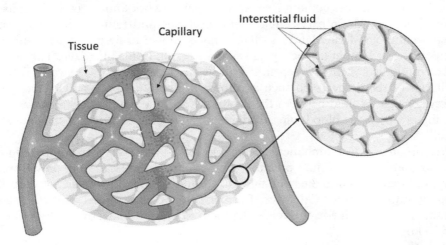

Figure 6.7. Existence of the interstitial fluid inside the pores of the tissue. Copyright © smart.servier.com. The figure was partly generated using Servier Medical Art, provided by Servier, licensed under a Creative Commons Attribution 3.0.

It is important to note that equation (6.13) assumes the pores of the porous medium to be the interstitial space and contains only the interstitial fluid, and not the vasculature, as in the analysis of blood flow in capillaries (see section 5.6).

6.5.2 Contributions from transvascular fluid exchange

Equation (6.13) describes the interstitial fluid pressure inside tissue that is completely free of the vasculature. In the presence of vasculature, there will be fluid exchange between the interstitial space and the vasculature, which can affect the interstitial fluid pressure distribution. To account for the transvascular fluid exchange, the Starling forces must be incorporated into equation (6.13), such that (Baxter and Jain 1989):

$$\nabla \cdot \left(-\frac{\kappa_i}{\mu} \nabla p_i \right) = \frac{J_v}{V}, \qquad (6.14)$$

where J_v ($m^3\,s^{-1}$) is the expression from Starling law (see equation (6.11)) and V (m^3) is the tissue volume. When $J_v > 0$, fluid flows from the vasculature to the interstitial space (see section 6.4.1), which contributes to the increase in the interstitial fluid pressure. Hence, the right-hand side of equation (6.14) becomes a mass source. On the other hand, when $J_v < 0$, fluid flows from the interstitial space to the vasculature, such that the right-hand side becomes a mass sink. In expressing the transvascular fluid exchange as a source or a sink term in the Darcy equation, we have assumed the vasculature to be homogeneously distributed within the tissue, which prevents the need to explicitly model the individual vessels within the capillary network.

6.5.3 Contribution from lymphatics

Some biological tissues contain a separate vessel network known as the lymphatics. Its function is to drain excess fluid from the tissue and return it into the venous system of the blood circulatory system. This is shown in figure 6.8(a). Unlike the vasculature, the lymphatics occupy a smaller fraction inside the tissue. The network of the lymphatic system is independent of the vasculature and is separated from the capillaries at the tissue level, such as shown in figure 6.8(b). As such, there is no direct exchange of fluid between the capillaries and the lymphatics. However, fluid that filters out from blood can still enter the lymphatics through the interstitial space.

Pressure inside the lymphatics is usually lower (~1 mmHg) when compared to the vascular and interstitial fluid pressure. Consequently, fluid can only flow from the interstitial space and into the lymphatics as the low lymphatic pressure prevents fluid backflow into the interstitial space. Furthermore, vessels in the lymphatics system contain valves, just like in the veins, that help to prevent backflow of fluid (Shayan *et al* 2006).

In tissues containing the lymphatics, the loss of fluid from the interstitial space to the lymphatics can be accounted for by introducing a sink term to equation (6.14), such that (Baxter and Jain 1990):

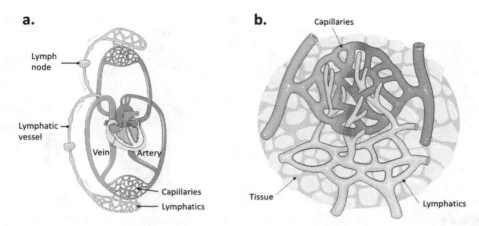

Figure 6.8. Schematic of the (a) lymphatic network as the third circulatory system and (b) lymphatic vessels within the tissue-capillaries structure. Copyright © smart.servier.com. The figure was partly generated using Servier Medical Art, provided by Servier, licensed under a Creative Commons Attribution 3.0.

$$\nabla \cdot \left(-\frac{\kappa_i}{\mu} \nabla p_i \right) = \frac{J_v}{V} - \frac{J_L}{V}, \qquad (6.15)$$

where J_L (m^3 s^{-1}) is the rate of fluid transfer from the interstitial space to the lymphatics through walls of lymphatic vessels and is mathematically given by:

$$J_L = L_{pL} S_L (p_i - p_L), \qquad (6.16)$$

where L_{pL} (m (Pa·s)$^{-1}$) is the hydraulic conductivity of the lymphatic vessel wall, S_L (m^2) is the surface area of the lymphatic vessel wall and p_L (Pa) is the lymphatics pressure.

6.5.3.1 Case study 6.1: increase in interstitial fluid pressure due to fluid retention in tissues

This case study[2] demonstrates how fluid retention in tissues can result in an increase in the interstitial fluid pressure. Knowing the elevation in the interstitial fluid pressure is vital in understanding the risk of cerebral oedema. Cerebral oedema is a pathological condition defined by the swelling of the brain due to fluid accumulation inside the brain (Koenig 2018). Several conditions can cause cerebral oedema, including traumatic brain injury, infection, presence of brain tumour and brain haemorrhage (Ho *et al* 2012). Cerebral oedema is potentially fatal as the swelling can restrict blood flow into the brain. Moreover, the retention of fluid inside the brain can raise the interstitial fluid pressure and subsequently the intracranial pressure. Clinical studies have shown that an elevation in the intracranial pressure

---

[2] Source files for case study 6.1 are available at https://doi.org/10.1088/978-0-7503-4016-8.

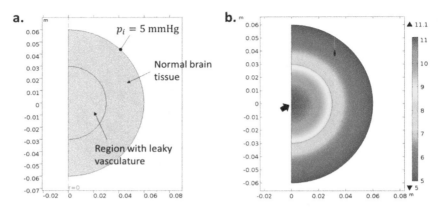

Figure 6.9. (a) Model of the brain tissue with a region of leaky vasculature in case study 6.1 and (b) contours of the interstitial fluid pressure (mmHg) for the model with $L_p = 1.04 \times 10^{-10}$ m (Pa·s)$^{-1}$ in the leaky vasculature region.

by 5 mmHg is abnormal and anything above 10 mmHg requires immediate medical attention (Czosnyka and Pickard 2014).

To simulate the formation of oedema, the case of leaky vasculature (see section 6.4.2) is considered. For simplicity, the brain is assumed to be a sphere of radius 6 cm. The region of leaky vasculature is located at the centre of the brain and is localised to a spherical region 3 cm in radius. Lymphatics is assumed to be absent from the brain tissue. Pressure inside the capillaries is assumed to be constant at 30 mmHg, while osmotic pressure difference is 20 mmHg. Under these assumptions, the interstitial fluid pressure inside the brain can be described using equation (6.13).

The model of the brain was constructed as a semicircle in 2D axisymmetry. This is shown in figure 6.9(a). At the outer boundary of the model, interstitial fluid pressure was set to 5 mmHg, which is equivalent to that at basal level. Table 6.3 summarises the material properties required to carry out the simulation in this case study. To simulate leaky vasculature, five values of the capillary hydraulic conductivity were investigated, namely 1.06×10^{-14}, 1.06×10^{-13}, 1.06×10^{-12}, 1.06×10^{-11} and 1.06×10^{-10} m (Pa·s)$^{-1}$. These values represent magnitudes that are one to five orders higher than the hydraulic conductivity under normal conditions.

Figure 6.9(b) presents the contours of the interstitial fluid pressure obtained for the case where the hydraulic conductivity of the leaky vasculature is 1.06×10^{-10} m (Pa·s)$^{-1}$. The elevation in the hydraulic conductivity causes excess fluid to be filtered out from the capillaries and into the surrounding tissue. Since no lymphatics are present, fluid is retained inside the tissue and this leads to a build-up of the interstitial fluid pressure, see black arrow in figure 6.9(b).

Figure 6.10(a) plots the variation of the interstitial fluid pressure along the $z = 0$ axis. The region with leaky vasculature ($r < 0.03$ m) showed a larger elevation in interstitial fluid pressure, which is not surprising due to the greater retention of fluid in this region. Plot of the maximum interstitial fluid pressure against the hydraulic conductivity of the leaky vasculature is shown in figure 6.10(b).

Table 6.3. Values of the material properties used in case study 6.1.

Parameter	Value
Pressure in capillaries, p_v (kPa)	3.5
Osmotic pressure difference, $\Delta\pi$ (kPa)	2.7
Tissue porosity, φ	0.35
Hydraulic conductivity in healthy tissue, L_p (m (Pa·s)$^{-1}$)	1.06×10^{-15}
Hydraulic conductivity in tissue with leaky vasculature, L_p (m (Pa·s)$^{-1}$)	1.06×10^{-14}–1.06×10^{-10}
Osmotic reflection coefficient, σ_s	0.8
Surface area to volume ratio, S/V (m^{-1})	7000
Interstitial space permeability, κ_i (m^2)	1×10^{-13}
Dynamic viscosity of interstitial fluid, μ (Pa·s)	0.0007
Density of interstitial fluid, ρ_i (kg m^{-3})	996

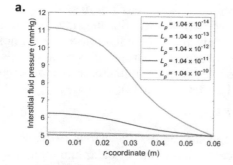 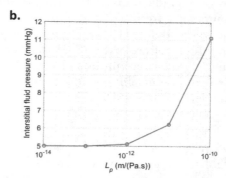

Figure 6.10. Plots of the (a) interstitial fluid pressure along the $z = 0$ coordinate and (b) maximum interstitial fluid pressure against the hydraulic conductivity in the leaky vasculature region.

The interstitial fluid pressure increases exponentially with the hydraulic conductivity. This suggests that an increase in vascular permeability below a certain critical threshold is tolerable. Beyond this threshold, there will be a rapid elevation in the interstitial fluid pressure.

Case study 6.1 demonstrates how the retention of fluid in tissues can cause the interstitial fluid pressure to increase. In the brain, the increase in the interstitial fluid pressure can induce adverse effects that can potentially be fatal. The contiguous nature and the ability of the interstitial fluid and cerebrospinal fluid to exchange freely meant that an increase in interstitial fluid pressure can result in an increase in the cerebrospinal fluid (Rosenberg *et al* 2022). The latter causes an increase in intracranial pressure, which if left untreated, can lead to pathological conditions such as stroke, coma and even death (Rangel-Castillo *et al* 2008).

6.6 Drug delivery

Drug delivery is the transport of pharmaceutical components (drugs) inside the human body. Various forms of drug delivery methods are available including oral ingestion tablets and pills (Tiwari *et al* 2012), nasal spray (Djupesland 2013), eye drops and contact lenses (Patel *et al* 2013), percutaneous injection (Smits *et al* 2002), intravenous infusion (Peterfreund and Philip 2013), transdermal patch (Alkilani *et al* 2015), and vaginal/rectal tablets (Purohit *et al* 2018, Osmalek *et al* 2021). Almost all these methods involve the transport of drugs in the blood stream to the targeted site. At the targeted site, drugs are transferred from blood to tissue at the capillary bed, where the effectiveness of the process is governed by the drug transport through the capillary walls and the absorption of the drug components inside the tissue. Hence, the ability to describe drug transport between the vasculature and the interstitium can facilitate better understanding and the development of more efficient drug delivery mechanism.

Under normal circumstances, pressure inside the capillaries is higher than the surrounding interstitial fluid. As described by Starling's law in section 6.4.1, this pressure gradient drives the efflux of fluid, which carries with it the solutes or drug compounds from blood into the tissue. This process is the basis of drug delivery in biological tissues. However, equation (6.11) describing the Starling law accounts only for pressure-driven fluid transfer. Not only that, the equation alone cannot quantify the concentration of drugs that are transported across the capillary walls. To quantify the efflux of drugs, one may use the following mathematical expression (Baxter and Jain 1989, Erbertseder *et al* 2012, Ooi *et al* 2018):

$$\Theta_s = J_v(1 - \sigma_f)c_v + PS(c_v - c_i), \tag{6.17}$$

where Θ_s (mol s^{-1}) is the rate of solute transfer across the capillary walls, c_v (mol m^{-3}) and c_i (mol m^{-3}) are the drug concentration in the vascular and interstitial space, respectively, σ_f (dimensionless) is the solute retardation coefficient, P (m s^{-1}) is the solute permeability of the capillary walls, S (m^2) is the surface area of the capillary walls, and J_v (m^3 s^{-1}) is the expression from Starling's law, see equation (6.11).

The first term on the right-hand side of equation (6.17) represents the pressure-driven solute transport across the capillary wall, while the second term on the right-hand side represents solute transport due to the concentration difference between blood and the surrounding tissue. The second term effectively describes diffusion across the capillary wall and the effectiveness of the diffusion process is determined by the concentration gradient and the capillary wall permeability, P. One may view the pressure-driven and concentration-driven transport as convection and diffusion, respectively. Just like convection and diffusion, transport driven by the pressure gradient is usually greater than that of concentration gradient.

In tissues where lymphatics are present, the pressure difference between the interstitial space and the lymphatics may cause some of the drugs inside the tissue to be the drained into the lymphatics. In this case, the rate of mass transfer from the interstitial space to the lymphatics can be expressed as:

$$\Theta_L = J_L(c_i - c_L), \tag{6.18}$$

where Θ_L (mol s^{-1}) is the rate of solute transfer across the walls of the lymphatic vessels, c_L (mol m^{-3}) is the drug concentration inside the lymphatics and J_L (m^3 s^{-1}) is the rate of fluid flow from the interstitial space into the lymphatics, as expressed in equation (6.16).

Equations (6.17) and (6.18) can be combined with the convection–diffusion equation (see equation (6.9)) to obtain a differential equation that describes the spatio-temporal concentration inside the interstitial space:

$$\frac{\partial c_i}{\partial t} + \mathbf{v}_i \cdot \nabla c_i = D_i \nabla^2 c_i + \frac{\Theta_s}{V} - \frac{\Theta_L}{V}, \tag{6.19}$$

where $\mathbf{v}_i$ (m s^{-1}) is the velocity of the fluid inside the interstitial space and D_i (m^2 s^{-1}) is the diffusion coefficient of drugs in the interstitial space. Note that the positive sign preceding the term Θ_s implies that it is a source term, while the negative sign preceding the Θ_L term implies that it is a sink term. Equation (6.19) assumes the capillaries and lymphatics to be homogeneously distributed across the tissue such that the solute transport can be expressed as source and sink terms within the convection–diffusion equation. The fluid velocity inside the interstitial space $\mathbf{v}_i$ can be estimated from equation (6.12) after solving equations (6.13) or (6.15) (if lymphatics are present) for the interstitial fluid pressure distribution.

6.6.1 Case study 6.2: drug delivery in solid tumours

Successful chemotherapy of cancer relies on an efficient delivery of therapeutic agents to the tumour sites (van der Wall et al 1995). Solid tumours, which are often treated using chemotherapy, are typically separated into two regions: a necrotic core that is avascular (lack of vasculature) and a vascularized periphery (Jiao et al 2018). The efficiency of drug delivery to solid tumours can be understood from a fluid and mass transfer analysis carried out across the region of interest (Jang et al 2003). This will be the demonstrated in this case study[3].

Consider a spherical solid tumour with a radius of 1 cm. The core of the tumour is necrotic and is 1 cm in diameter. The tumour is surrounded by healthy tissues, also spherical, with a diameter of 5 cm. For simplicity, the model of the tumour and the surrounding tissue is developed in 2D axisymmetry and is shown in figure 6.11(a).

In accordance with equations (6.13) and (6.19), the capillaries in the tumour periphery and in the normal tissues are assumed to be homogeneously distributed. It is assumed that both the tumour and the surrounding healthy tissue do not possess a lymphatic system. Drugs enter the system through the capillaries of both the tumour periphery and the surrounding normal tissue. Since the tumour core is avascular, different governing equations must be prescribed for the core, the tumour periphery, and the surrounding healthy tissues. At the core, the lack of blood vessels permits the

---

[3] Source files for case study 6.2 are available at https://doi.org/10.1088/978-0-7503-4016-8.

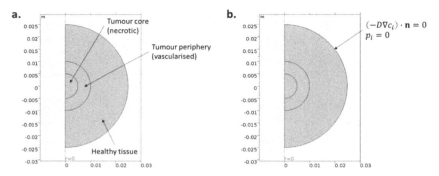

Figure 6.11. Illustration of the (a) model geometry of the tumour (core and periphery) and the surrounding healthy tissues and (b) boundary condition employed.

omission of the source (right-hand side) terms from equations (6.14) and (6.19). The equations governing the pressure and concentration distribution inside the tumour core are thus given by:

$$\nabla \cdot \left(-\frac{\kappa_i}{\mu} \nabla p_i \right) = 0,$$

and

$$\frac{\partial c_i}{\partial t} + \mathbf{v}_i \cdot \nabla c_i = D_i \nabla^2 c_i,$$

respectively. For the tumour periphery and healthy tissues, the governing equations are identical to equations (6.14) and (6.19).

The initial drug concentration inside the tumour and surrounding healthy tissue was set to zero to mimic the absence of drugs at the initial state. At the outer boundary of the model, a pressure of 5 mmHg and an outflow condition (see table 6.2) were prescribed. These are shown in figure 6.11(b). The drugs that enter the capillaries were set to have a concentration of 0.05 mol m^{-3}. Values of the material properties used in this case study are summarised in table 6.4. When carrying out the simulations, the equations for pressure were solved first in steady state to obtain the interstitial fluid pressure distribution across the solution domain. The pressure distribution is then used to estimate the velocity $\mathbf{v}_i$ and the results were used as inputs into the convection–diffusion equations. These were solved for 6 h of drug exposure.

Figure 6.12 plots the contours of the interstitial fluid pressure distribution across the tumour and surrounding healthy tissues. Arrows representing the velocity of the interstitial fluid flow are also shown. The contours indicate that the pressure inside the tumour is higher than the surrounding healthy tissue, which causes interstitial fluid to be driven out of the tumour, as depicted by the arrow plots. The high interstitial fluid pressure inside the tumour may be explained by its low permeability, which increases the flow resistance inside the tumour and ultimately elevating the

Table 6.4. Values of the material properties used in case study 6.2.

Parameter	Value		
	Tumour core	Tumour periphery	Healthy tissue
Hydraulic conductivity, L_p (m (Pa·s)$^{-1}$)	2.1×10^{-11}	2.1×10^{-11}	2.7×10^{-12}
Permeability, κ_i (m^2)	2.2×10^{-17}	2.2×10^{-17}	4.5×10^{-18}
Capillary surface area to volume ratio, S/V (m^{-1})	—	20 000	7000
Vessel pressure, p_v (mmHg)	—	15.6	15.6
Vessel osmotic pressure, π_v (mmHg)	—	20	20
Interstitial osmotic pressure, π_v (mmHg)	—	15	10
Osmotic reflection coefficient, σ_f	—	0.82	0.91
Solute retardation coefficient, σ_s	—	0.9	0.9
Capillary wall permeability, P (m s^{-1})	—	4×10^{-9}	2.4×10^{-9}
Porosity, φ	0.2	0.2	0.24
Diffusion coefficient, D (m^2 s^{-1})	1×10^{-10}	1×10^{-10}	1×10^{-10}
Drug concentration, c_v (mol m^{-3})	0.05		
Interstitial fluid dynamic viscosity, μ_s (Pa·s)	0.0007		

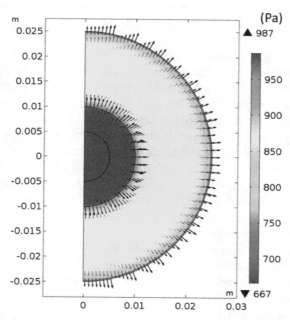

Figure 6.12. Contours of the interstitial fluid pressure (Pa) inside the tumour and surrounding healthy tissue. Arrows represent the velocity vector of the interstitial fluid flow. The high interstitial fluid pressure of solid tumours is clearly depicted by the pressure contours.

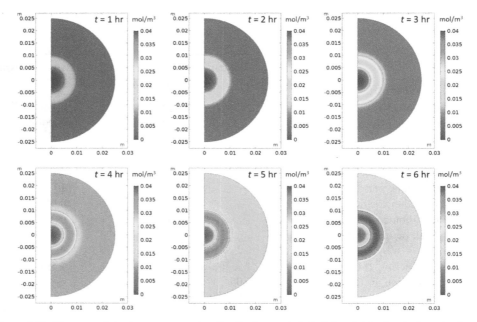

Figure 6.13. Contours of the drug concentration distribution $t = 1, 2, 3, 4, 5$ and 6 h after the introduction of drugs into the tumour periphery and surrounding tissue.

interstitial fluid pressure. The latter explains why drug delivery into solid tumour through the conventional route, i.e., through the vasculature, is very difficult (Jain 1994, Sriraman *et al* 2014).

Contours of the drug concentration distribution at $t = 1, 2, 3, 4, 5$ and 6 h after drugs were introduced into the capillaries are presented in figure 6.13. Drug concentration increases in the tumour periphery more prominently than the surrounding tissue despite the transfer of drugs from the capillaries into both domains. This may be explained by the higher fluid efflux from the capillaries in the tumour periphery due to its higher hydraulic conductivity. Moreover, the higher capillary wall permeability, P inside the tumour and the larger surface area to volume ratio, S/V allowed greater drug transfer from the capillaries to the tumour. In the surrounding tissue, most of the drugs that are transferred from the capillaries to the tissue are transported out of the domain. Since the pressure inside the tumour core is the highest, it is not possible for the drugs from the healthy tissue to flow against the potential gradient and into the tumour. Consequently, at the tumour core, the drug concentration remains low even after 6 h of infusion.

The results presented above were obtained under the assumption that drugs are delivered to the tissue through the vasculature of both the tumour periphery and the surrounding tissue. If drugs are introduced into the system only through the surrounding tissue, which is more likely the case, then drugs that can enter the tumour (both tumour periphery and core) are significantly reduced. This is shown in figure 6.14, where simulations were carried for the case where drugs only enter the

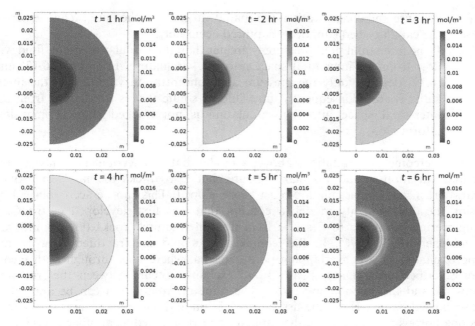

Figure 6.14. Contours of the drug concentration distribution $t = 1, 2, 3, 4, 5$ and 6 h after the introduction of drugs only into the surrounding tissue.

system from the vasculature of the surrounding tissues. One may observe that even after 6 h of drug exposure, the concentration inside the tumour remains very low and close to zero. This demonstrates the difficulty in drug delivery to solid tumours.

In this case study, we have assumed that the drugs concentration inside the capillaries remained constant throughout the 6 h of observation. Unless there is a continuous supply of drugs to the system, this assumption is a gross simplification that overestimates the concentration of drugs that are delivered to the tissue. During actual treatment, the concentration of drugs will diminish with time, further reducing the concentration of drugs that is delivered into the tumour.

6.7 Dual porosity model

When solving equation (6.12) in case studies 6.1 and 6.2, the vascular pressure, p_v in the Starling law was assumed to be constant throughout the tissue. Likewise, the drug concentration inside the vasculature, c_v was set to constant when solving equation (6.19) in case study 6.2. The assumptions of constant vascular pressure and concentration may not accurately represent the actual transvascular fluid and solute exchange inside the tissue. The reason for this is two-fold (Ooi and Ooi 2017):

1. As demonstrated in section 6.4.1, a pressure gradient exists across the capillary bed, which is responsible for fluid efflux and influx across the arteriole and venule ends, respectively. By assuming a constant vascular

pressure and concentration, the spatial variation in the fluid exchange across the capillary bed cannot be captured accurately.

2. If the interstitial fluid pressure is greater than the vascular pressure, fluid will flow from the interstitial space into the vasculature. Equations (6.13) and (6.19) describe only the pressure and concentration variation in the interstitial space. Consequently, any fluid or solute that is transferred from the interstitial space into the vasculature is not tracked and becomes lost information.

To overcome the limitations above, a model that can account not only for the spatial variation in the vascular pressure, but also tracks the fluid and solute transport inside the vasculature must be developed. This can be accomplished by using the dual porosity model; a concept that was first developed in the Civil Engineering discipline to describe fluid flow in fractured rocks (Gerke and van Genutchen 1993, 1996). In this context, rocks and the fractured network are approximated as two overlapping porous media, where flow through both media are described using Darcy's law. Fluid exchange occurs between the fractured network and the surrounding rocks. The same approximation can be applied to vascularised tissues. Here, the tissue (interstitium and interstitial space) is assumed as one porous medium, while the capillary bed is assumed as another overlapping porous medium (Ooi and Ooi 2017). This is illustrated in figure 6.15. For the sake of argument, the models described by equations (6.13) and (6.19), where pressure and solute concentration in the vasculature are assumed to be constant, may be regarded as single porosity models, since the interstitium is the only porous medium considered (Ooi and Ooi 2017).

The dual porosity model treats the interstitium and the vasculature as two separate overlapping porous domains. Each domain occupies a certain fraction within the solution space. Fluid flow and mass transport in both domains become

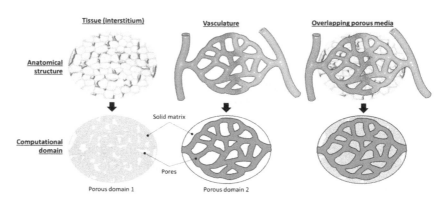

Figure 6.15. Conceptual framework of the dual porosity model applied to biological tissues. Copyright © smart.servier.com. The figure was partly generated using Servier Medical Art, provided by Servier, licensed under a Creative Commons Attribution 3.0 unported license.

the solution of interest. Following the porous medium assumption, fluid flow inside the interstitium and vasculature can be described using Darcy's law, such that:

$$\nabla \cdot \left(-\varphi_i \frac{\kappa_i}{\mu} \nabla p_i \right) = \frac{J_v}{V} - \frac{J_L}{V}, \tag{6.20}$$

in the interstitium and:

$$\nabla \cdot \left(-\varphi_v \frac{\kappa_v}{\mu} \nabla p_v \right) = -\frac{J_v}{V}, \tag{6.21}$$

in the vasculature, where p_v (Pa) is pressure inside the vasculature, κ_v (m^2) is the permeability of the vasculature, and φ_i (dimensionless) and φ_v (dimensionless) are the volume fractions of the interstitial space and vasculature, respectively, such that $\varphi_i + \varphi_v = 1$. The volume fraction of each domain is incorporated into the Darcy equations to account for the interstitium and vasculature occupying the same solution space.

The term J_v in equations (6.20) and (6.21) is obtained from Starling's law and is given by equation (6.11). Unlike the single porosity model, p_v in the dual porosity model is not a constant but a spatially varying unknown that is governed by equation (6.21). The opposing signs preceding J_v in equations (6.20) and (6.21) preserve mass conservation between the interstitium and vasculature. This can be demonstrated from a simple analysis of the equations. When $J_v > 0$, Starling's law states that fluid efflux occurs. The interstitial space gains fluid as a result and this is captured by the positive J_v term (mass source) in equation (6.20). Since the vasculature loses fluid, the corresponding term in equation (6.21) becomes negative (mass sink). A similar interpretation can be made when $J_v < 0$.

Note that equation (6.20) includes the presence of the lymphatics, which is represented by the term J_L (see equation (6.16)). This term however, does not appear in equation (6.21), implying that there is no direct fluid interaction between the vasculature and the lymphatics, as mentioned in section 6.5.3.

The dual porosity model can also be written to describe solute transport in both the interstitium and vasculature. The equations are based on the convection–diffusion equation and are given by (Ooi *et al* 2018):

$$\varphi_i \frac{\partial c_i}{\partial t} + \varphi_i (\mathbf{v}_i \cdot \nabla c_i) = \varphi_i D_i \nabla^2 c_i + \frac{\Theta_s}{V} - \frac{\Theta_L}{V}, \tag{6.22}$$

for the interstitium, and:

$$\varphi_v \frac{\partial c_v}{\partial t} + \varphi_v (\mathbf{v}_v \cdot \nabla c_v) = \varphi_v D_v \nabla^2 c_v - \frac{\Theta_s}{V}, \tag{6.23}$$

for the vasculature, where c_v (mol m^{-3}) is the solute concentration inside the vasculature, D_v (m^2 s^{-1}) is the diffusion coefficient in the vasculature, and $\mathbf{v}_i$ (m s^{-1}) and $\mathbf{v}_v$ (m s^{-1}) are the velocities in the interstitial and vascular spaces, respectively, which can be obtained from Darcy's law:

$$\mathbf{v}_i = -\frac{\kappa_i}{\mu}\nabla p_i \text{ and } \mathbf{v}_v = -\frac{\kappa_v}{\mu}\nabla p_v.$$

The term Θ_s (mol s^{-1}) represents the transvascular solute exchange between the vasculature and the interstitium, which for the dual porosity model, is given by (Erbertseder *et al* 2012):

$$\Theta_s = J_v(1 - \sigma_f)\bar{c} + PS(c_v - c_i), \tag{6.24}$$

where $\bar{c}$ is the mean mole fraction of the drugs, which may be calculated using the logarithmic mean (Erbertseder *et al* 2012):

$$\bar{c} = \frac{c_v - c_i}{\ln(c_v/c_i)}, \tag{6.25}$$

or approximated using:

$$\bar{c} = \left|\frac{c_v - c_i}{2}\right|. \tag{6.26}$$

The opposing signs preceding the term Θ_s ensure mass conservation between the two domains, similar to equations (6.20) and (6.21).

6.7.1 Case study 6.3: comparison between single porosity and dual porosity models

This case study[4] compares the numerical predictions of the pressure and solute concentration distribution obtained using the dual porosity model against those using the single porosity model. Consider a 1D tissue domain defined by $x \in [0, 0.05]$ m. The tissue consists of both the interstitium and the vasculature. Fluid enters the vascular domain at $x = 0$ at a constant pressure of $p_{v,\,in}$ and carries with it drugs at a concentration of 100 mol m^{-3}. Fluid exits the tissue at $x = 0.05$ m carrying with it any solutes that remain. The vascular pressure here is constant at 15 mmHg. Interstitial pressures at $x = 0$ and $x = 0.05$ m are constants at 0 mmHg. When solving the single porosity model, the vascular pressure and concentration were assumed to be constant with values given by $p_{v,\,in}$ and 100 mol m^{-3}, respectively. The initial drug concentration inside both the interstitium and vasculature was set to zero. The 1D model and their corresponding boundary conditions are illustrated in figure 6.16. The material properties used for both the single porosity and dual porosity models are summarised in table 6.5. To examine the effects of different vascular pressure, simulations were carried out for four values of $p_{v,\,in}$ given by 20, 25, 30 and 35 mmHg. The interstitial fluid and vascular pressures at steady state, and the drug concentration distribution after 10 min of drug exposure are investigated.

Figure 6.17(a) plots the interstitial fluid pressure along the x coordinate obtained using the single porosity model. Corresponding plots obtained using the dual porosity for the interstitial fluid and vascular pressures are presented in

---

[4] Source files for case study 6.3 are available at https://doi.org/10.1088/978-0-7503-4016-8.

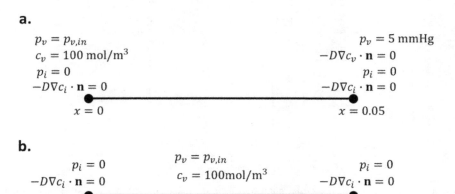

a.

$p_v = p_{v,in}$
$c_v = 100 \, \text{mol/m}^3$
$p_i = 0$
$-D\nabla c_i \cdot \mathbf{n} = 0$

$x = 0$

$p_v = 5 \, \text{mmHg}$
$-D\nabla c_v \cdot \mathbf{n} = 0$
$p_i = 0$
$-D\nabla c_i \cdot \mathbf{n} = 0$

$x = 0.05$

b.

$p_i = 0$
$-D\nabla c_i \cdot \mathbf{n} = 0$

$x = 0$

$p_v = p_{v,in}$
$c_v = 100 \, \text{mol/m}^3$

$p_i = 0$
$-D\nabla c_i \cdot \mathbf{n} = 0$

$x = 0.05$

Figure 6.16. Boundary conditions and model setup for the (a) dual porosity and (b) single porosity models.

Table 6.5. Values of the material properties used in case study 6.3.

Parameter	Value
Interstitial permeability, κ_i (m^2)	3.1×10^{-17}
Vascular permeability, κ_v (m^2)	3.6×10^{-12}
Fluid dynamic viscosity, μ (Pa·s)	0.0007
Fluid density, ρ (kg m^{-3})	998
Vasculature surface area to volume ration S/V (m^{-1})	7000
Interstitial osmotic pressure, π_i (mmHg)	10
Vascular osmotic pressure, π_v (mmHg)	20
Osmotic reflection coefficient, σ_f	0.91
Solute retardation coefficient, σ_s	0.9
Vascular surface permeability, P (m s^{-1})	7.3×10^{-12}
Interstitial volume fraction, φ_i	0.857
Vascular volume fraction, φ_v	0.143
Interstitial diffusion coefficient, D_i (m^2 s^{-1})	1×10^{-9}
Vascular diffusion coefficient, D_v (m^2 s^{-1})	4.2×10^{-10}

figure 6.17(b) and (c). The single porosity model predicted an almost uniform interstitial fluid pressure except near the domain end points, where it decreases to zero due to the prescribed boundary condition. The uniform interstitial fluid pressure may be explained by the constant vascular pressure assumption of the single porosity model, which results in uniform transvascular fluid exchange across the tissue domain. With the dual porosity model, the interstitial fluid pressure displays a linear decrease from $x = 0$ to $x = 0.05$ m, with enforced zero pressure at the end points. The linear decrease is in response to the linear variation in the vascular pressure, see figure 6.17(c).

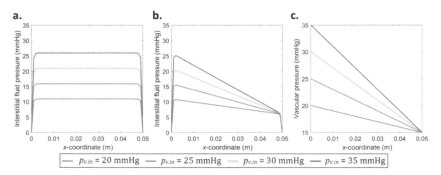

Figure 6.17. Plots of the (a) interstitial fluid pressure from the single porosity model, (b) interstitial fluid pressure from the dual porosity model, and (c) vascular pressure from the dual porosity model.

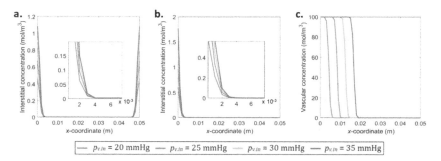

Figure 6.18. Plots of the (a) interstitial drug concentration from the single porosity model, (b) interstitial drug concentration from the dual porosity model, and (c) vascular drug concentration from the dual porosity model. Inset: enlarged view of the interstitial drug concentration.

Figure 6.18 plots the drug concentration distribution along the x coordinate obtained using the single (a) and dual porosity (b) models at $t = 10$ min. With the single porosity model, the drug concentration across the majority of the tissue remains very low except at the end points. This may be explained by the small pressure difference between the interstitial fluid pressure and the prescribed constant vascular pressure (see figure 6.17(a)). This explanation is supported by the observation of high concentration at the end points, where the pressure difference here is higher due to the enforced zero pressure boundary conditions, which led to a larger pressure difference between the interstitial fluid and the vasculature. The dual porosity model also predicted very low interstitial drug concentration. However, unlike the single porosity model, concentration at $x = 0.05$ m is zero. This can be explained by the absence of drugs in the vasculature at points $x > 0.02$ m (see figure 6.18(c)), which prevented transvascular solute transport from taking place. This is not the case with the single porosity model since the drug concentration across the entire vascular space is assumed to be constant at 100 mol m^{-3}.

6.7.2 Case study 6.4: saline-infused radiofrequency ablation

Saline-infused RFA is a cancer treatment technique that incorporates saline infusion into the tumour tissue either prior to or during the ablation procedure (Goldberg *et al* 2001). A brief explanation of the mechanisms of action during saline infused RFA has been presented in chapter 4. A key element that determines the success of saline infused RFA treatment is the knowledge of the saline distribution inside the tissue (Kho *et al* 2021a, 2021b). Distribution that are localised may not change the tissue electrical properties sufficiently to induce any significant effect. On the other hand, a widespread saline distribution may cause extravasation to nearby organs, potentially damaging them during the ablation process (Gilliams and Lees 2005).

In this case study[5], we will demonstrate the use of the single and dual porosity models to describe saline distribution following infusion into liver tissue. The predictions obtained using the single and dual porosity models will be compared, where we will show how the single porosity model tends to underestimate the distribution of saline inside liver tissue.

Liver tissue was assumed to be a sphere of radius 6 cm, which was modelled as a semi-circle in 2D axisymmetry. This is shown in figure 6.19(a). The vasculature inside the liver tissue was assumed to be homogeneously distributed. We assume the liver to be free of the lymphatic vessels. Saline enters the tissue domain through a spherical surface of radius 1 mm whose centre coincides with the tissue centre, mimicking the needle outlet.

At the infusion surface, the following boundary conditions were prescribed for the dual porosity model:

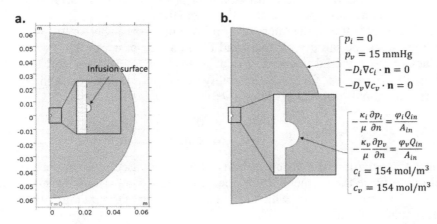

Figure 6.19. (a) Model geometry developed for case study 6.4 and (b) the boundary conditions prescribed to the model.

[5] Source files for case study 6.4 are available at https://doi.org/10.1088/978-0-7503-4016-8.

$$\begin{cases} -\dfrac{\kappa_i}{\mu}\dfrac{\partial p_i}{\partial n} = \dfrac{\varphi_i Q_{in}}{A} \\[2mm] -\dfrac{\kappa_v}{\mu}\dfrac{\partial p_v}{\partial n} = \dfrac{\varphi_v Q_{in}}{A}, \\[2mm] c_i = 154\,\text{mol/m}^3 \\[2mm] c_v = 154\,\text{mol/m}^3 \end{cases} \qquad (6.27)$$

where $Q_{in} = 0.5$ ml min^{-1} is the volumetric infusion rate of saline, A (m^2) is the surface area where infusion takes place and the value 154 mol m^{-3} represents the concentration of infused saline, which in this case study, is assumed to be isotonic (0.9%). The boundary conditions in equation (6.27) indicate that saline enters both the interstitial space and the vasculature at the point of infusion.

At the exterior boundary of the model, the following boundary conditions were applied:

$$\begin{cases} p_i = 0\,\text{mmHg} \\[2mm] p_v = 15\,\text{mmHg} \\[2mm] -D_i\dfrac{\partial c_i}{\partial n} = 0\,. \\[2mm] -D_v\dfrac{\partial c_v}{\partial n} = 0 \end{cases} \qquad (6.28)$$

The last two rows of equation (6.28) indicate outflow of saline from the solution domain. When solving the single porosity model, the second and fourth rows in equations (6.27) and (6.28) are omitted, and φ_i is set to 1. Figure 6.19(b) illustrates the boundary conditions prescribed in this case study.

Initial concentration of the interstitial and vascular space was set to 134 mol m^{-3}, which represents the salinity of tissue and blood at the basal level.

Values of the material properties used in this case study are identical to those listed in table 6.4, except for the permeability of the vasculature, which in this study, assumes a diagonal property given by (Debbaut *et al* 2012):

$$\kappa_v = \begin{bmatrix} 1.5 \times 10^{-14} & 0 \\ 0 & 3.64 \times 10^{-14} \end{bmatrix} \text{m}^2. \qquad (6.29)$$

According to equation (6.29), permeability of the liver vasculature in the z-direction is more than twice the permeability in the r-direction. Simulations were carried for an infusion duration of 6 min, which for an infusion rate of 0.5 ml min^{-1}, leads to an infused volume of 3 ml.

Figure 6.20(a) presents the contours of saline concentration inside the tissue interstitium obtained using the single porosity model. Contours representing the saline concentration inside the interstitial and vascular space obtained using the dual porosity model are presented figure 6.20(a) and (b), respectively. Using the single porosity model, the saline concentration inside the tissue interstitium is localised to a

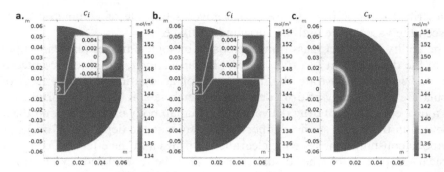

Figure 6.20. Contours of saline concentration across (a) the interstitial space obtained from the single porosity model; (b) the interstitial space and (c) the vascular space obtained from the dual porosity model. Inset: enlarged view of the concentration distribution across the interstitial space.

very small region near the infusion surface. A very similar distribution is observed when using the dual porosity model. The saline concentration distribution in the vasculature estimated using the dual porosity model is more widespread than in the interstitium. This may be explained by permeability of the vasculature, which is three orders higher than the permeability of the interstitium. There is also a greater spread of saline in the z-direction than in the r-direction due to the anisotropic permeability (see equation (6.29)).

The results above suggest that the use of the single porosity model to predict the saline concentration distribution will result in an underestimation of the saline distribution when compared to the dual porosity model. This is because any transport of saline into the vasculature is not tracked in the single porosity model and becomes information that is lost from the computational model. The larger distribution observed in the vasculature has in fact been reported by Burdío *et al* (2013), who found a tendency for saline to flow into and through the vasculature when injected into the liver. Although it is acknowledged that the experiments by Burdío *et al* (2013) were carried out on *ex vivo* liver, where the vasculature is voided and therefore presents the path of least resistance for saline to flow, this alone is not sufficient to explain the preferential flow into vasculature. The vascular permeability being three orders of magnitude higher than interstitial permeability is likely to also contribute to the greater saline flow inside the vasculature than the interstitium.

6.8 General summary

Some of the important physical concepts that describe mass transport in biological tissues have been presented in this chapter. The two main mechanisms involved in mass transfer in biological tissues are diffusion and convection, with the latter usually the dominant mode due to the small diffusion coefficients of biological molecules in biological media. An important element when describing mass transport in biological tissues is transvascular fluid exchange, i.e., the exchange of fluid and mass between the vasculature and the surrounding tissue. This phenomenon can be described using Starling's law, which governs the rate of volumetric fluid flow between the vasculature and the surrounding tissue.

The ability to predict mass transport inside biological tissues plays an important role in the development of drug delivery. In this chapter, we have presented a few case studies to demonstrate the importance of accounting for the effects of the vasculature in the study of drug delivery. Nevertheless, it is also important to note that a proper analysis of drug delivery in the human body extends beyond the scope presented in these case studies. Other factors, such as the depletion of drugs due to metabolic consumption, systemic clearance of drugs and the effects of drugs on the physical properties of the tissue, should also be considered in the analysis. Furthermore, whether the drug delivery process is diffusion-controlled, chemically controlled, dissolution-controlled or osmotically-controlled can play a role in how the drug delivery analysis is carried out (Peppas and Narasimhan 2014).

It is also noteworthy that not all drug delivery analysis is focused on the transvascular fluid and solute exchange between the tissue and the vasculature. For instance, ophthalmic drugs are typically delivered via topical eye drops and their delivery mechanism is primarily influenced by the flow of aqueous humour inside the anterior chamber (Loke *et al* 2018) instead of a tissue-vasculature interaction.

References

Alkilani A Z, McCrudden M T C and Donnelly R F 2015 Transdermal drug delivery: innovative pharmaceutical developments based on disruption of the barrier properties of the stratum corneum *Pharmaceutics* **7** 438–70

Baxter L T and Jain R K 1989 Transport of fluid and macromolecules in tumors I. Role of interstitial pressure and convection *Microvasc. Res.* **37** 77–104

Baxter L T and Jain R K 1990 Transport of fluid and macromolecules in tumors II. Role of heterogeneous perfusion and lymphatics *Microvasc. Res.* **40** 246–63

Burdío F, Berjano E, Millan O, Grande L, Poves I, Silva C, de la Fuente M D and Mojal S 2013 CT mapping of saline distribution after infusion of saline into the liver in an *ex vivo* model. How much tissue is actually infused in an image-guided procedure? *Phys. Med.* **29** 188–95

Czosnyka M and Pickard J 2014 Monitoring and interpretation of intracranial pressure *J. Neurol. Neurosurg. Psychiatry* **75** 813–21

Erbertseder K, Reichold J, Flemisch B, Jenny P and Helmig R 2012 A coupled discrete continuum model for describing cancer-therapeutic transport in the lung *PLoS One* **7** e31966

Fick A 1855 Ueber diffusion *Ann. Phys. (Berlin)* **170** 59–86

Debbaut C, Vierendeels J, Casteleyn C, Cornillie P, Loo D V, Simoens P, Hoorebeke L V, Monbaliu D and Segers P 2012 Perfusion characteristics of the human hepatic micro-circulation based on three-dimensional reconstructions and computational fluid dynamic analysis *J. Biomech. Eng.* **134** 011003

Djupesland P G 2013 Nasal drug delivery devices: characteristics and performance in a clinical perspective—a review *Drug Deliv. Transl. Res.* **3** 42–62

Duan C-Y, Zhang J, Wu H-L, Li T and Liu L-M 2017 Regulatory mechanisms, prophylaxis and treatment of vascular leakage following severe trauma and shock *Mil. Med. Res.* **4** 11

Gerke H H and van Genutchen M T 1993 Evaluation of a first-order water transfer term for variably saturated dual-porosity flow models *Water Resour. Res.* **29** 1225–38

Gerke H H and van Genutchen M 1996 Macroscopic representation of structural geometry for simulating water and solute movement in dual-porosity media *Adv. Water Resour.* **19** 343–57

Gilliams A R and Lees W R 2005 CT mapping of the distribution of saline during radiofrequency ablation with perfusion electrodes *Cardiovasc. Intervent. Radiol.* **28** 476–80

Goldberg S N, Ahmed M, Gazelle G S, Kruskal J B, Huertas J C, Halpern E F, Oliver B S and Lenkinski R E 2001 Radio-frequency thermal ablation with NaCl solution injection: effect of electrical conductivity on tissue heating and coagulation-phantom and porcine liver study *Radiology* **219** 157–65

Hinghofer-Szalkay H 2011 Gravity, the hydrostatic indifference concept and the cardiovascular system *Eur. J. Appl. Physiol.* **111** 163–74

Ho M L, Rojas R and Eisenberg R L 2012 Cerebral edema *Am. J. Roentgenol.* **199** W258–73

Incropera F P, DeWitt D P, Bergman T L and Lavine A S 2006 *Fundamentals of Heat and Mass Transfer* 6th edn (Hoboken, NJ: Wiley)

Jain R K 1994 Barriers to drug delivery in solid tumors *Sci. Am.* **271** 58–65

Jang S H, Wientjes M G, Lu D and Au J L S 2003 Drug delivery and transport to solid tumors *Pharm. Res.* **20** 1337–50

Jiao D, Cai Z, Choksi S, Ma D, Choe M, Kwon H-J, Baik J Y, Rowan B G, Liu C and Liu Z 2018 Necroptosis of tumor cells leads to tumor necrosis and promotes tumor metastasis *Cell Res.* **28** 868–70

Kho A S K, Ooi E H, Foo J J and Ooi E T 2021a Role of saline concentration during saline-infused radiofrequency ablation: observation of secondary Joule heating along the saline-tissue interface *Comput. Biol. Med.* **128** 104112

Kho A S K, Ooi E H, Foo J J and Ooi E T 2021b How does saline backflow affect the treatment of saline-infused radiofrequency ablation? *Comput. Methods Programs Biomed.* **211** 106436

Koenig M A 2018 Cerebral edema and elevated intracranial pressure *Neurocrit. Care* **24** 1588–602

Levick J R and Michel C C 2010 Microvascular fluid exchange and the revised Starling principle *Cardiovasc. Res.* **87** 198–210

Loke C Y, Ooi E H, Salahudeen M S, Ramli N and Samsudin A 2018 Segmental aqueous humour outflow and eye orientation have strong influence on ocular drug delivery *Appl. Math. Model.* **57** 474–91

Michel C C, Woodcock T E and Curry F E 2020 Understsanding and extending the Starling principle *Acta Anaesthesiol. Scand.* **64** 1032–37

Ong E S, Gao X-P, Xu N, Predescu D, Rahman A, Broman M T, Jho D H and Malik A B 2003 *E. coli* pneumonia induces CD18-independent airway neutrophil migration in the absence of increased lung vascular permeability *Am. J. Physiol. Lung Cell. Mol. Physiol.* **285** L879–88

Ooi E H and Ooi E T 2017 Mass transport in biological tissues: comparisons between single- and dual-porosity models in the context of saline-infused radiofrequency ablation *Appl. Math. Model* **41** 271–84

Ooi E H, Chia N J Y, Ooi E T, Foo J J, Liao I Y, Nair S R and Mohd Ali A F 2018 Comparison between single- and dual-porosity models for fluid transport in predicting lesion volume following saline-infused radiofrequency ablation *Int. J. Hyperthermia* **34** 1142–56

Osmalek T *et al* 2021 Recent advances in polymer-based vaginal drug delivery systems *Pharmaceutics* **13** 884

Patel A, CHolkar K, Agrahari V and Mitra A K 2013 Ocular drug delivery systems: an overview *World J. Pharmacol.* **2** 47–64

Peppas N A and Narasimhan B 2014 Mathematical models in drug delivery: how modeling has shaped the way we design new drug delivery systems *J. Control. Release* **190** 75–81

Peterfreund R A and Philip J H 2013 Critical parameters in drug delivery by intravenous infusion *Expert Opin. Drug Deliv.* **10** 1095–108

Purohit T J, Hanning S and Wu Z 2018 Advances in rectal drug delivery systems *Pharm. Dev. Technol.* **23** 942–52

Rangel-Castillo L, Gopinanth S and Robertson C S 2008 Management of intracranial hypertension *Neurol. Clin.* **26** 521–41

Reed R K, Lidén A and Rubin K 2010 Edema and fluid dynamics in connective tissue remodeling *J. Mol. Cell. Cardiol.* **48** 518–23

Rosenberg G A, Maki T, Arai K and Lo E H 2022 Gliovascular mechanisms and white matter injury in vascular cognitive impairment and dementia ed J C Grotta, G W Albers, J P Broderick, A L Day, S E Kasner, E H Lo, R L Sacco and L K S Wong *Stroke: Pathophysiology, Diagnosis, and Management* 7th edn (Philadelphia, PA: Elsevier)

Shayan R, Achen M G and Stacker S A 2006 Lymphatic vessels in cancer metastasis: bridging the gaps *Carcinogenesis* **27** 1729–38

Smits P C, van Langenhove G, Schaar M, Reijs A, Bakker W H, van der Giessen W J, Verdouw P D, Krenning E P and Serruys P W 2002 Efficacy of percutaneous intramyocardial injections using a nonfluoroscoping 3-D mapping based catheter system *Cardiovasc. Drugs Ther.* **16** 527–33

Sriraman S K, Aryasomayaiula B and Torchilin V P 2014 Barriers to drug delivery in solid tumors *Tissue Barriers* **2** e29528

Starling E 1896 On the absorption of fluids from the connective tissue spaces *J. Physiol.* **19** 312–26

Tiwari G, Tiwari R, Sriwastawa B, Bhati L, Pandey S, Pandey P and Bannerjee S K 2012 Drug delivery systems: an updated review *Int. J. Pharm. Investig.* **2** 2–11

van der Wall E, Beijnen J H and Rodenhuis S 1995 High-dose chemotherapy regimens for solid tumors *Cancer Treat. Rev.* **21** 105–32

Watkins L Jr, Burton J A, Haber E, Cant J R, Smith J W and Barger A C 1976 The renin-angiotensin-aldosterone system in congestive failure in conscious dogs *J. Clin. Invest.* **57** 1606–17

IOP Publishing

Model-Based Approaches in Biomedical Engineering

Ean Hin Ooi and Yeong Shiong Chiew

Chapter 7

Physiological modelling and data analytics

7.1 Fundamentals of physiological modelling

Physiological modelling, by definition, is to use mathematical models to describe a specific or the whole characteristic of a physiological system. Physiological models are essentially mathematical models defined by a set of equations and model variables to characterise a physiology. A physiological system is a complex system that can be described with various considerations and assumptions but it is (or almost) mathematically impossible to describe the physiological system fully. Nevertheless, these systems can be simplified to capture certain physiology or dynamic by making appropriate assumptions that reflect the system.

The primary aim of physiological modelling is to study, model and understand the biological process of the physiological system. With proper understanding, it is then possible to apply identification and control strategies to the system for treatment purposes. It is a big challenge to combine individualised control therapies with physiological models. This process requires a combination of mathematical knowledge, control engineering, computer engineering and biomedical engineering. In the following chapters, we will introduce a few physiological models, namely the glucose–insulin model, respiratory model and cardiovascular model.

To perform physiological modelling, a wide range of disciplines must be covered. Some of the main disciplines include:

7.1.1 Data acquisition

Data acquisition encompasses the data collection process, using the appropriate tools, equipment and/or specialised devices to gather data that are useful to describe the physiological system. For example, in a glucose–insulin model, the key data used in the model are the blood glucose levels that one can obtain through blood sample collection. A glucometer can then be used to measure blood glucose level.

7.1.2 Data processing

Data processing is the process of conversion of data into usable and desired information. The data collected from the acquisition stage is processed via filtering, data segmentation, alteration, or performing signal processing to convert the original data into forms that are useful for the application. An example is measuring airflow during respiration. Airflow can be derived via measuring pressure difference along the respiratory tract. These pressure measurements are also derived from original voltage signals that were initially measured using pressure sensors.

7.1.3 Model-based analysis

Model-based analysis is about how a physiological model is generated from the data via parameter identification, which are methods used to find optimal parameter values to fit the models to measured data. The model can then be fitted to the data to describe the physiological condition, provide forward simulation to pre-determine the extreme condition *in-silico*, and help to determine a control strategy of the system based on the prediction.

7.1.4 Data analytics

Data analytics cover the techniques to analyse the data collected and processed from experiments or clinical trials. These may include error analyses that help to determine the accuracy and reliability of the data obtained, and statistical tests that inform about the distribution and significance of the data.

7.1.5 Data presentation

Data presentation is important in demonstrating the performance of the model with respect to the prediction of the physiological system. Data presentation is not limited to one approach and often, various techniques are required to present and demonstrate the results.

Ultimately, physiological modelling and its data analytics are very broad topics. Hence, it will not be possible within the scope of this book to go in-depth into how to solve the complex problems pertaining to specific subtopics of physiological modelling. Instead, we will introduce the basics on how to perform model fitting and provide some general guidance on performing data analytics commonly used for physiological modelling. Over time, you will develop a foundation on the topics related to physiological modelling and use them in your application.

7.2 Theories of model fitting and linear regression

Model fitting involves the fitting of a physiological model to the data it is trying to describe. This is one of the key important aspects of performing model-based analysis. The model captures the dynamics of the measured data and thus, is capable of describing the physiology. A simple example of model fitting is the fitting of a set of data with a linear equation, $y = mx + C$. The mathematical equation in this case is the model, while measurements of the dependent variable y at x are the data, and *m* (the slope) and *C* (the offset) are the model parameters. Fitting the equation to the dataset will thus allow the characteristic of the measured data to be described.

In an ideal world, model fitting should be perfect, where the model can capture the dynamics of the data. However, due to the complex nature of the human physiology, data sparsity, and challenges in parameter identification, most models may not truly capture the observed behaviour due to their incapability to distinguish between actual modelled and unmodelled dynamics. Dickson *et al* (2014) noted that the human physiology is complex and clinical data is often highly variable in nature, with outcomes dependant on several different clinical and patient specific aspects. They attempted to model the relation between insulin secretion and other measurements in a neonatal population. However, they found that it was easier to play dot-to-dot cartoonish drawings than to generate meaningful models of physiology. Figure 7.1 shows the cartoon drawings presented by Dickson *et al* (2014), where they attempted to perform model fitting. While comedic, there is certainly truth behind the challenges faced in physiological modelling.

One of the simplest approaches to perform model fitting is to perform linear regression. Linear regression is a linear approach to model the relationship between a scalar response and with one or more explanatory variables. In essence, it attempts to model the relation between dependent and independent variables by fitting a linear equation to the observed data. One can easily perform regression using proprietary engineering software such as **MATLAB** (Natick, MA) and their built-in functions. We will be exploring two case studies on model fitting. All case study codes are available for download.

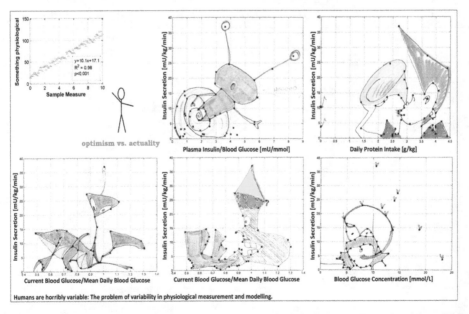

Figure 7.1. A fun attempt in model fitting of complex human physiological data. Reproduced from Dickson *et al* (2014). Copyright © 2014 International Journal of Clinical & Medical Images All Rights Reserved.

Case study 7.1: Parameter identification (inverse simulation)

To demonstrate the concepts behind model fitting and linear regression, consider the dataset shown in table 7.1, where the variation of y with respect to x is shown in figure 7.2. From this dataset, we wish to determine the value of y when x is at 12, i.e., $y(x = 12)$. Suppose that we want to describe the measured data in table 7.1 using a linear model, i.e.:

$$y = mx + C, \qquad (7.1)$$

where m is the slope (or gradient) of the straight line and C is the intercept of the straight line with the y-axis. Both m and C are known as model parameters, and in physiological models, they represent physiological constants, or some *a priori* knowledge of the model. These constants are important as they can be used to describe the physiological condition and how it affects the model response with a given input.

Performing model fitting to the given data will determine the model parameters. In this case, the values of m and C can be determined by applying equation (7.1) to each of the data point in table 7.1, such that:

Table 7.1. Dataset for x and y considered in case study 7.1.

i	1	2	3	4	5	6	7	8
x	0.5	1.0	2.2	3.2	4.8	7.0	10.0	14.0
y	6.73	7.37	8.52	9.37	10.19	11.48	12.69	14.02

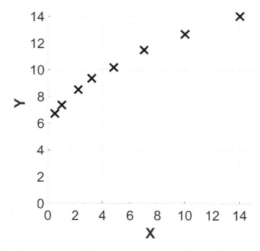

Figure 7.2. Changes in y with respect to x plotted from the data in table 7.1.

$$mx_1 + C = y_1,$$
$$mx_2 + C = y_2,$$
$$\vdots$$
$$mx_8 + C = y_8,$$

(7.2)

where $x_1, x_2, ..., x_8$, and $y_1, y_2, ..., y_8$ are the dataset values of x and y in table 7.1. Equation (7.2) can be re-written in the following matrix equation:

$$A\theta = b,$$

(7.3)

where A is a coefficient matrix, b is a vector of known values and θ is a vector of unknowns to be solved given by:

$$A = \begin{bmatrix} x_1 & 1 \\ x_2 & 1 \\ \vdots & \vdots \\ x_8 & 1 \end{bmatrix}, \theta = \begin{Bmatrix} m \\ C \end{Bmatrix}, b = \begin{bmatrix} y_1 \\ y_2 \\ \vdots \\ y_8 \end{bmatrix}.$$

(7.4)

Equation (7.3) can be re-arranged to solve for m and C, such that:

$$\theta = (A^T A)^{-1} A^T b,$$

(7.5)

which can be solved in **MATLAB** using built-in functions such as `lsqlin.m` or the backslash operator (\).

These MATLAB functions perform different variations of linear least squares to obtain θ by minimising the objective function. In mathematical optimisation, an objective function is a function that is to be maximised or minimised. For the linear regression problem here, the parameter of interest is the sum of squared residuals (SSR) for y_i, i.e.:

$$SSR = \sum_{i=1}^{N}(y_i - \hat{y}_i)^2,$$

(7.6)

where i is the ith data with a total of N data points, y_i is the measured y at the ith data and $\hat{y}_i$ is the value of y fitted to the ith data. Hence, for equation (7.1), SSR can be written as:

$$SSR = \sum_{i=1}^{N}(y_i - mx_i - C)^2.$$

(7.7)

Since we are interested in minimising the SSR with respect to the model parameters, we can derive the objective functions to be:

$$\frac{\partial SSR}{\partial m} = 0, \text{ and } \frac{\partial SSR}{\partial C} = 0.$$

(7.8)

Solving equation (7.3) for the dataset in table 7.1 yields $m = 0.5302$ and $C = 7.2158$. The linear model fitted to the dataset is shown in figure 7.3(a). Thus, substituting $x = 12$ into the linear model results in $y = 13.58$. The process of model fitting, obtaining the coefficient matrix is also known as inverse simulation, where

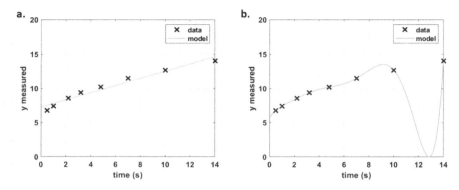

Figure 7.3. Model fitting to the data in table 7.1 using (a) linear and (b) 7th order polynomial.

one attempts to construct a mathematical model of a system from measurements of inputs to and outputs from the system.

The estimated value of $y(12)$ appears to be reasonable with the model fitting well to the data and capturing well the dynamics of the data. However, is the linear model the best model representation to describe the measured data? How do we know it is correct? The answers to these questions are not as straightforward, unfortunately. One may argue that the model is correct simply based on the observation that the model matches well with the overall dynamics of the measured data. Equally, it is also possible to argue that the model is incorrect as some data points were not fully captured by the model.

We can instil some confidence in our results by conducting additional model fittings to the data. For example, we can use a higher order model such as a 7th order polynomial model to fit the data, i.e.:

$$y(x) = a_1x^7 + a_2x^6 + a_3x^5 + a_4x^4 + a_5x^3 + a_6x^2 + a_7x + a_8, \quad (7.9)$$

where the coefficients a_1 to a_8 are the model parameters that can be determined using established interpolation techniques, such as the Lagrange interpolation or Newton's method. Alternatively, one may use the built-in function `polyfit` in MATLAB. Doing so yields the following:

$$a_1 = 5.53 \times 10^{-5}, a_2 = -2.18 \times 10^{-4}, a_3 = 0.0327,$$
$$a_4 = -0.2378, \quad a_5 = 0.8998, \quad a_6 = -1.8288, \quad (7.10)$$
$$a_7 = 2.8343, \quad a_8 = 5.6723.$$

The seventh-order polynomial when fitted to the data from table 7.1 is shown in figure 7.3(b). Evaluating the value of $y(12)$ using the seventh-order polynomial yields a value of -0.128, which clearly deviates from the overall trend of the data.

Perhaps another model, such as the square root model of $y = a_1\sqrt{x} + a_2$, may be more suitable in fitting the dataset and estimating the value of $y(x = 12)$. Repeating the model fitting steps above to estimate a_1 and a_2, and using the fitted square root model to estimate $y(x = 12)$ yields a value of 3.02, which seems more reasonable compared to the 7th order polynomial model. The fitting of the square root model is shown in figure 7.4.

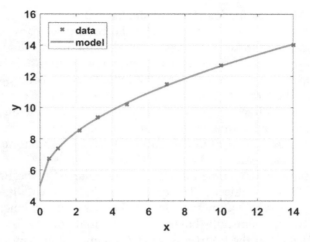

Figure 7.4. Model fitting of the square root model to the data in table 7.1.

All three linear, 7th order polynomial and square root models can capture the measured data, and the quality of model fitting plots appears to be reasonable. However, they can be deceiving at times with model formulations. Many physiological models contain non-linear characteristics that cannot be easily defined using proprietary software. We can, however, evaluate the models using the objective function by looking at the SSR. For this dataset, we obtained the SSR to be 1.834, $<10^{-6}$ and 0.0298 for the linear, 7th order polynomial and square root models, respectively. Clearly, the 7th order polynomial model has the lowest SSR; however, it gives an estimation of $y(12)$ that deviates significantly from the trend of datasets. The small SSR of the 7th order polynomial model is somewhat expected since its parameterisation is greater than the linear and square root models. However, deciding the level of model parameterisation is a very difficult and somewhat specialised task. Experience has shown that keeping the number of parameters to a minimum is the best way to capture the true underlying behaviours of phenomena. Therefore, in this case, we may choose the square root model as it balances between the degree of model parameterisation and having a reasonably low SSR.

In this case, if we look back at the original model[1] data was indeed generated from a square root model and were imposed with 1% measurement noise. With the effect of measurement noise, it is possible that the higher order model will produce a model fitting with lower SSR compared to the original square root model. Over-parameterisation runs the risk of assigning characteristics to a model that are simply artefacts of measurement error. This can cause false predictions via extrapolations of mode responses and thus, introduce the potential for unnecessary harm or cost. We are unable to really distinguish the efficacy of various model formulations when we have only one noisy dataset. However, when we have several datasets, we can generate the summary statistics of residuals to see if an observable trend in error is found.

---

[1] Source code for this model (Chapter07a.m) is available at https://doi.org/10.1088/978-0-7503-4016-8.

Case study 7.2: Model prediction (forward simulation)

In this second case study, we take a look at the concept of forward simulation in physiological modelling through the urea clearance model of the renal system. The renal system, also known as the urinary system in humans, includes a pair of kidneys, where urine is produced. Aside from kidneys, the other major organs of the renal system are the ureters, bladder, and urethra for the passage, storage, and voiding of urine, respectively. This is shown in figure 7.5(a). The human kidneys act as a filter to remove metabolic waste products (e.g., urea and uric acid) from the body and they are also involved in the reabsorptions of essential nutrients from the blood to maintain the health of the body (Depner 1994).

Kidneys regulate fluid volume and electrolyte balance in the body to ensure a steady-state condition is achieved. To achieve that, kidneys will filter out any excess fluid and electrolytes, which allows the body to be chemically balanced and maintain its osmolality. Being chemically balanced is essential for the body as failure to maintain the pH level in the body will cause proteins and enzymes to break down, which may lead to fatality in extreme cases.

Chronic kidney disease (CKD) is commonly used to indicate patients with any abnormalities of the kidneys or the presence of kidney damage which leads to a decrease in kidney function for more than three months. Once a patient is diagnosed with CKD, there are some treatment modalities available for renal function replacement, which are dialysis or kidney transplant for cases that are too severe, such as a patient with end-stage kidney disease. However, kidney transplant is not always available for patients due to the limited availability of the donor's kidneys. As such, haemodialysis as renal function replacement becomes the next best option for most patients.

Haemodialysis is a type of dialysis treatment for patients with CKD (Himmelfarb and Ikizler 2010). Haemodialysis is a procedure where a dialysis machine and a special filter, known as a dialyser (or an artificial kidney), are used to clean the patient's blood. Figure 7.5(b) shows an illustration of a patient who is undergoing

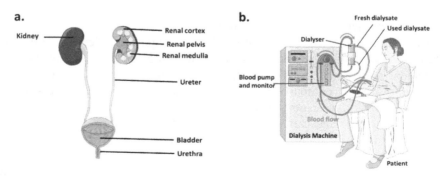

Figure 7.5. (a) Schematic of the urinary system and its organs. (b) Patient undergoing haemodialysis treatment. Patient's blood is drawn out from the body into the dialyser to clean the patient's blood before returning to the body. Copyright © smart.servier.com. The figure was partly generated using Servier Medical Art, provided by Servier, licensed under a Creative Commons Attribution 3.0 unported license.

haemodialysis. Apart from taking medications and diet restrictions, patients must undergo dialysis periodically to remove excess fluid and toxin waste accumulated from the metabolic processes in the body.

In the physiological modelling of the human kidney, we can model how waste is generated and how it is discharged from the body (Depner 1994, 2012). In this case study, we attempt to model the discharge of urea. Urea is a waste product of metabolism and is generated from protein breakdown. When your kidneys are functioning normally, they filter urea and other waste products from your blood. These waste products are then removed from your body through urination. Modelling of human kidneys can provide a fundamental understanding of kidney performance as well as guide haemodialysis treatment.

Urea is produced at a relatively consistent rate and cleared by the kidney. The urea concentration can be used to evaluate kidney function. A simple urea clearance model is the single pool urea kinetics model, which can be defined as (Grzegorzewska *et al* 2013):

$$\frac{dC(t)}{dt} = -\frac{k}{V}C(t) + \frac{G}{V}, \qquad (7.11)$$

where $C(t)$ (mg ml^{-1}) is the urea concentration, k (ml min^{-1}) is the combined urea clearance rate, G (mg min^{-1}) is the rate of urea generation and V (ml) is the total body compartment volume. Equation (7.11) can be solved using forward simulation to understand the patient's condition. Equally, if we acquire $C(t)$ and V through measurements, we can determine the values of k and G through inverse simulation (as in case study 7.1), and hence, determine how much urea is being generated and if the kidney is functioning properly. The most preferable method in forward simulation is to solve the ODE analytically, which for equation (7.11), yields:

$$C(t) = C_0 e^{-\frac{kt}{V}} + \frac{G}{k}\left(1 - e^{-\frac{kt}{V}}\right), \qquad (7.12)$$

where C_0 (mg ml^{-1}) is the initial urea concentration. Analytical solutions are very quick and are usually accurate. However, not all model formulations allow stable forward simulation with analytical solutions. In MATLAB, one can solve the ODE using time-stepping numerical integration such as the Runge–Kutta method (available as `ode45.m` in MATLAB).

Alternatively, one may opt for an error stepping algorithm known as Picard's iteration to solve the ODE in equation (7.11). To carry out Picard's iteration, the ODE is first re-arranged and integrated at both the left-hand and right-hand sides, such that:

$$\int_{C_0}^{C} dC = \int_{t_0}^{t} \left(-\frac{k}{V}C(t) + \frac{G}{V}\right)dt, \qquad (7.13)$$

where t_0 is the initial time. Integrating the left-hand side and re-arranging the terms leads to:

$$C(t) = C_0 + \int_{t_0}^{t} \left(-\frac{k}{V}C(t) + \frac{G}{V} \right) dt. \tag{7.14}$$

Note that it is not possible to integrate the right-hand side due to the presence of the $C(t)$ term inside the integral. It is possible, however, to make an initial assumption of the value of $C(t)$ to make possible the evaluation of this integral. This step can then be repeated and iterated until the difference in the solution $C(t)$ between two consecutive iterations is smaller than a pre-defined threshold. At this point, it is said that convergence has been achieved. This process is known as Picard's iteration and the pseudocode demonstrating this process is given by:

```
for i = 1:n
```
$$C(t) = C_0 + \int_{t_0}^{t_i} \left(-\frac{k}{V}C(t) + \frac{G}{V} \right) dt$$
```
end
```

where n is the number of pre-defined iterations.

As mentioned earlier, an initial value of $C(t)$ must be assumed before the initiation of Picard's iteration. A simple choice is to set $C(t)$ to zero initially. Suppose that the values of k, G, V and C_0 are known and are given by 200 ml min^{-1}, 7 mg min^{-1}, 40 000 ml and 80 mg ml^{-1}, respectively. Figure 7.6(a) shows the forward simulation of the urea clearance model using analytical solution and

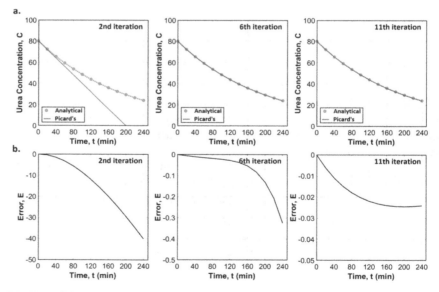

Figure 7.6. Plots of the (a) urea concentration against time obtained using Picard's iteration (blue) and the analytical solution (red dashed) and (b) the error between the Picard's iteration and analytical solutions for $C(t)$.

Picard's iteration. The error between analytical solution and Picard's iteration is shown in figure 7.6(b). One may observe that by the 6th iteration, the difference between the analytical and Picard's iteration solution is almost negligible. When the iteration is allowed the continue to the 11th iteration, no discernible difference in the urea concentration with the 6th iteration was found, suggesting that the iteration has reached convergence.

In the urea clearance model, each model parameter plays an important role in describing the dynamics of how urea is cleared from the kidney. Obviously, an increase in C_0 will change the baseline or starting point of the model simulation, while an increase in k will see a larger exponential drop in the urea concentration $C(t)$. The parameter V is aimed at capturing a subject's compartment volume that affects the magnitude clearance k. The parameter G is the urea generation rate and thus, an increase in G will instead decrease the rate of the drop in urea concentration. You can perform the simulation in the provided MATLAB m-file[2]. The model can be used to forward simulate the dynamics of the urea clearance given a set of model parameters. Similarly, when given the model and we have the measurements of $C(t)$, and V, we can perform model fitting to obtain the urea clearance rate and urea generation rate via linear regression.

Case study 7.3: Effects of noise on parameter identification
The presence of noise can influence the accuracy of the parameter identification process. In fact, clinical and laboratory measurements are bound to be affected by various uncontrollable factors that can contribute to errors in the measured data. These errors usually manifest themselves as noise. In this case study, we will examine the effects of noise on the parameter identification process. We shall use the urea clearance model from case study 7.2, which is reproduced here as:

$$\frac{dC(t)}{dt} = -\frac{k}{V}C(t) + \frac{G}{V}. \tag{7.15}$$

The model parameters to be identified are k and G.

The data for $C(t)$ was generated based on the analytical solution of the urea clearance model, see equation (7.12), for $k = 200$ ml min^{-1} and $G = 7$ mg min^{-1}. Obviously, the data generated from the analytical solution is ideal and free from noise. Hence, 5%, 10% and 15% of random noise were added to each data point of the original dataset. This added noise causes fluctuations to the data, such as shown in figure 7.7. As the percentage of noise added increases, the data deviates from the original value and this will affect the model estimates of the parameters k and G.

A Monte-Carlo simulation was carried out. For each noise level (5%, 10% and 15%), 1000 datasets were randomly generated. For each dataset with the added noise, inverse simulation was carried out to determine the values of k and G. Table 7.2 summarises the estimated values of k and G averaged across the 1000 randomly generated datasets. At 5% noise level, the mean identified k value (201.4 ml min^{-1}) is close to the correct value of 200 ml min^{-1}, which is the exact value set in

---

[2] Source code for this model (Chapter07b) is available at https://doi.org/10.1088/978-0-7503-4016-8.

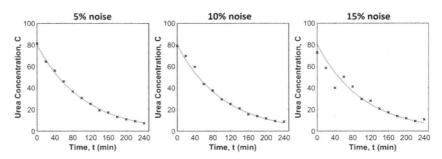

Figure 7.7. Solutions for urea clearance model added noise. Red line shows the original dataset and the 'x' markers are the data points with added noise levels.

Table 7.2. Estimation of k and G using the Monte-Carlo simulation for dataset with induced 5%, 10% and 15% noise.

Model parameters	Noise levels		
Without noise	5% noise	10% noise	15% noise
$k = 200$ ml min^{-1}	201.4 ± 38.3	204.1 ± 74.15	207.9 ± 113.88
$G = 7$ mg min^{-1}	56.7 ± 1814	109.5 ± 3475	157.1 ± 5313

the original noiseless dataset. However, G deviates far from its original value (56.7 vs 7 mg min^{-1}). This shows that the model parameter G may not have been estimated correctly due to the added noise. At 10% and 15% noise levels, the deviation of the estimated k from the correct value increases, although the difference is still considered to be acceptable. The same cannot be said for the estimation of G, however.

To explain why the estimation of k is not sensitive to the presence of noise but not G, one must first understand the physical meaning of these parameters. The parameter k can be seen as an exponential decay for the model, acting to describe the decrease in the rate of urea clearance, and thus, can still be observed easily from the noisy data. As for G, it describes the urea generation rate, where its value usually does not vary significantly during the period of urea clearance. As such, the estimation of this parameter becomes sensitive to the addition of noise to the data.

7.3 Data analytics and interpretation

Data analysis and presentation play important roles in the field of physiological modelling as they are vital in demonstrating the model's performance. They are also used to infer findings of the physiological model in the designated application. The applications range from evaluating the model's ability to capture the data, the quality of model fitting, the physiology that it captures, and even the performance of the model's diagnostic and predictive capability.

There are numerous approaches to physiological modelling results can be presented and they are not limited to one standardised method. In most cases, if the work is significant with an appropriate methodology, there is often no 'bad' results, but only badly presented results. Thus, it is important to choose the appropriate data analytics and presentation method that is suitable for the application.

7.3.1 Error analysis

Error measurement is one of the most used measurements during model-based analysis. They are used to represent the performance of the physiological model, where the model fittings residuals, or error is a measure of how good the model is at capturing the measured dataset. There is a wide range of measurement errors that can be derived from the data and model fittings. Table 7.3 shows a list of measurement errors, with their short descriptions and how they are calculated.

Table 7.3. Commonly used measurement errors in model-based analysis.

Measurement errors	Descriptions	Equation
Error, or residual	• A measure of the difference between two data points.	$E = X_i - X$
Absolute error	• Measurement of the absolute error between two data points.	$AE = \mid X_i - X \mid$
Mean absolute error	• The average of the absolute errors between two datasets.	$MAE = \frac{1}{N}\sum_{i}^{N}\mid X_i - X \mid$ where N is the number of data points
Square error, or square residual	• The square of error.	$SE = (X_i - X)^2$
Percentage error	• The percentage error in relation to the original data.	$PE = \frac{X_i - X}{X} \times 100\%$
Absolute percentage error	• The absolute of percentage error.	$APE = \frac{\mid X_i - X \mid}{X} \times 100\%$
Mean absolute percentage error	• The average of absolute percentage errors.	$MAPE = \frac{1}{N}\frac{\mid X_i - X \mid}{X} \times 100\%$
Sum square error or residual	• The sum of squared errors.	$SSE = \sum_{i}^{N}(X_i - X)^2$
Mean square error	• The mean of squared errors.	$MSE = \frac{1}{N}\sum_{i}^{N}(X_i - X)^2$
Root mean square error	• The root of mean square errors.	$RMSE = \sqrt{\frac{1}{N}\sum_{i}^{N}(X_i - X)^2}$

All errors presented in table 7.3 are possible representations of an error analysis. However, it is important to note that different error measurements can infer different meanings, and they are used differently. The type of measurement error selected must provide sufficient information to illustrate the actual condition. Below are two case examples of looking at application of different measurement errors.

Example A: If we are investigating how good the urea clearance model is at capturing the actual clinical data, we can use the measurement of absolute error, AE to quantify the difference between the model fitting and the actual clinical values. In this case, we can also measure the absolute percentage error, APE for each data point. The APE will enable us to identify weaknesses in the model or how the measured data deviate from the model interpretation as a percentage of the original data. The APE considers the magnitude of the quantity itself and thus, allows an equal comparison for data point irrespective of its magnitude. For example, if the initial urea concentration data is 80 mg ml^{-1} and the model estimate is at 84 mg ml^{-1}, the AE is then 4 mg ml^{-1}, while the APE is 5%. However, if the original urea data is 40 mg ml^{-1}, with a model estimate of 44 mg ml^{-1}, then the AE remains at 4 mg ml^{-1}, but the APE is now increased to 10%. Hence, while both error measurements can be used in this scenario, APE would show that 10% is a larger deviation, whereas presenting AE will somewhat give an impression that there is no difference between the two.

Example B: Consider two different mathematical models that describe respiratory mechanics, namely Model A and Model B. Both models are used to fit one dataset. For each model, we can measure the APE for every data point. However, as APE is unique to each data point, it may not truly reflect the overall performance of the model in capturing the data. APE alone may not be suitable if we wish to compare the performance of between two models. It will be better if one distinctive overall error value, such as the MAPE is used to represent each dataset. The MAPE for both models A and B can be compared. Equally, using SSE, MSE or RSME to compare the performance of the two models may also be possible.

While there is a wide range of possibilities of how error measurements can be presented, it is important to adapt the specific error application to a specific scenario. More importantly, they should be used consistently throughout an analysis to avoid confusion. Finally, if one error measurement is not sufficient to fully represent the results, it is always advisable to use more to represent the different conditions. However, one must be wary of over-presenting different error measurements that have the same meaning.

7.3.2 Model results presentation

7.3.2.1 Mean, median, standard deviation and ranges
Presentation of results derived from the physiological model or model-based analysis plays an important role in elucidating the findings of physiological modelling

analysis. Whether it is presenting results of the model fitting, model prediction or any values derived from the physiological model, data are presented using some common statistical approaches. Typically, when given a set of data or results, the data can be summarised using mean, standard deviation, median and interquartile range.

Mean and median are used to capture the centre of the dataset. Mean is simply the average of the given dataset. It provides an average value of the given dataset and thus, one can draw a conclusion of comparison from there. In general, the mathematical formula for mean can be written as:

$$\text{Mean, } \bar{x} = \frac{1}{n}\sum_{i=1}^{n} x_i, \tag{7.16}$$

where x_i is the ith value of x across the n data points.

The median represents the middle data among a dataset. It is also known as the 50th percentile. This value is used when the dataset or data distribution is not normally distributed. The normal distribution, also known as the *Gaussian* distribution, is a theoretical probability distribution that is perfectly symmetric about its mean (median and mode) and has a 'bell' like shape. Since median gives the middle value of the dataset, it is robust against extreme values within a dataset. For example, the data in table 7.4 are samples of systolic blood pressures taken from seven subjects. The mean of this dataset $\bar{x}$ is 111 mmHg, and one see that the $\bar{x}$ is somewhat skewed by the large value of 169 mmHg. On the other hand, the median of this dataset is 101 mmHg. As it is the 50th percentile of the dataset, it is not affected by the large value (169 mmHg) in the dataset.

When describing the variability of the dataset, we can use sample variance s^2, standard deviation s or the interquartile range, IQR. The variance s^2 is the average of the square of the deviations about the mean, which is given by:

$$s^2 = \frac{1}{n-1}\sum_{i=1}^{n}(x_i - \bar{x})^2, \tag{7.17}$$

and the standard deviation s is the square root of variance given by:

$$s = \sqrt{\frac{1}{n-1}\sum_{i=1}^{n}(x_i - \bar{x})^2}. \tag{7.18}$$

For the presentation of IQR, it is usually defined by the 25th and 75th percentile data.

Table 7.4. Dataset representing systolic blood pressures taken from seven subjects.

Subject	1	2	3	4	5	6	7
Blood pressure (mmHg)	87	95	100	101	110	115	169

In most cases, a dataset collected through experimentation is the sample dataset. This means that this is a smaller dataset that is derived from a larger data group, usually due to the limited resources in conducting the experiment. When deriving the $\bar{x}$ and s from a population, the symbols are written as μ and σ, respectively, to represent the population mean and population standard deviation. For example, the data in table 7.4 are samples of the systolic blood pressure for 24-year-old students from the larger data group (a population) of 24-year-old students in the country. It is important for the sample dataset to be sufficiently large to represent the population or cohort of data that one is investigating. For example, the data in table 7.4 contain only seven samples. This may not be sufficient to represent the data of a significantly larger population. In such circumstances, it is crucial to note the limitation of small sample sizes. One needs to determine the appropriate sample size of a study to ensure sufficient power and significance.

7.3.2.2 Graphical results
In physiological model analysis, graphical tools or figure plots are commonly used for result presentation. Examples include but are not limited to scatter plot, line plot, stair, stem, the area under the curve, bar, histogram, cumulative distribution plot and box-whiskers plot. Each plot has its own unique interpretation of the result. Table 7.5 shows examples of some of the figure plots typically used in data

Table 7.5. Examples of figure plots and descriptions.

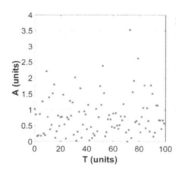

Scatter plot
- Scatter plots are typically used when the data are scattered without a clear relationship between A and T.
- Additional model fitting can be plotted on top of the scattered data to find the potential relationship between variable A and variable T.
- Example of fittings are linear, nth order, logarithmic, logistic, piecewise, exponential and etc.

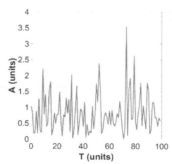

Line plot
- A line plot provides an opportunity to conduct a trend analysis between 2 variables.
- The relation between A and T is usually continuous.
- For example, the figure on the left shows how variable A changes with T.

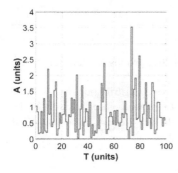

Stair plot

- Stair plot, similar to a line plot, is used for trend analysis.
- However, the changes of A with T are discrete rather than continuous.
- Thus, the A is represented as 'stair' or 'step' changes.

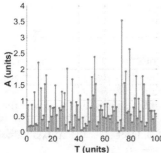

Stem plot

- Stem plots present a single line plot for each data point A at T.
- It plots the data sequence A, as stems that extend from a baseline along the T axis.
- The plot typically emphasises on the maximum values of A at each T value.

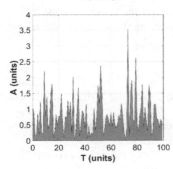

Area under the curve

- Area plots enable the area under the data points A to be filled or shaded.
- In this scenario, the values or coverage under the graph are more important.
- It usually represents the integral of the parameters.
- For example: If variable A is the rate of infection, area under the curve will indicate the number of infection.

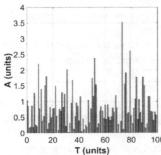

Bar chart

- Bar charts categorise data with rectangular bars with heights proportional to the values they represent.
- Bar charts in this scenario can be used to represent a summative value of A at each T.

- The focus is more on the occurrence of A at a specific T.
- Bar charts can also be plotted horizontally.

Table 7.5. (*Continued*)

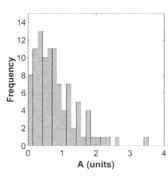

Histogram

- A histogram is a bar chart that groups the dataset *A* into smaller bins.
- It is used to represent a frequency distribution.
- In this scenario, it helps to provide information on the occurrence of a range of *A*, and we can infer that most values of *A* are less than 1.0.

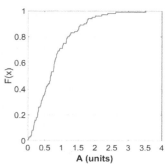

Cumulative distribution plot

- A cumulative distribution plot (CDF) is an empirical cumulative distribution function plot that is used to showcase the distribution of the data.
- The *Y*-axis is capped at 1.0, and the axis values represent the quantiles of variable *A*.
- For example, the median of dataset *A* is the *X*-axis value when *Y*-axis is 0.5, median *A* = ~0.75.
- CDF plot is suitable for comparison of two datasets with a different number of data points as the *Y*-axis is normalised to 1.0.

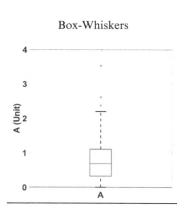

Box Whisker-plot

- The box whisker is a box plot used to summarise the dataset.
- The box values are the 25th percentile, 50th percentile and the 75th percentile.
- The whiskers are lines that extend above and below the box to showcase the range of the dataset.
- The whiskers are 1.5 ×IQR (when outliers are present), and the red points represent the outliers.
- Without outliers, then the whiskers would represent the minimum and maximum values.
- Similar to CDF plot, it is also suitable for the comparison of two datasets with a different number of data points.

presentation together with their application description of a randomly generated dataset with variable *A* against variable *T*[3].

Other commonly used plots to present data include contour plots, surface plots, logarithms, pie charts, percentage bars and, etc. Each plot can be used as a standalone or combined to convey the message of what the data represent. Thus,

---

[3] Source code to generate these data (Chapter07c) is available at https://doi.org/10.1088/978-0-7503-4016-8.

when working on the plots and results presentation, it is advisable to explore different methods to deliver the findings.

7.3.3 Statistical tests and data analysis

Statistical tests and analyses are commonly used to assess the dataset or results in physiological model analysis. Specifically, these tests and analyses enable researchers to draw a general conclusion from a limited amount of data. It is especially useful when there are considerable biological variability, imprecise measurements, and errors in physiological modelling. The following are some of the common tests used in physiological modelling analysis. Their descriptions and usage are shown in table 7.6.

These tests are some samples of statistical tests and analyses that can be carried out to help analyse results derived from physiological model. Data analysis is not a straightforward process. There are almost limitless data investigation methods that

Table 7.6. Some commonly used statistical tests.

Pearson coefficient of relation	• It is also known as *Pearson's r*, where it measures the linear correlation between two datasets. • The analysis is often used together with coefficient of determination, r^2, where it is the proportion of the variation in the dependent variable from the independent variable.
Chi-square test	• A *chi-square test* compares two categorical variables in a contingency table to check if they have any relationship. • *Chi-square test* is also used as a goodness of fit test to determine if the sample data is within the sample population.
Student t-test	• Also known as the *t-test*, the s*tudent t-test* is the most used significance test to check if there is any significant difference between two datasets. • A *p*-value of <0.05 is typically considered statistically significant, which means two datasets are significantly different from each other.
Wilcoxon ranksum test	• *Wilcoxon ranksum* test (also known as the *Mann–Whitney U-test*) is carried out to check if two datasets are significantly different. • It is a non-parametric test carried out in datasets that are not normally distributed. • It can also be used in normally distributed data and will typically yield similar results to the *t*-test, but *t*-test is not suitable for non-normal distribution.
Kolmogorov–Smirnov test	• The Kolmogorov–Smirnov test (*K–S* test) compares a dataset with a known distribution if they have the same distribution. • It is used as a test for normality, to check if the dataset is normally distributed.

Table 7.6. (*Continued*)

Analysis of variance	• The analysis of variance (ANOVA) is carried out on datasets to see if there is a difference between them. • There ANOVA test can be divided into one-way or two-way ANOVA. • The one- or two-way refers to the number of independent variables that you are carrying out.
Kruskal–Wallis test	• The Kruskal–Wallis test is a non-parametric alternative to ANOVA. • It is a rank-based test that can be used to determine if there are statistically significant differences between two or more datasets of independent variables.
Odds ratio	• Odds ratio (OR) is carried out to measure the association between a certain characteristic to another characteristic in a sample dataset. • It provides information on if a characteristic has an effect on the other characteristic.
Survival analysis	• One of the most used survival analyses is the Kaplan–Meier estimate. • It measures the survival time from a start time to the time of death, failure or another significant event.

can be performed on the data. During the analysis, assumptions must be made, and the statistical analysis results can have a very different outcome depending on the said analysis. The following are two case studies carried out by researchers, highlighting the challenges and considerations during data analysis.

Case study 7.4: Silberzahn *et al*'s dilemma
In a study by Silberzahn *et al* (2018), they asked 29 groups of researchers to perform statistical analysis on the same dataset. They were all tasked to address the question of 'whether referees are more likely to give red cards to dark-skin-toned players than to light-skin-toned players'. Typically, we would expect all research groups will come to a consensus, and one conclusive result can be derived from the analysis.

To their surprise, Silberzahn *et al* (2018) reported that 20 groups of researchers found that there is a significance where they are likely to give red cards, whereas the remaining nine groups yielded a different result. There were also 21 unique analyses being carried out and presented by different groups of researchers. The study by Silberzahn *et al* (2018) showed that there is variation in performing statistical analysis, and it is possible that during the analysis process, an individual would have influenced how the analysis is being conducted and potentially how results could vary. At the end of the study, Silberzahn *et al* (2018) suggested that having multiple groups to perform analysis of the same dataset would instil more confidence when drawing the conclusion.

Case study 7.5: Wald *et al*'s survivorship bias

Another interesting view on statistics and data analysis is the survivorship bias introduced by Abraham Wald (Mangel and Samaniego 1984). His research group was tasked to examine World War II fighter aircraft that had returned safely from missions. From the damage sustained by the aircraft, they were required to provide recommendations on where throughout the aircraft additional armour could be added on to the planes to minimise damage. An example of collective damage sustained by all aircraft returned from missions is shown in the illustration in figure 7.8. It was found that the damage sustained by the aircraft were distributed on their wings, tail and centre body.

Typically, from the data collected from returned aircraft, analysis resulted in adding armour plating to most-hit areas as shown in the yellow-coloured areas in figure 7.9 (left). However, contrary to common understanding, Wald and his group of researchers recommended adding armour to the least damaged area as shown in the green-coloured areas figure 7.9 (right). Wald noted the damaged areas marked in yellow were an indication that the fighter aircraft could take damage and still be able

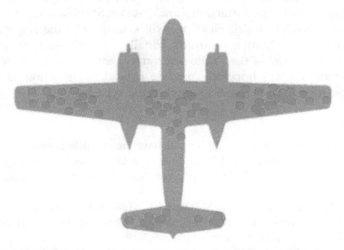

Figure 7.8. Collective damage data from fighter aircraft that returned safely from missions.

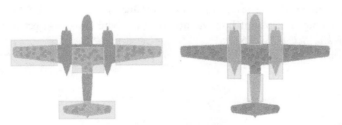

Figure 7.9. The most damaged areas (left) and areas which were recommended for additional armour plating (right).

to return safely from the mission. Other aircraft that sustained damage (marked green) had been shot down and did not return for data collection. Thus, there is a significant difference, as no data had been collected in those areas. In this analysis, Wald and his co-researchers introduced a concept of survival bias, and that data analysis and conclusion drawn based on observed data are influenced by the availability of data.

7.4 Summary

Physiological modelling is a mathematical modelling approach which aims to describe human physiology for the purpose of better understanding, improvement of care and providing medical support. It comprises multi-disciplinary aspects from data acquisition, data processing, model-based analysis and data interpretation. Performing linear regression is one of the simplest forms of model fitting. Data can be presented in various forms and equally, various statistical tests can be conducted to draw a general conclusion from the analysis. It is a field with vast exploration and can take a decade to master and investigate.

In the following chapters, we will explore a few physiological systems and how model-based analysis are performed in these systems. Specifically, we will be looking into the glucose–insulin model. Next, we will venture into the respiratory system, looking into models for human breathing. Finally, we will also look briefly into the lumped parameter model of the cardiovascular system. These few systems and their application examples will hopefully provide a brief introduction to model-based approaches performed in biomedical engineering systems.

References

Depner T A 1994 Assessing adequacy of hemodialysis: urea modeling *Kidney Int.* **45** 1522–35

Depner T A 2012 *Prescribing Hemodialysis: A Guide to Urea Modeling* (New York: Springer)

Dickson J, Gunn C and Chase J G 2014 Humans are horribly variable *Int. J. Clin. Med. Imag.* **12** 1000142

Grzegorzewska A E, Azar A T, Roa L M, Oliva J S, Milán J A and Palma A 2013 Single pool urea kinetic modeling ed A T Azar *Modelling and Control of Dialysis Systems: Volume 1: Modeling Techniques of Hemodialysis Systems* (Berlin: Springer)

Himmelfarb J and Ikizler T A 2010 Hemodialysis *New Engl. J. Med.* **363** 1833–45

Mangel M and Samaniego F J 1984 Abraham Wald's work on aircraft survivability *J. Am. Stat. Assoc.* **79** 259–67

Silberzahn R, Uhlmann E L, Martin D P, Anselmi P and Aust F *et al* 2018 Many analysts, one data set: making transparent how variations in analytic choices affect results *Adv. Meth. Pract. Psychol. Sci.* **1** 337–56

IOP Publishing

Model-Based Approaches in Biomedical Engineering

Ean Hin Ooi and Yeong Shiong Chiew

Chapter 8

Glucose–insulin system

8.1 Human endocrine system and the pancreas

The human endocrine system is a fascinating system that works together with the nervous system to coordinate bodily functions. This system controls the body's activities by releasing hormones. These hormones are excreted by the endocrine glands to regulate cell activities in other parts of the body. Hormones are typically secreted into the interstitial space, where they are absorbed into the blood and transported to other parts of the body to regulate cell activities.

The major glands of the endocrine system include the hypothalamus, pituitary gland, parathyroid glands, pancreas, thyroid glands, adrenal glands, pineal gland and ovaries or testes. These glands are responsible for secreting hormones to control body temperature, sleep, growth, heart rate and even sex drive. The endocrine gland that is our topic of interest is the pancreas. The pancreas is also a major human organ of the digestive system, and it controls the blood sugar level within the body. The pancreas sits behind the stomach, above the intestines, and controls the glucose–insulin interaction within the human body. The location of the pancreas within the human digestive system is shown in figure 8.1.

The pancreas contains millions of tiny tissues known as *pancreatic islets* or *islets of Langerhans* as shown in figure 8.1. Within the pancreas, the islets of Langerhans secrete four different types of hormones listed below:

- *Insulin*—Around 60%–70% of pancreatic islet cells are Beta or B cells that secrete insulin. This hormone is vital for blood sugar level regulation.
- *Glucagon*—Similar to insulin, it is an essential hormone that regulates blood sugar level. It is produced by the Alpha cells (A cells) in the islet. Approximately 15% of pancreatic islet cells are Alpha cells.
- *Somatostatin*—Somatostatin is produced by the Delta cells (D cells) in the pancreas. They act as circulating hormones that slow the absorption of nutrients and inhibit the release of insulin and glucagon. Approximately 7% of pancreatic islet cells are the Delta cells

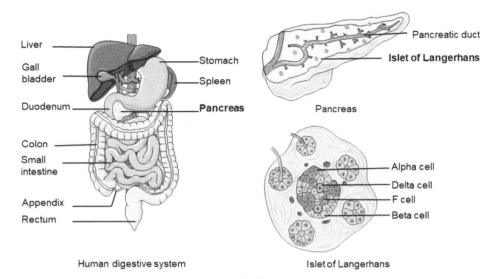

Figure 8.1. Digestive system, the pancreas, and the islet of Langerhans. Copyright © smart.servier.com. The figure was partly generated using Servier Medical Art, provided by Servier, licensed under a Creative Commons Attribution 3.0 unported license.

- *Pancreatic polypeptide*—The other remaining pancreatic cells are F cells, which secrete pancreatic polypeptide to inhibit somatostatin secretion.

The interactions between these four hormones are complex as they work together to maintain balance. In this chapter, we will only be focusing on insulin (and a bit on glucagon) and its role in regulating the blood glucose level in the human body.

8.2 Glucose level regulation and diabetes mellitus

8.2.1 Glucose level regulation

The word glucose is derived from the ancient Greek word '*glykys*', which means 'sweet'. Glucose in the human body is called blood sugar (blood glucose), and it is the major free sugar circulating in the human blood. Glucose comes from the food one eats and drinks, where they are broken down from complex carbohydrates. Glucose is the body's main source of energy for cells to function. And thus, regulation of its metabolism is of great importance to maintain homeostasis. If glucose levels are too high or too low, serious health problems can arise.

Abnormal glucose levels can be categorised as either hypoglycaemia or hyperglycaemia, the former describing abnormally low blood glucose levels and the latter describing it as being too high. Hypoglycaemia is a condition when the human body's blood glucose is lower than expected (less than ~70 mg dL^{-1} or less than ~3.9 mmol L^{-1} during fasting). Abnormally low blood glucose levels can be caused by critical illness, medication, treatment, or hormone deficiencies. If a person is

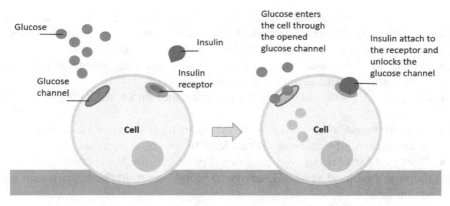

Figure 8.2. Insulin's role in glucose transport in cells.

hypoglycaemic, they may experience fatigue, irregular heartbeat, anxiety, hunger, anxiousness and dizziness. In more severe cases, symptoms can extend to blurred vision, seizures and even loss of consciousness.

On the other hand, hyperglycaemia is an excess of blood glucose in the human body (greater than ~126 mg dl^{-1} or 7.0 mmol L^{-1} during fasting). The leading cause of hyperglycaemia is the inability of the body to produce sufficient insulin or if the body is resistant to the effects of insulin. Other possible causes include but are not limited to excessive carbohydrate intake, stressed-induced hyperglycaemia and infection. Those afflicted may experience tiredness or weakness, increased urination, thirst and vision impairment. In more severe cases, where those afflicted have experienced hyperglycaemia for an extended period, diabetes mellitus can develop. The patients can suffer from other complications of diabetes, such as the risk of heart disease, high blood pressure, stroke, loss of consciousness, cataracts, glaucoma, organ failure, etc.

Insulin plays a crucial role in keeping blood glucose at the proper levels. Insulin was first named by Edward Albert Sharpey-Schafer after he theorised the cause of diabetes mellitus was the absence of a hormone produced by the pancreas. Later in the 1920s, Dr Frederick Banting, Charles Best, James Collip, and John Macleod successfully extracted insulin from the animal pancreas and later used it in a clinical trial to treat diabetes. Insulin is a hormone that helps move glucose from your bloodstream into your cells. Figure 8.2 shows a schematic of how insulin functions as a key to open glucose channels for a cell to receive glucose.

8.2.2 Diabetes mellitus

Under normal circumstances, the pancreas will produce insulin that opens glucose channels in the cell to receive glucose. However, some people cannot produce sufficient insulin, or their cells do not respond to insulin properly. These people are diabetic or have diabetes mellitus, also commonly abbreviated as DM. Diabetes mellitus is a metabolic disorder characterised by high blood sugar levels over a prolonged period. Symptoms include frequent urination, increased thirst, and an increase in appetite. If left untreated, diabetes can cause many complications. The complications and risks involved in diabetic patients are as follows:

- *Feeling of thirst and frequent urination*—A diabetic patient will often feel thirsty and need to urinate frequently.
- *Fatigue*—Diabetic patients often feel tired and find it difficult to concentrate on work.
- *Diabetic ketoacidosis*—The body produces high levels of blood acids known as ketones due to diabetes. It can lead to loss of consciousness.
- *Damaged blood vessels*—A prolonged period of the hyperglycaemic state can damage the blood vessels. Damage to blood vessels in the eye can also lead to vision loss.
- *Nerve damage*—Diabetes can cause diabetic neuropathy.
- *Cataracts and glaucoma*—Increased risk of cataracts and glaucoma.
- *High blood pressure and heart disease*—Diabetic patients are at risk of developing high blood pressure, which increases the risk of cardiovascular diseases.
- *Stroke*—Diabetic patients have a four-fold increased risk of stroke compared to healthy humans.

There are three main types of diabetes mellitus, namely Type 1, Type 2 and gestational diabetes.

8.2.2.1 Type 1 diabetes

Type 1 diabetes results from the failure of the pancreas to produce sufficient insulin due to a loss of beta cells within the pancreas. This form of diabetes was referred to as 'juvenile diabetes' or more commonly known as 'insulin-dependent diabetes mellitus (IDDM)'. The loss of beta cells is caused by an autoimmune response. The cause of this autoimmune response is unknown. Patients with Type 1 diabetes must be managed with insulin injections.

8.2.2.2 Type 2 diabetes

Type 2 diabetes begins with a person developing insulin resistance in the body. It is a condition in which the human body cells fail to respond to insulin properly or are insulin resistant. As the disease progresses, a lack of insulin may also develop. This form was previously referred to as 'adult-onset diabetes' or 'noninsulin-dependent diabetes mellitus (NIDDM)'. The most common cause of Type 2 diabetes is a combination of excessive body weight, insufficient exercise and a possibly unhealthy lifestyle. Thus, the best course of prevention and treatment of Type 2 diabetes involves maintaining a healthy diet, regular physical exercise, an appropriate body weight, and avoiding the use of tobacco. Type 2 diabetes may also be treated with medication such as insulin sensitisers and insulin. Figure 8.3 shows the difference between Type 1 and Type 2 diabetes. In essence, Type 1 diabetes means no insulin production, whereas Type 2 means insulin resistance.

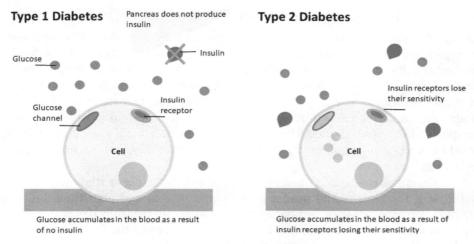

Figure 8.3. (Left) Type 1 diabetes and (right) Type 2 diabetes.

8.2.2.3 Gestational diabetes

The third form of diabetes is gestational diabetes. It is the third main form of diabetes and occurs in pregnant women. In gestational diabetes, pregnant women without a history of diabetes develop high blood sugar levels as they become insulin resistant during pregnancy. Being overweight or obese is also linked to gestational diabetes. Gestational diabetes usually resolves on its own after pregnancy, but it may increase the risk of developing Type 2 diabetes in the future. However, as gestational diabetes can have significant consequences to pregnant women and their babies, it is important to seek treatment and maintain a healthy diet with regular physical exercise.

As of 2019, the World Health Organisation (WHO) estimated that around 463 million people or 8.8% of the global adult population, had diabetes, with Type 2 diabetes making up about 90% of the cases. In the same year, diabetes resulted in approximately 4.2 million deaths. It is the seventh leading cause of death globally, and the current trend suggests that mortality rates will continue to rise. Aside from that, there is a significant economic cost for diabetes-related health expenditures. In a recent study, Williams *et al* (2020) reported that the estimated global direct health expenditure on diabetes in 2019 was USD 760 billion. This number is expected to increase to a projected USD 825 billion by 2030 and USD 845 billion by 2045.

In summary, diabetes has a significant impact on health and imposes an increasing economic burden on national healthcare systems worldwide. More prevention efforts are needed to reduce this burden, and equally, treatment for these patients needs to be more efficient and improved. Thus, studies to model the human body's glucose–insulin system to better understand glucose–insulin dynamics, help monitor and regulate blood glucose, and improve patient treatment have always been a continuous effort and of great interest.

8.3 Model for human glucose–insulin interaction

As diabetic patients rely on insulin treatment to control their blood glucose levels, it is imperative to understand how glucose and insulin interact with each other mathematically. A glucose–insulin model attempts to provide a basic outline of the fundamental physiology of glucose sources, insulin sources and their utilisation to regulate glucose levels. To develop a model, one can perform mechanistic modelling, combining the function of every cell. However, this will increase the complexity of the overall model, rendering it non-identifiable if there is insufficient *a priori* knowledge or input to the model. It would take days before any simulation results can be obtained.

One simplified method to model glucose–insulin system is to study the dynamics and flow of the glucose and insulin in the blood plasma and interstitial fluid. One example is how glucose or insulin appears and disappears from the blood. This is shown in figure 8.4, which presents a schematic of the potential flow of glucose and insulin in the blood plasma and interstitial fluid. The insulin input to the blood plasma and interstitial fluids can be sourced either from the pancreas or from an external intake. An external insulin source can be administered to the body intravenously via bolus injection or continuous infusion. As for the glucose input, glucose can enter from meal intake, where the glucose appears via absorption from the gut or intravenous nutrition. The glucose uptake is relatively straightforward, whereas insulin reacts to the cells allowing glucose to enter the body's cells to provide energy. Finally, the clearance and degradation of circulating or unused insulin will occur in the liver and kidney.

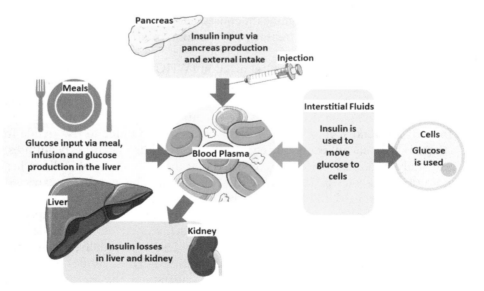

Figure 8.4. Schematic of glucose and insulin interaction in the human. Copyright © smart.servier.com. The figure was partly generated using Servier Medical Art, provided by Servier, licensed under a Creative Commons Attribution 3.0 unported license.

Efforts to model the glucose–insulin system have led to various research studies being carried out to investigate the pharmacokinetics of both glucose and insulin. They are studies of the time course of both insulin and glucose's appearance, absorption, distribution, metabolism, and excretion. In addition, the glucose–insulin pharmacodynamics or the study of a drug's molecular, biochemical, and physiologic effects or actions, is vital to derive the relationship of how glucose interacts with insulin inside the human body.

8.3.1 Single-compartment model

A simple model of glucose–insulin dynamics can be described as a single compartment such as shown in figure 8.6. This single-compartment model describes the change in glucose level (or concentration) inside the compartment (in this case, blood) $G(t)$ as a result of glucose production at a rate $P(t)$ and disappearance at a rate of k_1. A simple differential equation describing the rate of change of $G(t)$ in the single-compartment model can thus be written as:

$$\frac{dG}{dt} = -k_1 G(t) + P(t). \tag{8.1}$$

Note that $G(t)$ has an SI unit of kg m^{-3} but is commonly quantified in mg L^{-1} or g h^{-1}, k_1 is typically expressed as 1/h and $P(t)$ has a unit of mg (L·h)$^{-1}$.

8.3.2 Two-compartment model

The single-compartment model shown in figure 8.5 is clearly too simplified to correctly describe the glucose dynamics inside the human body. Hence, one may choose to add more compartments into the model to account for other contributing factors, such as the dynamics of insulin within the system. Furthermore, one may opt to describe the glucose levels at the extracellular space instead of blood.

An example of a two-compartment model describing the glucose–insulin dynamics is shown in figure 8.6, where G_{ex} and I_{ex} describe the glucose and insulin levels in the extracellular space, which are both modelled as single compartments. The clearance and disappearance of the glucose are dependent on the blood plasma glucose and insulin entering the compartment space (Bolie 1961). We can assume that the equilibrium values of the glucose and insulin concentrations within the compartment to be $I(t)$ and $G(t)$, respectively. The changes in glucose and insulin are introduced by the rates of external intravenous glucose and insulin injection given by $\dot{G}_{in}$ and $\dot{I}_{in}$, respectively.

In addition, the model includes how glucose and insulin appear, and are utilised in the compartment. These are captured in the terms I_1, I_2, G_3 and G_4, where I_1 is the

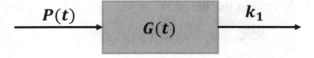

Figure 8.5. A simple single-compartment glucose model.

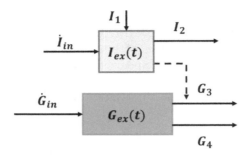

Figure 8.6. A two-compartment model of glucose–insulin interaction.

rate of insulin production, I_2 is the rate of insulin disappearance, G_3 is the rate of glucose accumulation in the liver, and G_4 is the rate of glucose usage by tissues.

The differential equations describing the rate of change of the glucose and insulin concentration in the extracellular space in the two-compartment model can be written as:

$$V_e \frac{dI_{ex}(t)}{dt} = \dot{I}_{in}(t) + I_1 - I_2, \tag{8.2}$$

$$V_e \frac{dG_{ex}(t)}{dt} = \dot{G}_{in}(t) - G_3 - G_4, \tag{8.3}$$

where t is time and V_e is the extracellular fluid volume. This simplified model and its iterations were later used for monitoring and diagnosis.

8.3.3 Minimal model for glucose–insulin modelling

Although several glucose–insulin models have been developed over the past decades to model glucose–insulin interaction, the Bergman minimal model is by far the most well-known. It has been frequently adopted in clinical and research environments to provide basic understanding of the interaction between glucose and insulin in the human body. Despite its simplification and neglected dynamics, the parameters and variables in the Bergman minimal model are able to capture clear and significant physiological information. In addition, these parameters are readily identified from measured clinical data (Bergman *et al* 1979, 1981, Bergman 2021).

The Bergman minimal model, or in short, the minimal model, is a three-compartment non-linear system that includes ODEs as shown in figure 8.7. This model consists of one glucose compartment and two insulin compartments: one the plasma compartment and the other a remote compartment.

The equations describing the Bergman minimal model are given by:

$$\frac{dG}{dt} = -(k_1 + k_5 + X(t))G(t) + B_0, \tag{8.4}$$

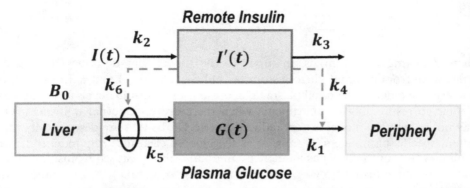

Figure 8.7. Schematic of the Bergman minimal model. © IEEE. Reprinted, with permission from Khodaei *et al* (2020).

Table 8.1. Bergman's minimal model parameters.

Parameters	Unit	Description
k_1	min^{-1}	Glucose ability to increase uptake by the peripheral
k_2	min^{-1}	Insulin transport rate to remote compartment
k_3	min^{-1}	Active insulin clearance rate
k_4	L (min mU)^{-1}	Active insulin effect on uptate by the peripheral
k_5	min^{-1}	Glucose ability to change net hepatic glucose balance
k_6	L (min mU)^{-1}	Active insulin effect on net hepatic glucose balance

$$\frac{dX}{dt} = -k_3 X(t) + k_2(k_4 + k_6)I(t), \qquad (8.5)$$

$$X(t) = (k_4 + k_6)I'(t), \qquad (8.6)$$

where $G(t)$ (mg dL^{-1}) is the total plasma glucose concentration in the glucose compartment, $X(t)$ (min^{-1}) is the insulin action in the remote compartment, $I(t)$ (mU L^{-1}) is the plasma insulin concentration, $I'(t)$ (mU L^{-1}) is the remote insulin concentration, B_0 (mgdL^{-1}·min^{-1}) is the hepatic glucose production at zero plasma glucose concentration, and k_1 to k_6 are patient-specific model parameters to describe the glucose–insulin kinetics. The descriptions of k_1 to k_6 are show in table 8.1. Note that the term mU (or simply U) represents International Unit, which is the unit typically used to quantify insulin doses (Knopp *et al* 2019).

A simplified Bergman minimal model that describes the changes in plasma glucose concentration and interstitial insulin concentration can be expressed as:

$$\frac{dG}{dt} = -(X(t) + k_1)G(t) + k_1 G_b + P(t), \qquad (8.7)$$

$$\frac{dX}{dt} = -k_3 X(t) + k_2(I(t) - I_b), \tag{8.8}$$

where $P(t)$ (mg dL^{-1}·min) is an input to the model that describes the glucose appearance from external glucose sources, and G_b (mg dL^{-1}) and I_b (mU L^{-1}) are two terms that define the basal plasma glucose and basal insulin levels at steady state in their corresponding compartments when there are no external influences. One may notice that the model is now reduced to two ODEs that are described by three patient-specific parameters, k_1 (min^{-1}) as the glucose clearance rate independent of insulin, k_2 (L (min^2·mU)$^{-1}$) as an increase in uptake ability caused by insulin, and k_3 (min^{-1}) is active insulin rate of clearance (decrease of uptake). A schematic of the three parameters Bergman model is illustrated in figure 8.8.

Within the interstitial compartment, the kinetics of the insulin is very similar to the plasma glucose kinetics. The insulin enters and exits the compartment at a rate k_2 that is proportional to the difference between the plasma insulin level, $I(t)$ and the basal plasma insulin, I_b. If the plasma insulin level falls below the basal level, insulin leaves the interstitial compartment. Conversely, if the plasma insulin level rises above the basal level, insulin enters the interstitial tissue compartment. Insulin exits from the interstitial compartment via a secondary pathway at a rate k_3, which is proportional to the amount of insulin in the interstitial tissue compartment. k_1 is the glucose utilisation rate (S_g), and the ratio k_2/k_3 is the insulin sensitivity index (S_I). When given a set of blood glucose and insulin measurements during a clinical test, one can solve for the model parameters k_1, k_2 and k_3 to better understand the model's behaviour. The normal values for S_I and S_g, when identified using the minimal model, are approximately in the range of 4.0×10^{-4} to 8.0×10^{-4} L (min·mU)$^{-1}$ and 0.01 to 0.03 1 min^{-1} (Pacini and Bergman 1986).

8.3.3.1 Forward simulation
Forward simulation using Picard's iteration (see chapter 7) can be used to solve the Bergman minimal model defined by equations (8.7) and (8.8) simultaneously to obtain $G(t)$ and $X(t)$ for a given set of model parameters. First, a recap of Picard's iteration. If the right-hand side of a differential equation does not contain the

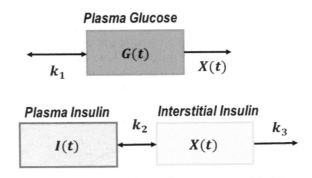

Figure 8.8. Three parameter glucose disappearance model of Bergman.

unknown variable, we can solve the equation by integrating both sides of the equations, such as shown below:

$$\frac{dx}{dt} = F(t), \; x(t_0) = x_0,$$

$$x(t) = x_0 + \int_{t_0}^{t} f(t)dt.$$

However, this approach is no longer applicable if the function on the right-hand side of the ODE is expressed in terms of x. In calculus, we learn some tricks that allow us to solve differential equations with more complicated right-hand sides. These tricks involve some manipulation of the differential equation that turns it into the simplest case, as shown above, so we can solve it by integrating both sides. The most important cases are separable differential equations and first-order linear differential equations.

For equation (8.7), we can substitute k_1 with S_g, thus yielding:

$$\frac{dG}{dt} = S_g(G_b - G(t)) - X(t)G(t) + P(t). \tag{8.9}$$

Equations (8.8) and (8.9) can thus be solved using Picard's iteration, where a pseudocode of this technique in MATLAB is given by:

```
for i = 1:n
```

$$G(t) = G_0 + \int_{t_0}^{t_f} \left(S_g(G_b - G(t)) - X(t)G(t) + P(t) \right)dt, \tag{8.10}$$

$$X(t) = X_0 + \int_{t_0}^{t_f} \left(-k_3 X(t) + k_2(I(t) - I_b) \right)dt, \tag{8.11}$$

```
end
```

where t_0 is the start time, t_f is the time when the data is last collected, and n is set at a value until the simulation converges.

To initiate Picard's iteration, we will need to first define some unknown variables. For the case above, S_g, k_2, k_3, G_b, I_b, $P(t)$, and $I(t)$ are parameters that define the dynamics of the output, $G(t)$. They are typically given or *a priori* inputs for the model. As for other variables G_0, $G(t)$, X_0 and $X(t)$, they are neither measured nor usually given. Initial values for these variables, typically set to zeros, must be defined prior to the iteration to simulate $G(t)$. As the simulation progresses, $G(t)$ and $X(t)$ are updated at every iteration until the solution converges. An excerpt of MATLAB code to perform Picard's iteration to determine $G(t)$ and $X(t)$ is shown in figure 8.9. In the MATLAB excerpt below, cumtrapz is a built-in MATLAB function that

```
G = G0 + Sg*cumtrapz(tspan, Gb-G)-cumtrapz(tspan, X.*G);
X = X0 + k2*cumtrapz(tspan,(Inew-Ib)) - k3*cumtrapz(tspan,X);
```

Figure 8.9. Excerpt of MATLAB code on Picard's iteration.

performs the cumulative trapezoidal rule integration and is used to evaluate the integrals in the right-hand side of equations (8.10) and (8.11).

8.3.3.2 Inverse simulation

Similarly, if we were given the data of $G(t)$ and $I(t)$, we can perform a linear regression (see chapter 7) to obtain S_g, k_2 and k_3 with Picard's iteration. Firstly, by expanding the right-hand side of equations (8.10) and (8.11), one obtains:

$$G(t) = G_0 + S_g \int_{t_0}^{t_f} (G_b - G(t))dt - \int_{t_0}^{t_f} X(t)G(t)dt + \int_{t_0}^{t_f} P(t)dt, \qquad (8.12)$$

$$X(t) = X_0 - k_3 \int_{t_0}^{t_f} X(t)dt + k_2 \int_{t_0}^{t_f} (I(t) - I_b)dt. \qquad (8.13)$$

Replacing $X(t)$ in equation (8.12) with (8.13) yields:

$$G(t) = G_0 + S_g \int_{t_0}^{t_f} (G_b - G(t))dt$$

$$- \int_{t_0}^{t_f} \left[X_0 - k_3 \int_{t_0}^{t_f} X(t)dt + k_2 \int_{t_0}^{t_f} (I(t) - I_b)dt \right] G(t)dt \qquad (8.14)$$

$$+ \int_{t_0}^{t_f} P(t)dt,$$

which upon expansion of the term in the square bracket, leads to:

$$G(t) = G_0 + S_g \int_{t_0}^{t_f} (G_b - G(t))dt - \int_{t_0}^{t_f} X_0 G(t)dt$$

$$+ k_3 \int_{t_0}^{t_f} \left[\int_{t_0}^{t_f} X(t)dt \right] G(t)dt - k_2 \int_{t_0}^{t_f} \left[\int_{t_0}^{t_f} (I(t) - I_b)dt \right] G(t)dt \qquad (8.15)$$

$$+ \int_{t_0}^{t_f} P(t)dt.$$

To perform parameter identification, equation (8.15) must be re-arranged in the form of $A\theta = b$. Doing so, we obtain:

$$S_g \int_{t_0}^{t_f} (G_b - G(t))dt + k_3 \int_{t_0}^{t_f} \left(\int_{t_0}^{t_f} X(t)dt \right) G(t)dt \cdots - k_2 \int_{t_0}^{t_f} \left(\int_{t_0}^{t_f} (I(t) - I_b)dt \right) G(t)dt$$

$$= G(t) - G_0 + \int_{t_0}^{t_f} X_0 G(t)dt - \int_{t_0}^{t_f} P(t)dt, \qquad (8.16)$$

where S_g, k_3 and k_2 are the unknown parameters that can be determined by applying equation (8.16) to each of the data point of $G(t)$ and $I(t)$, while the integrals represent the coefficients of the matrix evaluated at each data point. This sets up a system matrix that can be written as:

$$\begin{bmatrix} A_{11} & A_{12} & A_{13} \\ A_{21} & A_{22} & A_{23} \\ \vdots & \vdots & \vdots \\ A_{n1} & A_{n2} & A_{n3} \end{bmatrix} \begin{Bmatrix} S_g \\ k_3 \\ k_2 \end{Bmatrix} = \begin{Bmatrix} b_1 \\ b_2 \\ \vdots \\ b_n \end{Bmatrix}, \qquad (8.17)$$

where the coefficients A_{i1}, A_{i2}, A_{i3} and b_i are expressed as:

$$A_{i1} = \int_{t_0}^{t_i} (G_b - G(t))dt,$$

$$A_{i2} = \int_{t_0}^{t_i} \left(\int_{t_0}^{t_i} X(t)dt \right) G(t)dt,$$

$$A_{i3} = -\int_{t_0}^{t_i} \left(\int_{t_0}^{t_i} (I(t) - I_b)dt \right) G(t)dt,$$

$$b_i = G(t_i) - G_0 + \int_{t_0}^{t_i} X_0 G(t)dt - \int_{t_0}^{t_i} P(t)dt, \qquad (8.18)$$

and i represents the ith data point of $G(t)$ and $I(t)$. Equation (8.17) can be solved for the unknown parameters S_g, k_2 and k_3 using the backslash (\) operator in MATLAB. Equally, MATLAB functions such as lsqlin.m, which solves constrained linear least-squares problems, can be used to obtain S_g, k_2 and k_3.

So far, we have only looked at the equations describing glucose disappearance from the blood plasma and tissue interstitial compartments. It is also possible to model the kinetics of insulin $I(t)$ in the Bergman minimal model by treating insulin in blood plasma as another compartment, such as shown in figure 8.10. Accordingly, the rate of change of insulin in this compartment is governed by the entry via exogeneous insulin and removal via utilisation within the human body.

The equation describing insulin kinetics is thus given by:

$$\frac{dI}{dt} = -nI(t) + \frac{u(t)}{V}, \tag{8.19}$$

where n (min^{-1}) is the time constant for insulin disappearance rate, $u(t)$ (mU min^{-1}) is a model input that describes the exogenous insulin intake with time and V (L) is the distribution volume. Combining equations (8.7), (8.8) and (8.19) sets up the minimal model of glucose disappearance and minimal model of insulin kinetics, which is known as the Bergman minimal model.

8.3.3.3 Case study 8.1: forward simulation performed on glucose tolerance test data

During a glucose tolerance test, test subjects are required to consume a fixed amount of glucose, where changes in the glucose and insulin levels with time are monitored. Table 8.2 presents the data obtained from a subject following a glucose–insulin test. It is of interest to determine how fast the glucose and insulin level decreases with time. To do so, we can use Picard's iteration to solve equations (8.10) and (8.11).

To solve equations (8.10) and (8.11), several *a priori* values must be set. Firstly, G_0 was set to the maximum value of $G(t)$ observed in table 8.2, which assumes that

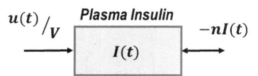

Figure 8.10. Minimal model of insulin kinetics.

Table 8.2. Sample of blood glucose and insulin level measured during glucose tolerance test. Adapted from Hariri and Wang (2011) Copyright © 2011 by authors and Scientific Research Publishing Inc.

Time (min)	0	2	4	6	8	10	12	14
Glucose level, $G(t)$ (mg dL^{-1})	92	350	287	251	240	216	211	205
Insulin level, $I(t)$ (μU mL^{-1})	11	26	130	85	51	49	45	41

Time (min)	16	19	22	27	32	42	52	62
Glucose level, $G(t)$ (mg dL^{-1})	196	192	172	163	142	124	105	92
Insulin level, $I(t)$ (μU mL^{-1})	35	30	30	27	30	22	15	15

Time (min)	72	82	92	102	122	142	162	182
Glucose level, $G(t)$ (mg dL^{-1})	84	77	82	81	82	82	85	92
Insulin level, $I(t)$ (μU mL^{-1})	11	10	8	11	7	8	8	7

glucose level is at its maximum after glucose intake. Secondly, G_b was set to the baseline value of $G(t)$ from table 8.2, i.e., the value of $G(t)$ at $t = 0$ or prior to the intake of exogenous glucose. Finally, the values $P(t)$ are set to be zeros, with the assumption that there is no intake of glucose during the measuring period. This way, the drop in glucose, $G(t)$ is primarily influenced by the glucose utilisation rate S_g.

Once these *a priori* values have been set, equations (8.10) and (8.11) can be solved with Picard's iteration by making an initial guess of the values of $G(t)$ and $X(t)$. Here, we set them to zero, although other appropriate values may be chosen. Using the MATLAB code that accompanies this chapter[1] and with the maximum iteration number set to 1000, the solutions for $G(t)$ at various iteration levels are shown in figure 8.11. At the first iteration, the solution for $G(t)$ can be seen as a straight line with a positive slope. As the iteration continues within the MATLAB for loop, $G(t)$ slowly converges to the value close to the actual data in table 8.2. At iteration number 30, most of the $G(t)$ values are very close to those at iteration 25. This suggests that the simulation has started to converge. During Picard's iteration, convergence can be determined by providing a threshold error value that compares the $G(t)$ values obtained at the n th iteration and $(n - 1)$th iteration. It may also be possible to limit the number of iterations to stop the simulation.

Figure 8.12 plots the converged solutions of $G(t)$ and $X(t)$ obtained from Picard's iteration.

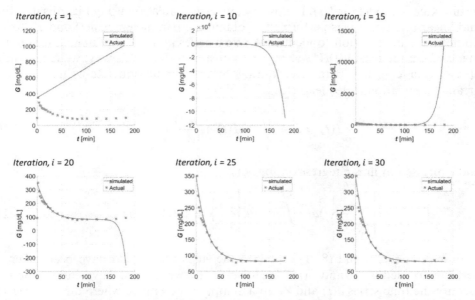

Figure 8.11. Picard's iteration performed on the data in table 8.2 to solve for $G(t)$. Each plot represents the solution of $G(t)$ at various iteration levels.

---

[1] Source code for this model (Chapter08a) is available at https://doi.org/10.1088/978-0-7503-4016-8.

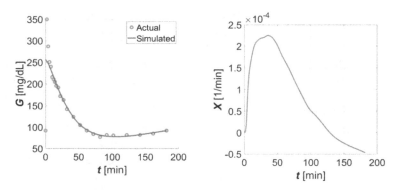

Figure 8.12. Model estimated $G(t)$ and $X(t)$ obtained from Picard's iteration.

8.3.3.4 Case study 8.2: inverse simulation performed on glucose tolerance test data

In this case study, an inverse simulation is carried out to identify the parameters S_g, k_2, k_3 and G_0 based on the glucose and insulin data in table 8.2. This is achieved by solving equations (8.17) and (8.18)[2]. As demonstrated in figure 8.10 and equation (8.19), the Bergman minimal model includes modelling of the insulin kinetics. Thus, when given insulin measurements, as shown in table 8.2, we can also identify the insulin kinetic model for $I(t)$. In this case, inverse simulation using Picard's iteration and linear regression was performed to obtain the parameters n, $u(t)$ and V. As we do not have information to identify the time series $u(t)$ and V, an assumption was made where the term $u(t)/V$ was set to a constant value. This way, we can identify $u(t)/V$ as a constant parameter during inverse simulation. Re-writing and re-arranging equation (8.19) leads to:

$$I(t) = I_0 + \int\limits_0^t -nI(t) + \frac{u(t)}{V} dt, \tag{8.20}$$

and expressed in linear regression form as:

$$\left[\int\limits_0^{t_i} -I(t)dt \quad \int\limits_0^{t_i} u(t)dt \right] \begin{Bmatrix} n \\ \frac{1}{V} \end{Bmatrix} = \{I(t) - I_0\}. \tag{8.21}$$

Equations (8.20) and (8.21) represent the steps that would have been taken to perform to identify n and $u(t)/V$. However, as we do not have information to identify the time series $u(t)$ and V, an assumption was made where the term $u(t)/V$ was set to a constant during inverse simulation. Hence, equations (8.20) and (8.21) becomes

---

[2] Source code for this model (Chapter08b) is available at https://doi.org/10.1088/978-0-7503-4016-8.

$$I(t) = I_0 + \int_0^t -nI(t) + \frac{u}{V}dt, \tag{8.22}$$

and

$$\left[\int_0^{t_i} -I(t)dt \quad \int_0^{t_i} 1dt \right] \left\{ \begin{matrix} n \\ \frac{u}{V} \end{matrix} \right\} = \{I - I_0\}, \tag{8.23}$$

respectively.

By carrying out Picard's iteration and linear regression (see MATLAB codes for this case study[3]), the values of n and u/V are found to be -1.1×10^{-4} s^{-1} and -4.21×10^{-6} μU (mL·s)$^{-1}$, respectively. With these values, the variation of $I(t)$ can be modelled and used to perform parameter identification of the glucose model.

Figure 8.13 plots the solution for $G(t)$ and $X(t)$ obtained using the simulated values of $I(t)$ based on the insulin kinetic model, The solutions for both $G(t)$ and $X(t)$ using simulated $I(t)$, are different from solutions for $G(t)$ and $X(t)$ when using the actual $I(t)$ (see figure 8.12). One may observe that the solution of $X(t)$ using simulated values of $I(t)$ has a smoother trend and a smaller decreasing slope than those obtained with actual $I(t)$ values. The actual $I(t)$ and simulated $I(t)$ are shown in figure 8.14, where the smoothness of the simulated $I(t)$ explains the smoothness of the estimated $X(t)$ values.

Using the MATLAB code for case study 8.2, the values of S_g, k_2, k_3 and G_0 estimated when using actual and simulated values of $I(t)$ are summarised in table 8.3. Comparing the parameters identified using the glucose model only (i.e., with actual values of $I(t)$) and the glucose–insulin model, the identified parameters for both methods are different, with errors of up to 21.98%. Clearly, the choice of

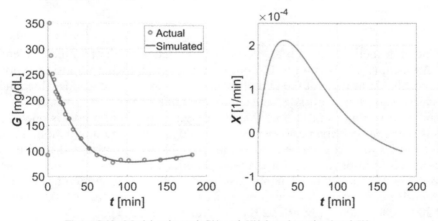

Figure 8.13. Model estimated $G(t)$ and $X(t)$ based on simulated $I(t)$.

---

[3] Source code for this model (Chapter08c) is available at https://doi.org/10.1088/978-0-7503-4016-8.

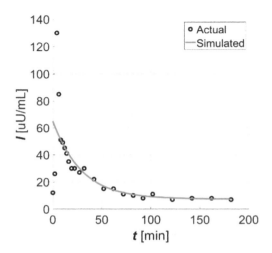

Figure 8.14. Plots of the actual $I(t)$ from table 8.2 and simulated $I(t)$ based on Picard's iteration of equations (8.10), (8.11) and (8.22).

Table 8.3. Comparison between the model parameters identified from the Bergman's minimal model based on actual and simulated values of $I(t)$.

Model parameters	Unit	Identified using actual $I(t)$	Identified using simulated $I(t)$	Difference (%)
S_g	s^{-1}	2.32×10^{-4}	2.83×10^{-4}	21.98
k_2	mL $(s^2 \cdot \mu U)^{-1}$	5.85×10^{-9}	5.32×10^{-9}	9.06
k_3	s^{-1}	3.86×10^{-4}	3.46×10^{-4}	10.36
S_I	mL $(s\ \mu U)^{-1}$	1.52×10^{-5}	1.53×10^{-5}	1.00
G_0	mg dL^{-1}	257	259	0.78

identification method, as well as the model used affected the parameter identification. As such, it is important to be consistent and careful when choosing a model to represent the data. It is not the aim of this book to discuss and decide which method is correct or more appropriate, as each method has its pros and cons.

Finally, it is important to note that the Bergman minimal model is one of many models that can describe basic glucose–insulin dynamics and interaction. There are more complex and descriptive models that have been developed and used throughout research to improve care for diabetic patients. Some examples include the oral glucose minimal model, the dynamic insulin sensitivity and secretion test model, and the intensive control insulin–nutrition–glucose model (Arleth et al 2000, Dalla Man et al 2002, 2006, 2007, Lin et al 2011, McAuley et al 2011).

To further understand these models, it will be good to explore different models and how they behave. More importantly, the models should be uniquely identifiable and capable of capturing the dynamics that are required for the application.

Glucose model parameters such as S_g and S_I are important parameters in capturing the behaviour of the glucose–insulin system of an individual. In particular, S_g indicates how fast glucose is being metabolised in the system while S_I denotes how sensitive an individual is towards insulin. However, these values are dependent on the complexity of the models, as well as the methods of measurement. The parameter values may vary in range and/or magnitude depending on the models or methods used. For example, quantification of insulin sensitivity have been carried out using several methods aside from using model-based methods (Gutch *et al* 2015). There is a wide range of insulin sensitivity metrics, and each metric has its own unique clinical procedure and how the metric can be calculated. It is difficult to determine which metric is the most appropriate as the metric depends on the available resources and clinical practices. This uncertainty also means that having a unified model or a method to select a 'global equivalent' insulin sensitivity metric that can potentially benefit clinical practice.

8.4 Application of glucose–insulin models in regulating glucose level

8.4.1 Diabetic patient glucose monitoring

Blood glucose management among diabetic patients requires the tracking of any fluctuations in their blood glucose levels. Aside from taking care of their nutrition intake and exercise, they will need to perform self-testing of their blood glucose regularly and manage their medication. Typically, this process is done through self-testing several times, from 4 to 10 times a day, such as before and after meals, before and after exercise, and before bed.

Patients can use either a glucose meter (glucometer) or a continuous glucose monitor (CGM) for this blood glucose monitoring process. First, the subject draws a blood sample from their fingers tip using a lancet device. The lancet is also known as a finger stick blood sampler, which consists of two parts: a lancet holder that houses a lancet (a sharp needle for drawing the blood) and a compressed spring mechanism within the lancet holder. When the lancet is activated, the spring is released, and the needle is launched to penetrate the subject's fingertip at a safe distance to draw a blood sample.

The blood sample is then collected using a blood glucose test strip. The test strip is placed into the glucometer for blood glucose level reading. Once the reading is known, the subject may take insulin injections or other medication to control their blood glucose level. Figure 8.15 shows the typical process flow of blood glucose monitoring using a lancet device and a glucometer.

Alternatively, this process can be automated, where the process is replaced with a continuous glucose monitor (CGM) (Ribet *et al* 2018). The CGM measures the patient's blood sugar every few minutes using a sensor inserted under the skin, as illustrated in figure 8.16. A sensor is placed under the patient's skin (subcutaneously) and measures the glucose in the fluid around the cells (interstitial fluid). This glucose information is associated with glucose levels in the blood and thus can be used to monitor the patient's blood glucose. A small transmitter then sends the information to a receiver. The sensor is typically worn by the patient for a week or two before

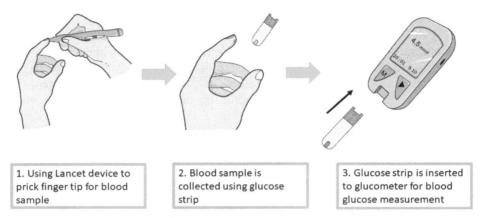

| 1. Using Lancet device to prick finger tip for blood sample | 2. Blood sample is collected using glucose strip | 3. Glucose strip is inserted to glucometer for blood glucose measurement |

Figure 8.15. How a subject measures blood glucose using a glucometer. Copyright © smart.servier.com. The figure was partly generated using Servier Medical Art, provided by Servier, licensed under a Creative Commons Attribution 3.0 unported license.

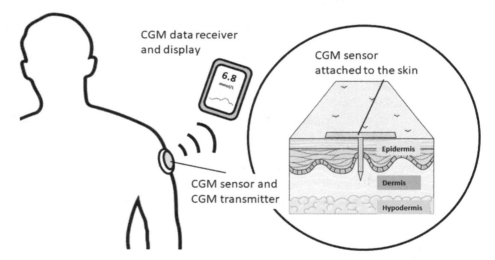

Figure 8.16. Illustration of a typical CGM system. The CGM sensor is attached to the skin to monitor the blood glucose levels in the interstitial fluid. The CGM sensor then transmits interstitial glucose level to the CGM data receiver for display. Copyright © smart.servier.com. The figure was partly generated using Servier Medical Art, provided by Servier, licensed under a Creative Commons Attribution 3.0 unported license.

they are replaced. While CGM is capable of continuously providing estimates of a patient's blood glucose level, most devices still require calibration using a lancet device and glucometer.

Once the patient knows the blood glucose level, they can take their medication according to their doctor's advice. The patient's blood glucose can be regulated through oral intake of medication or onsite injection of insulin into their body. As this process is disruptive to patient's daily routine, an artificial pancreas can be used to automate this process. It potentially provides better control and treatment to the patient.

8.4.2 Artificial pancreas

The artificial pancreas, as it is named, is a medical device that replaces the function of the human pancreas. An artificial pancreas device system (APDS) will not only monitor glucose levels in the body but also automatically adjusts the delivery of insulin to reduce high blood glucose levels (hyperglycaemia) and minimise the incidence of low blood glucose (hypoglycaemia) with little or no input from the patient.

One would imagine an artificial pancreas as a robotic-like pancreas system implanted into the human body replacing the human pancreas organ. It can perform the normal functions of a pancreas organ, such as detecting the blood glucose level automatically and producing insulin and other hormones on its own through an internal insulin generator. However, in reality, the current form of an artificial pancreas is a system containing not one but multiple devices that closely mimic the glucose regulating function of a healthy human pancreas.

There are two main functions that the artificial pancreas needs to fulfil. First, the artificial pancreas needs to be able to continuously measure the patient's blood glucose level. Next, an insulin infusion device is required to deliver the right amount of insulin into the body to regulate blood glucose levels. The current artificial pancreas technology consists of a combination of three device types, mainly a blood glucose meter, a continuous glucose monitoring system (CGM) and an insulin infusion pump, as shown in figure 8.17.

8.4.2.1 Continuous glucose monitor (CGM)
The CGM provides a steady stream of information that reflects the patient's blood glucose levels. This CGM continuously displays an estimate of blood glucose levels and their direction and rate of change in these estimates. This information will be used in the controller of the insulin infusion pump.

8.4.2.2 Blood glucose meter or glucometer
In order to get an accurate estimate of blood glucose from a CGM, the patient needs to periodically calibrate the CGM using a blood glucose measurement from a glucometer. Therefore, while an artificial pancreas takes over the measurements, monitoring and insulin infusion, the glucometer still plays a critical role in the proper management of diabetic patients. However, over time, we anticipate that improved CGM performance may do away with the need for periodic blood glucose checks with a glucometer.

8.4.2.3 Control algorithm and controller
The controller is the heart of the artificial pancreas delivery system. The control algorithm can be run from any device of the artificial pancreas delivery system, including an insulin pump, computer or cellular phone. The controller is an external

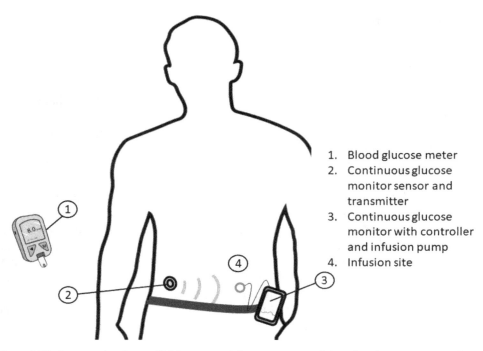

Figure 8.17. An example of an artificial pancreas delivery system consisting of a glucose meter, continuous glucose monitor, controller and infusion pump. Copyright © smart.servier.com. The figure was partly generated using Servier Medical Art, provided by Servier, licensed under a Creative Commons Attribution 3.0 unported license.

processor that houses the software that is programmed with a control algorithm and mathematical model. The controller receives information from the CGM and performs calculations with a mathematical model and control algorithm. Based on the model estimation, the controller sends dosing instructions to the infusion pump.

A computer-controlled algorithm connects the CGM and insulin infusion pump to allow continuous communication between the two devices. Sometimes an artificial pancreas device system is a 'closed-loop' system, an 'automated insulin delivery' system, or an 'autonomous system for glycaemic control.' There are numerous published works on the control algorithm, including the classic feedback proportional–integral–derivative (PID) controller (Steil *et al* 2006), the model predictive controller (Plank *et al* 2006, Thabit and Hovorka 2016), sliding mode controller, observer state feedback and the list goes on. We will discuss some of the basic control algorithms in the later section of the chapter.

8.4.2.4 Insulin infusion pump and insulin types
Based on the instructions sent by the controller, an infusion pump adjusts the insulin delivery to the tissue under the skin. Insulin is usually injected into the abdomen, but it can also be injected into the upper arms, thighs, or buttocks. There are also different types of insulin used in the infusion pump. These include:

- Rapid-acting insulin reaches the bloodstream within 15 min and keeps working for up to 4 h.
- Short-acting insulin enters the bloodstream within 30 min and works for up to 6 h.
- Intermediate-acting insulin finds its way into your bloodstream within 2–4 h and is effective for about 18 h.
- Long-acting insulin starts working within a few hours and keeps glucose levels even for about 24 h.

Aside from the artificial pancreas delivery system, the patient also plays a vital role in it. In particular, the concentration of glucose circulating in the patient's blood is constantly changing. It is affected by the patient's diet, activity level, and how his or her body metabolises insulin and other substances. Thus, the control algorithm needs to account for patient variability, and more clinical trials are being carried out to study the feasibility and performance of these artificial pancreas systems in actual patients. Equally, new approaches have been adopted to provide better control, minaturisation of the device, as well as improve the ease of clinical adoption of these artificial pancreas systems (Cobelli *et al* 2009, 2011, Lunze *et al* 2013, Peyser *et al* 2014).

While this research seems to be maturing, there are more research areas in model-based glycaemic control. In particular, there should be more enhanced models of glucose–insulin kinetics, particularly concerning injection delivery area and how it gets absorbed in the human body. Equally, patients will also respond differently to the types of insulin. Adding these considerations would add robustness to the overall control algorithm development. There should also be better methods of managing measurement errors, either via improved sensor design or signal processing methods. Finally, more clinical trials are required to test these methods and their performance.

8.4.3 Intensive care hyperglycaemia patients

Within hospital intensive care, hyperglycaemia can occur in critically ill patients with no history of diabetes mellitus (Capes *et al* 2000, McCowen *et al* 2001, Esposito *et al* 2003, Finney *et al* 2003, Christiansen *et al* 2004). The patient's acute illness and critical condition in the intensive care unit (ICU) can cause their bodies to experience stress-induced hyperglycaemia. Acute hyperglycaemia is common in critically ill patients, with an estimated 30% or more patients suffering from hyperglycaemia. The causes of hyperglycaemia in these patients vary. Both physiological and emotional stress experienced by the patients lead to an intense activation of stress hormones such as cortisol and epinephrine. The release of inflammatory cytokines causes an increase in peripheral insulin resistance and hepatic glucose production, leading to hyperglycaemia. In addition, some patients will undergo steroid-based therapies, which affect insulin action and production, further exacerbating the problem.

Patients with stressed-induced hyperglycaemia have been associated with adverse outcomes, such as an increased risk of severe infection, acute myocardial infarction, sepsis, septic shock, polyneuropathy, multiple organ failure and etc. Thus, during the treatment of patients with stress-induced hyperglycaemia, these ICU patients need to be treated as if they are diabetic patients, and it is important to implement blood glucose control to improve patient outcomes. Studies found that control of blood glucose levels using insulin has significantly reduced the need for dialysis, bacteraemia testing (for sepsis) and the number of blood transfusions. In studies by Van den Berghe *et al* (2001, 2003) and Krinsley (2004), tight blood glucose control within 6.1–7.75 mmol L^{-1} in critically ill patients has seen a reduction in mortality.

However, tight control of patients' blood glucose levels is difficult. This process is difficult due to the difference in patients' conditions, and their response to insulin therapy varies from one another. For example, highly insulin-resistant patients require significantly more insulin to achieve the desired glucose reductions, whereas an insulin-sensitive patient will only require lesser insulin intake. Furthermore, the effect of insulin therapy saturates at high doses, which leads to excessive insulin administration. Finally, the patient conditions may also evolve over time. All these confounding patient-dependent factors have made tight glycaemic control a very challenging task.

In addition to patient-specificity, due to the nature of the ICU environment and clinicians' workload, there can be infrequent measurements of patient blood glucose levels and delivery of insulin treatment. During insulin therapy, insulin must be injected to regulate the blood glucose concentration in order to decrease the glucose level in the blood so that the glucose concentration can be kept near to the normal glycaemic level. It is very crucial to inject a suitable amount because if too much insulin is injected, blood glucose concentration levels may decrease too much and cause hypoglycaemia. If too little insulin is given, there is no control, and blood glucose levels remain high. Equally, the therapy needs to be administered timely for optimal control. Thus, a lack of clinical resources to support patient treatment can also impact the control of blood glucose. As a result, tight glycaemic control is not easily achieved. Thus, attempts have been made to have better glycaemic control, not fully tight glycaemic control, such as an example shown in figure 8.17, where a patient's blood glucose level is controlled within a clinical target of 4 mmol L^{-1} to 7.8 mmol L^{-1} in the 24 h period.

As shown in figure 8.18, there are unpredictable and significant fluctuations in blood glucose levels. Insulin therapy risks adverse clinical outcomes if not controlled. Insulin, as mentioned earlier, is a hormone that is critical to the regulation of glucose concentration in the blood. Without it, blood glucose levels are often too high (hyperglycaemia), which can cause long-term problems like eye, nerve, kidney diseases, and strokes. On the other hand, overdosage of insulin will cause low blood glucose (hypoglycaemia), resulting in the patient falling into a coma or having other immediate consequences.

8.4.4 Sliding scale insulin infusion protocol

The current standard of glycemic control adopted in most hospital ICUs is the sliding scale insulin infusion protocol (Donihi *et al* 2006, Hui *et al* 2012). A sliding

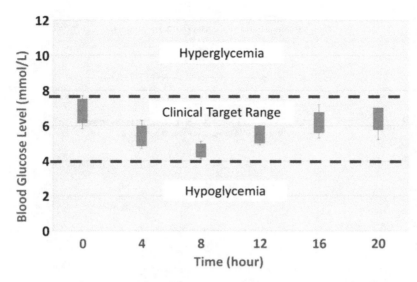

Figure 8.18. Tight glycaemic control for critically ill patients.

scale protocol is an umbrella term that describes most typical protocols currently implemented. These protocols follow a logical thought process. If glucose levels get too high, provide more insulin to the patient. If blood glucose levels get too low, reduce or stop insulin input altogether. Hence the name sliding scale. Figure 8.19 shows an example of an insulin infusion protocol based on a sliding scale protocol. It aims to maintain the patient's blood glucose level between 4 mmol L^{-1} to 10 mmol L^{-1}.

The overall general procedure of this example protocol is as follows:

- Under this protocol, upon administration to the ICU, the patient's blood glucose levels are measured on an hourly basis.
- If two consecutive blood glucose readings are above 10 mmol L^{-1}, the insulin infusion protocol is started according to the scale at Scale 2.
- Based on the current blood glucose level, if the blood glucose level is lower than the previously measured blood glucose level, the insulin infusion rate is maintained the same as the previous rate.
- If the blood glucose level is the same or higher, the infusion rate is increased to the first right column with a higher infusion, as shown on the scale.
- When the blood glucose level is within the target range, the infusion is maintained the same.
- Finally, when blood glucose is within 4–6 mmol L^{-1}, the infusion rate is decreased to the first left column.
- If the blood glucose drops below 4 mmol L^{-1}, the insulin infusion is ceased.

The slide scale protocol is a common and easy-to-follow insulin infusion protocol. These protocols and the way they were designed were mainly based on clinical experience. This meant it could not capture the unpredictable metabolic changes within the body and was only very general. It cannot cater to patient-specific needs.

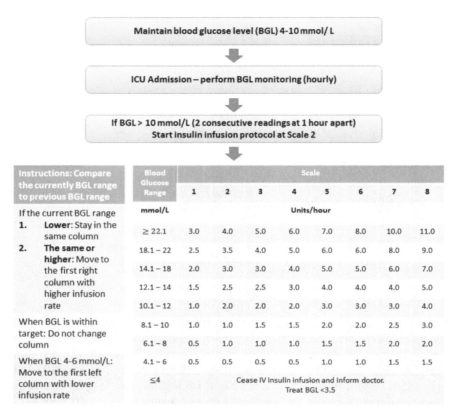

Figure 8.19. Example of a sliding scale insulin infusion protocol.

In addition, glucose measurements for most sliding scale protocols were usually taken every 4-hourly or less, depending on the state of the patient, to reduce labour-intensiveness. These factors contributed to highly variable blood glucose levels, which potentially threaten patient morbidity.

8.4.5 Model-based insulin protocol

Computational physiological models can help overcome this by using patient-specific data to create personalised solutions for highly variable ICU patients (Chase *et al* 2018). Some patient physiological data also cannot be directly measured or are simply too impractical to do so. Direct testing on human subjects for the development and evaluation of an adaptive system to deliver insulin treatment to patients is time-consuming, costly, and confounded by ethical issues. Therefore, blood glucose control is being managed via *in silico* experiments through mathematical modelling of the glucose–insulin system, which brings us to model the glucose–insulin interaction of the patient. Utilising these models in glycemic control creates a huge potential for improving outcomes for patients in the ICU.

In the past decade, much research has been carried out to investigate model-based methods that can be used in the clinical examination of critical care patients and glycaemic control. There are several mathematical models capable of capturing patient glucose–insulin interaction. Equally, studies have also been carried out to determine control algorithms to provide robust and tight glycaemic control. The model-based methods are different in terms of how the models were constructed or the control algorithms used. For example, Andreassen *et al* (1994) presented a probabilistic approach to glucose prediction and insulin dose adjustment. Chee *et al* (2003a, 2003b) adopted a proportional–integral–derivative (PID) control together with an active sliding table according to patient condition. Hovorka *et al* (2004) and Plank *et al* (2006) conducted model-based treatment in critical care glycaemic control trials. Others used non-linear models, based on Bergman's minimal model for glycemic control (Parker *et al* 1999, 2001, Doran *et al* 2004, Wong *et al* 2006, Chase *et al* 2008).

In these model-based methods, the glucose–insulin models are integrated with control algorithms to regulate the insulin input and glucose intake to manage the patient blood glucose range. Through models, researchers can perform parameter identification to obtain information about the behaviour of diabetic patients. Specifically, information such as patient-specific nutrition absorption, how a patient utilises glucose, what is the patient's insulin sensitivity, or the patient's insulin production rate, can help in determining a suitable way of administrating insulin injections (Chase *et al* 2006). Next, the control algorithm will perform its wonders to regulate the patient's blood glucose output when given a set of inputs.

The following list shows one possible scenario of how model-based methods are implemented in glucose control:

- A glucose–insulin model is selected/developed to better understand the patients' physiologic glucose–insulin interaction and how they respond to treatment.
- Using measured blood glucose data from a clinical trial, parameter identification is performed using the glucose–insulin model for the patient. Here, patient-specific parameters such as rate of glucose utilisation and insulin sensitivity are identified.
- Using the identified patient-specific parameters, forward simulation of the glucose–insulin model is carried out to predict future blood glucose levels. This process is performed using model inputs such as current blood glucose level, insulin treatment and nutrition.
- The predictions for the development of a control algorithm and/or insulin and nutrition recommendations are tabulated.
- The recommendations are then documented as treatment plans and can be tested *in silico* and in clinical trials.

Generally, the control process used for regulating blood glucose levels for critically ill patients can be similar to that of diabetic patients. The major differences are how glucose–insulin interaction and patients' responses are modelled. The control algorithms are also different in some ways, but all will have a common goal, which is to provide optimal control for blood glucose management.

Different control algorithms have been proposed in the literature for closed-loop administration of insulin so far, but two of the most used algorithms are the proportional–integral–derivative controller (PID) and the model predictive control (MPC).

8.4.5.1 PID control

One conventional control algorithm used in model-based glucose control is the proportional–integral–derivative controller, in short, the PID controller. For the application of blood glucose control, a PID controller is used to estimate the amount of insulin input into the human system based on system feedback. The insulin input to the patient is dependent on the difference between the measured blood glucose level from the feedback loop and desired blood glucose concentration from the glucose reference input. This difference, also known as the error signal, is then fed into the PID controller system to estimate the amount of insulin input into the glucose–insulin model to regulate the patient's blood glucose level within a set target.

A general schematic flow of a PID controller applied in blood glucose level control is shown in figure 8.20, which represents the human glucose–insulin interaction system. A mathematical model or the actual system can be used to produce the patients' response (output, or glucose level) when it is given a specific input (control signal/insulin input) and disturbance (nutrition, meal intake). The output glucose signal is then compared to the glucose level set point. The difference between the output glucose level and a glucose set point is used as an error for the control algorithm to determine how insulin or other medication should be administered to the patient. In essence, the PID controller regulates insulin by noticing variations from the target glucose levels.

8.4.5.2 Model predictive control

Model predictive control is a different class of control algorithm from conventional control approaches. It is a class of control algorithms that relies heavily on the modelling of the process in order to make predictions at each known time point

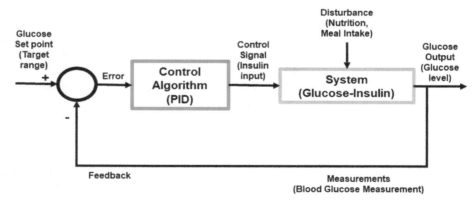

Figure 8.20. A simple diagram on how the glucose–insulin model is used with a PID control algorithm to manage patients' blood glucose level.

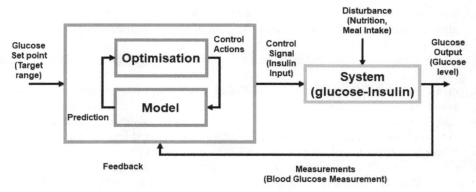

Figure 8.21. Simple diagram of a model predictive control in glucose control.

about future outputs, while satisfying a set of constraints (Jelsch *et al* 2021, Schwenzer *et al* 2021). Thus, MPC in glucose control is a control algorithm where a physiological glucose–insulin model is used for predicting the future behaviour of the system over a finite time window.

The patient glucose level predictions are made based on the current measured/state of the system and the input given to the system. Based on these predictions, the optimal control signal (insulin inputs) with respect to a defined control objective and subject to system constraints are computed. After a specific interval, the measurement, estimation and computation process is repeated with a shifted finite time window.

In summary, MPC regulates the insulin by minimising the difference of forecasted and target glucose levels. Figure 8.21 shows a simple diagram of a model predictive control that can be used for glucose control. The application of MPC strategy in blood glucose control has recently gained popularity among researchers. It has been widely used in blood glucose control clinical trials, more so than PID controllers (Mehmood *et al* 2020).

8.5 Summary

Overall, hyperglycaemia is prevalent and has a significant impact on the subject's livelihood. Tight regulation can significantly reduce these negative outcomes, but achieving it remains clinically challenging. Model-based treatments have provided unique opportunities to understand the physiology of glucose–insulin interactions and how a patient would respond to medication. With ever increasing published studies, it is very much an emerging field rather than a mature area of research. This chapter has presented a general introduction to the glucose–insulin model and its applications around it. Perhaps more importantly, the state of the model-based control of hyperglycaemia in patient care and opportunities for future studies.

References

Andreassen S, Benn J J, Hovorka R, Olesen K G and Carson E R 1994 A probabilistic approach to glucose prediction and insulin dose adjustment: description of metabolic model and pilot evaluation study *Comput. Methods Programs Biomed.* **41** 153–65

Arleth T, Andreassen S, Federici M O and Benedetti M M 2000 A model of the endogenous glucose balance incorporating the characteristics of glucose transporters *Comput. Methods Programs Biomed.* **62** 219–34

Bergman R N 2021 Origins and history of the minimal model of glucose regulation *Front. Endocrin.* **11** 1151

Bergman R N, Ider Y Z, Bowden C R and Cobelli C 1979 Quantitative estimation of insulin sensitivity *Am. J. Physiol.* **236** E667

Bergman R N, Phillips L S and Cobelli C 1981 Physiologic evaluation of factors controlling glucose tolerance in man: measurement of insulin sensitivity and beta-cell glucose sensitivity from the response to intravenous glucose *J. Clin. Invest.* **68** 1456–67

Bolie V W 1961 Coefficients of normal blood glucose regulation *J. Appl. Physiol.* **16** 783–8

Capes S E, Hunt D, Malmberg K and Gerstein H C 2000 Stress hyperglycaemia and increased risk of death after myocardial infarction in patients with and without diabetes: a systematic overview *Lancet* **355** 773–8

Chase J G *et al* 2018 Next-generation, personalised, model-based critical care medicine: a state-of-the art review of in silico virtual patient models, methods, and cohorts, and how to validation them *Biomed. Eng. Online* **17** 24

Chase J G, Shaw G, Le Compte A, Lonergan T, Willacy M, Wong X-W, Lin J, Lotz T, Lee D and Hann C 2008 Implementation and evaluation of the SPRINT protocol for tight glycaemic control in critically ill patients: a clinical practice change *Crit. Care* **12** R49

Chase J G, Shaw G M, Wong X W, Lotz T, Lin J and Hann C E 2006 Model-based glycaemic control in critical care-A review of the state of the possible *Biomed. Signal Process. Control* **1** 3–21

Chee F, Fernando T and van Heerden P V 2003a Closed-loop glucose control in critically ill patients using continuous glucose monitoring system (CGMS) in real time *IEEE Trans. Inf. Technol. Biomed.* **7** 43–53

Chee F, Fernando T L, Savkin A V and van Heerden V 2003b Expert PID control system for blood glucose control in critically ill patients *IEEE Trans. Inf. Technol. Biomed.* **7** 419–25

Christiansen C, Toft P, Jørgensen H S, Andersen S K and Tønnesen E 2004 Hyperglycaemia and mortality in critically ill patients *Inten. Care Med.* **30** 1685–8

Cobelli C, Man C D, Sparacino G, Magni L, Nicolao G D and Kovatchev B P 2009 Diabetes: models, signals, and control *IEEE Rev. Biomed. Eng.* **2** 54–96

Cobelli C, Renard E and Kovatchev B 2011 Artificial pancreas: past, present, future *Diabetes* **60** 2672–82

Dalla Man C, Caumo A and Cobelli C 2002 The oral glucose minimal model: estimation of insulin sensitivity from a meal test *IEEE Trans. Biomed. Eng.* **49** 419–29

Dalla Man C, Camilleri M and Cobelli C 2006 A system model of oral glucose absorption: validation on gold standard data *IEEE Trans. Biomed. Eng.* **53** 2472–8

Dalla Man C, Rizza R A and Cobelli C 2007 Meal simulation model of the glucose–insulin system *IEEE Trans. Biomed. Eng.* **54** 1740–9

Donihi A C, DiNardo M M, DeVita M A and Korytkowski M T 2006 Use of a standardized protocol to decrease medication errors and adverse events related to sliding scale insulin *Qual. Safe. Health Care* **15** 89

Doran C V, Hudson N H, Moorhead K T, Chase J G, Shaw G M and Hann C E 2004 Derivative weighted active insulin control modelling and clinical trials for ICU patients *Med. Eng. Phys.* **26** 855–66

Esposito K, Marfella R and Giugliano D 2003 Stress hyperglycemia, inflammation, and cardiovascular events *Diabetes Care* **26** 1650–1

Finney S J, Zekveld C, Elia A and Evans T W 2003 Glucose control and mortality in critically ill patients *JAMA* **290** 2041–7

Gutch M, Kumar S, Razi S M, Gupta K K and Gupta A 2015 Assessment of insulin sensitivity/resistance *Indian J. Endocrinol. Metab.* **19** 160–4

Hariri A and Wang L 2011 Identification and low-complexity regime-switching insulin control of type I diabetic patients *J. Biomed. Sci. Eng.* **4** 297–314

Hovorka R *et al* 2004 Nonlinear model predictive control of glucose concentration in subjects with type 1 diabetes *Physiol. Meas.* **25** 905–20

Hui M L, Kumar A and Adams G G 2012 Protocol-directed insulin infusion sliding scales improve perioperative hyperglycaemia in critical care *Periop. Med.* **1** 7

Jelsch M, Roggo Y, Kleinebudde P and Krumme M 2021 Model predictive control in pharmaceutical continuous manufacturing: a review from a user's perspective *Eur. J. Pharm. Biopharm.* **159** 137–42

Khodaei M J, Candelino N, Mehrvarz A and Jalili N 2020 Physiological closed-loop control (PCLC) systems: review of a modern frontier in automation *IEEE Access* **8** 23965

Knopp J L, Holder-Pearson L and Chase J G 2019 Insulin units and conversion factors: a story of truth, boots, and aster half-truths *J. Diabetes Sci. Technol.* **13** 597–600

Krinsley J S 2004 Effect of an intensive glucose management protocol on the mortality of critically ill adult patients *Mayo Clin. Proc.* **79** 992–1000

Lin J, Razak N N, Pretty C G, Le Compte A, Docherty P, Parente J D, Shaw G M, Hann C E and Chase J G 2011 A physiological Intensive Control Insulin-Nutrition-Glucose (ICING) model validated in critically ill patients *Comput. Methods Programs Biomed.* **102** 192–205

Lunze K, Singh T, Walter M, Brendel M D and Leonhardt S 2013 Blood glucose control algorithms for type 1 diabetic patients: a methodological review *Biomed. Signal Proc. Control* **8** 107–19

McAuley K A, Berkeley J E, Docherty P D, Lotz T F, Te Morenga L A, Shaw G M, Williams S M, Chase J G and Mann J I 2011 The dynamic insulin sensitivity and secretion test: a novel measure of insulin sensitivity *Metabolism* **60** 1748–56

McCowen K C, Malhotra A and Bistrian B R 2001 Stress-induced hyperglycemia *Crit. Care Clin.* **17** 107–24

Mehmood S, Ahmad I, Arif H, Ammara U E and Majeed A 2020 Artificial pancreas control strategies used for type 1 diabetes control and treatment: a comprehensive analysis *Appl. Syst. Innov.* **3** 31

Pacini G and Bergman R N 1986 Minmod: a computer program to calculate insulin sensitivity and pancreatic responsivity from the frequently sampled intravenous glucose tolerance test *Comput. Methods Programs Biomed.* **23** 113–22

Parker R S, Doyle F J and Peppas N A 1999 A model-based algorithm for blood glucose control in Type I diabetic patients *IEEE Trans. Biomed. Eng.* **46** 148–57

Parker R S, Doyle F J and Peppas N A 2001 The intravenous route to blood glucose control *IEEE Eng. Med. Biol. Mag.* **20** 65–73

Peyser T, Dassau E, Breton M and Skyler J S 2014 The artificial pancreas: current status and future prospects in the management of diabetes *Ann. New York Acad. Sci.* **1311** 102–23

Plank J *et al* 2006 Multicentric, randomized, controlled trial to evaluate blood glucose control by the model predictive control algorithm versus routine glucose management protocols in intensive care unit patients *Diabetes Care* **29** 271–6

Ribet F, Stemme G and Roxhed N 2018 Real-time intradermal continuous glucose monitoring using a minimally invasive microneedle-based system *Biomed. Microdevices* **20** 101

Schwenzer M, Ay M, Bergs T and Abel D 2021 Review on model predictive control: an engineering perspective *Int. J. Adv. Manuf. Technol.* **117** 1327–49

Steil G M, Rebrin K, Darwin C, Hariri F and Saad M F 2006 Feasibility of automating insulin delivery for the treatment of type 1 diabetes *Diabetes* **55** 3344–50

Thabit H and Hovorka R 2016 Coming of age: the artificial pancreas for type 1 diabetes *Diabetologia* **59** 1795–805

Van den Berghe G, Wouters P, Weekers F, Verwaest C, Bruyninckx F, Schetz M, Vlasselaers D, Ferdinande P, Lauwers P and Bouillon R 2001 Intensive insulin therapy in critically ill patients *New Engl. J. Med.* **345** 1359–67

Van den Berghe G, Wouters P J, Bouillon R, Weekers F, Verwaest C, Schetz M, Vlasselaers D, Ferdinande P and Lauwers P 2003 Outcome benefit of intensive insulin therapy in the critically ill: Insulin dose versus glycemic control *Crit. Care Med.* **31** 359–66

Williams R *et al* 2020 Global and regional estimates and projections of diabetes-related health expenditure: results from the International Diabetes Federation Diabetes Atlas, 9th edition *Diabetes Res. Clin. Pract.* **162** 108072

Wong X W, Chase J G, Shaw G M, Hann C E, Lotz T, Lin J, Singh-Levett I, Hollingsworth L J, Wong O S W and Andreassen S 2006 Model predictive glycaemic regulation in critical illness using insulin and nutrition input: a pilot study *Med. Eng. Phys.* **28** 665–81

IOP Publishing

Model-Based Approaches in Biomedical Engineering

Ean Hin Ooi and Yeong Shiong Chiew

Chapter 9

Respiratory system

9.1 Function of the human respiratory system

The human respiratory system, also known as the pulmonary system, is a network of organs and tissues, which primary function is to breathe. The respiratory system consists of the chest cavity, airways, lungs and blood vessels. The intercostal muscles connecting to the rib cage to power the breathing process are also a part of the respiratory system. This network of organs works closely together to move oxygen throughout the body and clear out waste gases like carbon dioxide. Figure 9.1 shows the anatomy of the human respiratory system.

The primary function of the human lung is ventilation and perfusion matching, such that gas exchange between alveolar air and alveolar capillary blood is efficient. The process of transporting the air from the surrounding environment into the lung is known as ventilation. Oxygen (O_2) is delivered from surrounding air into the body tissues through the process of inspiration (breathing in). Carbon dioxide (CO_2) is then transferred out from the tissues via the blood and to the air through an expiration process (breathing out). Oxygen in the inspired air is absorbed into the blood at the alveolar level via gas exchange with the blood at the alveolar capillaries. This gas exchange process is known as perfusion. It provides the human body with a constant supply of oxygen to enable the conversion of glucose in the cells to energy. At the same time, the exchange of CO_2 and the other metabolism end products are also transported back to the air during expiration (Mason *et al* 2010). Aside from these two main functions, the human respiratory system also helps balance acid-base within the body and produce sound by controlling the air movement in the vocal cord.

9.2 The mechanics of breathing

9.2.1 Breathing process and gas exchange

During inspiration in normal breathing, the diaphragm moves down, and the intercostal muscle moves the rib cage outwards and upwards. This combined

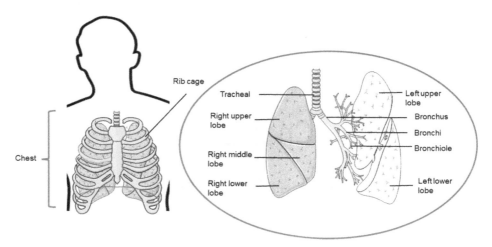

Figure 9.1. The human respiratory system. The airway consists of the tracheal, bronchus, bronchi and bronchiole. The end of the bronchiole connects to the alveoli, forming the lung lobes. Copyright © smart. servier.com. The figure was partly generated using Servier Medical Art, provided by Servier, licensed under a Creative Commons Attribution 3.0 unported license.

movement expands the chest cavity compartment and creates a negative pressure gradient in the lung with respect to atmospheric pressure. The negative pressure within the lung draws air into the lung through the airway passage, allowing the pressure inside the lung to equilibrate. The O_2 in the inspired air is then absorbed into the blood at the alveolar level via the gas exchange process. Figure 9.2 shows the mechanism of breathing during inspiration and expiration.

During inspiration, the air enters through the mouth or nose, where it is filtered and warmed. The air then passes into the pharynx and the larynx before entering the trachea. It then enters the bronchi and then the bronchioles. Eventually, it reaches the lung sacs and alveoli for gas exchange. The lung sacs or alveoli are hollow, porous bags that complete the airways. They are bubble-liked in shape with the presence of surfactant within the alveoli sac. These alveoli tend to collapse if there is no surfactant. Within the alveoli, the gas exchange process is performed through osmotic diffusion, where gas is transported from the area with higher concentrations to the area with lower concentrations. Figure 9.3 shows the alveoli structure and the perfusion process. O_2 from the inspired air is diffused into the alveolar capillary, and CO_2 from the surrounding body enters back into the air for expiration.

9.2.2 Respiratory diseases and failure

Respiratory diseases are pathological conditions that impair human lung functions. These respiratory diseases cause damage to the airway and alveoli, affecting the overall gas exchange process. Figure 9.4 shows three types of damage in the human respiratory system airway and alveoli.

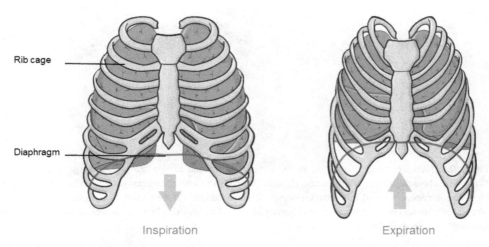

Figure 9.2. The diaphragm and rib cage movement during inspiration and expiration. (Left) During inspiration, the diaphragm contracts and the intercostal muscle moves upward, creating a negative pressure gradient in the lung. (Right) During expiration, the diaphragm relaxes, and the intercostal muscle moves down, pushing the air out from the lung. Copyright © smart.servier.com. The figure was partly generated using Servier Medical Art, provided by Servier, licensed under a Creative Commons Attribution 3.0 unported license.

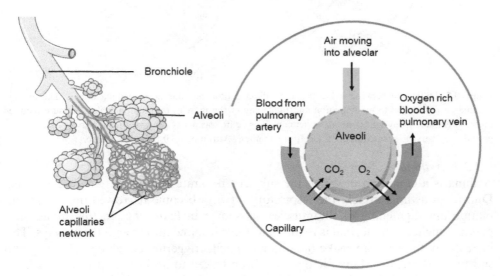

Figure 9.3. Alveoli structure is surrounded by capillaries for gas exchange. Blood is pumped from the heart to the pulmonary artery into the capillaries. The O_2 in the alveoli diffuses into the capillaries, and it is delivered to the body via the pulmonary vein. CO_2 is pumped from the surrounding body and is diffused into the alveoli to be expired out from the body. Copyright © smart.servier.com. The figure was partly generated using Servier Medical Art, provided by Servier, licensed under a Creative Commons Attribution 3.0 unported license.

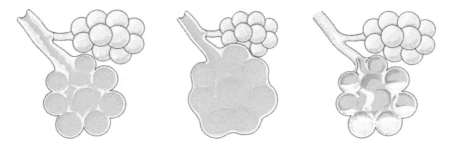

Figure 9.4. Different types of damage in the airway and alveoli impair the gas exchange process. (Left) Bronchitis where the airway is constricted. (Middle) Emphysema where the damaged alveoli merge and form a large alveolar space. (Right) Pulmonary oedema with fluid build-up in the alveoli. Copyright © smart.servier. com. The figure was partly generated using Servier Medical Art, provided by Servier, licensed under a Creative Commons Attribution 3.0 unported license.

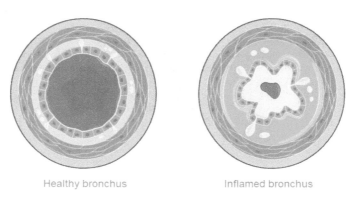

Healthy bronchus   Inflamed bronchus

Figure 9.5. Difference between a healthy and inflamed bronchus during an asthma attack. The airways become narrowed due to inflammation and tightening of the muscles resulting in higher pressure required during breathing. Copyright © smart.servier.com. The figure was partly generated using Servier Medical Art, provided by Servier, licensed under a Creative Commons Attribution 3.0 unported license.

9.2.2.1 Asthma

Asthma is a condition in which the subject's respiratory airways narrow and swell. During an asthma attack, the respiratory airways become narrowed due to inflammation and tightening of the muscles, as shown in figure 9.5. In this situation, a pressure higher than normal is required to force inspired air through the airways. This increase in pressure can make breathing difficult, triggering coughing, wheezing and shortness of breath. Many factors have been linked to an increased risk of asthma, such as genetic factors, allergies and air pollution. Asthma cannot be cured, but it can be managed with inhaled medications such as bronchodilators or steroids to control the disease and enable asthmatic patients to resume their everyday active life.

9.2.2.2 Emphysema

Emphysema is a lung condition that involves injury to the alveoli walls. The inner walls of the alveoli weaken and rupture. These ruptures create larger air space in the alveoli instead of many small ones as shown in the middle panel of figure 9.4. The overall larger air space reduces the surface area of the lungs and, in turn, the amount of oxygen that reaches the pulmonary capillaries during the gas exchange process. This reduction in the alveoli surface causes the subject to experience shortness of breath. Smoking or inhalation of air pollutants are the leading causes of emphysema, but genetic factors and respiratory infections can also play a role. There is no known cure for lung emphysema, and it can worsen over time if it is not managed. Thus, treatment focuses on slowing the speed of progressions, such as using a bronchodilator, anti-inflammatory medication, or oxygen therapy.

9.2.2.3 Pulmonary oedema

Pulmonary oedema occurs when excessive liquid accumulates in the alveoli. Pulmonary oedema is caused by either failure of the left heart ventricle to remove oxygenated blood adequately from the pulmonary circulation or injury to the lungs. The right panel in figure 9.4 shows pulmonary oedema, there is fluid build-up in the alveoli. The fluid increases the pressure within the lung and reduces alveoli surfactant, leading to impaired gas exchange and may cause hypoxemia and respiratory failure. The primary treatment for pulmonary oedema is oxygen therapy. In this therapy, oxygen supply is delivered via a facemask or a nasal cannula to the patient to ease their symptoms of respiratory failure. Other medications such as diuretics can help to reduce the pressure build-up in the heart and lungs, or blood pressure drugs to lower the blood pressure.

9.2.2.4 Chronic obstructive pulmonary disease

Chronic obstructive pulmonary disease (also known as COPD) is a chronic inflammatory lung disease that causes obstructed airflow to the lung. Symptoms of COPD patients include breathing difficulty, shortness of breath, cough, mucus (sputum) production and wheezing. COPD is usually caused by long-term exposure to the surrounding air pollution, irritating gases and, more often, cigarette smoke. Patients who suffer from COPD are at risk of developing heart disease, lung cancer, and various other conditions. COPD patients are treated with bronchodilators, anti-inflammatory medication, or oxygen therapy to ease their symptoms.

9.2.2.5 Acute respiratory failure

Respiratory failure is a serious lung condition when the human lungs are not able to receive enough O_2 into the blood. Respiratory failure patients often experience difficulties in breathing as their lung ventilation and perfusion matching are affected. The loss of ventilation-perfusion matching reduces O_2 supply intake and CO_2 removal. The build-up of CO_2 in the body can cause damage to the tissues and organs and further impair oxygenation, thus creating significant physiological stress in the human body (Ferring and Vincent 1997). These patients are admitted to the hospital intensive care and are normally treated with mechanical ventilation for breathing support.

Acute respiratory failure (ARF) happens quickly and without much warning, and thus the name acute. It is caused by a disease or injury, such as pneumonia, drug

Table 9.1. Clinical disorders associated with the development of ARDS.

	Direct lung injury	Indirect lung injury
Common causes	• Pneumonia • Aspiration of gastric contents	• Sepsis • Severe trauma with shock and multiple transfusions
Less common causes	• Pulmonary contusion • Fat emboli • Near-drowning • Inhalational injury • Reperfusion pulmonary oedema after lung transplantation or pulmonary embolectomy	• Cardiopulmonary bypass • Drug overdose • Acute pancreatitis • Transfusions of blood products

overdose, chest trauma, stroke, or lung or spinal cord injury. A more severe form of acute respiratory failure is called acute respiratory distress syndrome (ARDS) (Ashbaugh *et al* 1967, Ware and Matthay 2000, The ARDS Definition Task Force 2012). ARDS occurs due to severe inflammatory response of the lung, resulting in direct alveolar injury, pulmonary oedema and alveolar collapse. This lung injury occurs when fluid builds up in the patient's alveoli. The fluid prevents the patient lungs from filling with enough air, which means less oxygen reaches the blood bloodstream, depriving the organs of the oxygen they need to function (Bernard *et al* 1994, Kollef and Schuster 1995). This dynamic further reduces ventilation-perfusion matching and lung function.

The clinical disorders associated with the development of ARDS are shown in table 9.1 (Ware and Matthay 2000). Overall, these lung injuries significantly impair the breathing process, reducing alveolar gas exchange and resulting in an increased risk of organ failure and mortality if not treated (Mortelliti and Manning 2002, Ferguson *et al* 2005, Girard and Bernard 2007).

Aside from ARDS, another known respiratory disease is the severe acute respiratory syndrome (SARS). SARS is a respiratory disease of a zoonotic origin caused by severe acute respiratory syndrome coronavirus. It is an infectious disease caused by a pathogen (an infectious agent, such as a bacterium, virus, parasite or prion) that has jumped from an animal to a human. SARS-CoV-1 and SARS-CoV-2 Coronavirus disease 2019 (COVID-19) are some examples of SARS.

Respiratory failure patients have been associated with high morbidity and mortality. Acute respiratory failure is also relatively common, affecting around 30% of patients admitted to the hospital intensive care unit (Dasta *et al* 2005). It is estimated that in the United States of America, the mortality of ARDS patients can range from 30% up to 60% (Zambon and Vincent 2008, Phua *et al* 2009). ARDS also entail high medical costs (Dasta *et al* 2005, Kaier *et al* 2020). Therefore, giving the proper treatment to the respiratory failure patient is an important clinical and economic challenge.

9.2.3 Mechanical ventilation

Over the years, various treatments have been suggested for respiratory failure patients. These treatments can be divided into two categories: (a) pharmacological treatment and (b) non-pharmacological treatment. Pharmacological treatments are patient treatment using drugs. Some pharmacologic treatments were able to show improvement for respiratory failure patients (Ware and Matthay 2000). However, mechanical ventilation treatment, a non-pharmacological treatment, remains the primary treatment for patients with respiratory failure (Rouby *et al* 2004, Hasan 2010). Mechanical ventilation treatment has evolved from a supportive treatment to a treatment that can influence the progression of respiratory failure and patient outcomes (Esteban *et al* 2002, Girard and Bernard 2007).

Mechanical ventilation is fundamentally about delivering a supply of oxygen to a patient for breathing support using a mechanical ventilator. It is a form of therapeutic support in the hospital intensive care unit, supporting breathing work and function for respiratory failure patients until the underlying disease is resolved. The primary goal is to support breathing by applying external pressure during respiration to retain lung volume for gas exchange and provide flow to ensure sufficient air volume for oxygenation. The breathing support provided by the ventilator reduces the patient's work of breathing. It increases the lung's ability to recruit and retain lung units (alveoli), thus improving gas exchange (ventilation-perfusion matching) while also allowing a better chance for the diseased lung to recover.

There are two types of ventilation, one using negative pressure ventilation (iron lung) or positive pressure ventilation (modern ventilators), with the latter more commonly used. An illustration depicting negative pressure ventilation and positive pressure ventilation is shown in figure 9.6. As shown in figure 9.6 (left), the patient is encased in an iron lung, which generates negative pressure within the iron lung chamber. This negative pressure within the iron lung simulates a breathing environment similar to the human respiratory system and enables the air to be inhaled into

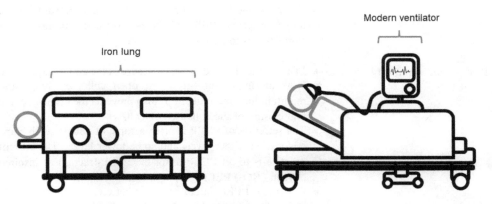

Figure 9.6. Illustration of negative pressure ventilation using the iron lung (left) and positive pressure ventilation using modern ventilators (right).

the patient's lung. A modern ventilator is shown in figure 9.6 (right). It is a mechanical pump applying external pressure to push the air into the patient's lung. The iron lungs are gradually being replaced with modern ventilators due lack of accessibility of the caregivers to the patients as well as patients' movements restriction.

For modern ventilators, ventilation is usually delivered invasively via an endotracheal tube or noninvasively using a facemask or nasal cannular. The positive pressure ventilation is delivered to the patients either in a partially assisted or fully ventilation mode, depending on the patient's breathing effort and level of sedation (Hasan 2010). If the patients can breathe on their own, partial assisted mode provides additional support on top of the patients breathing effort. In contrast, the ventilator can replace the patients' work of breathing completely during a full ventilation mode. Positive pressure ventilation can also be set in either pressure-targeted (pressure control or pressure support mode), volume-targeted (volume control or volume support mode) or other assisted modes (Hasan 2010). Aside from these major settings, there are also other key mechanical ventilator parameters, such as airway pressure, positive end-expiratory pressure, peak inspiratory pressure, plateau pressure, driving pressure, tidal volume, respiratory rate, inspiratory to expiratory ratio and the fraction of inspired oxygen (Major *et al* 2018). The descriptions of these ventilator parameters are shown in table 9.2. A sample of a square-waveform volume control ventilation mode airway pressure, flow and volume is also shown in the table to illustrate the ventilator parameters.

Table 9.2. Key parameters during mechanical ventilation.

Parameters	Descriptions
Airway pressure (P_{aw})	• P_{aw} is the pressure supplied to the patient during mechanical ventilation treatment to ensure sufficient air is delivered to the patient.
	• When setting the airway pressure, clinicians control the peak airway pressure (PIP) and the positive end-expiratory pressure (PEEP) to ensure patient safety.
Positive end-expiratory pressure (PEEP)	• PEEP is the elevated airway pressure at the end of expiration.
	• It is an important setting to open collapsed lungs and maintain lung recruitment. It also prevents the cyclic opening and closing of the collapsed alveoli.
	• The selection of PEEP is often a topic of debate, with some advocating higher levels and some lower levels. The current practice is to set PEEP using the PEEP-fraction of inspired oxygen (F_IO_2) PEEP – F_IO_2 table.
	• Generally, PEEP values can vary between 5 and 25 cmH$_2$O and at times, up to 45 cmH$_2$O during a recruitment manoeuvre to open collapsed alveoli.

Peak inspiratory pressure (PIP)	• PIP is the maximum airway pressure during mechanical ventilation treatment. • The PIP is limited to avoid excessive airway pressures that may cause further injury to the respiratory failure patient.
Plateau pressure (P_{plat})	• The plateau pressure (P_{plat}) is the airway pressure measured during a mechanical ventilation end-of-inspiratory pause. • This pressure level is lower than PIP as it is not influenced by the pressure differences due to airway resistance. It is used as a representation of the pressure in the alveoli. • During mechanical ventilation, the airway pressure is set so that P_{plat} is less than 30–35 cmH$_2$O to avoid pressure-induced injury (barotrauma).
Driving pressure (P_{drive})	• P_{drive} is the pressure difference between P_{plat} and PEEP. • Recent studies have suggested that driving pressure is an important ventilatory parameter that can affect patient outcomes. • Patient ventilated with higher P_{drive} have been associated with increased mortality.
Tidal volume (V_T)	• It is the air volume entering and exiting the lungs in each breathing cycle. • Higher V_T can assist with delivery of O$_2$ to patients with hypoxemia (low in O$_2$ level) and the removal of CO$_2$ in patients with hypercapnia (high CO$_2$). • V_T can be measured during inspiration, V_{TI} or expiration, V_{TE}. • V_T is set using predicted body weight, between 4 and 8 ml kg^{-1} to avoid overinflating the alveoli that may cause volume-induced injury (volutrauma).
Respiratory rate or frequency (f)	• f is the number of breathing cycles per minute. • It is commonly around 16–20 breaths per minute.
Minute ventilation (V_E)	• V_E is the volume of air displaced into and out of the lungs per minute. • It is a product of tidal volume and respiratory rate. • Common ventilation V_E is between 8 and 12 L min^{-1} for adults.
Flow rate ($\dot{V}$) and profile	• V is the rate of air entering the lungs to achieve the desired tidal volume. • It is generally set between 40 and 100 L min^{-1}, and it can be set in either square or reverse ramp profile. • A target V at higher levels for patients with COPD is generally administered, whereas a maximum value of 60 L min^{-1} is typical for ARDS patients.

(*Continued*)

Table 9.2. (*Continued*)

Parameters	Descriptions
Inspiration to expiration (IE) ratio	• Within each breathing cycle (corresponding to the *f*), the ratio of inspiration time to expiration time (IE) can be set to ensure the removal of CO_2 from the lung. • *f* is set together with V_T and IE to ensure adequate minute ventilation.
Fraction of inspired oxygen (F_IO_2)	• F_IO_2 is the O_2 concentration during mechanical ventilation. • F_IO_2 above 21% (O_2 concentration in the atmospheric air is around 21%) is used during mechanical ventilation to increase oxygenation. • Higher F_IO_2 increases the rate of diffusion (diffusion is the movement of gases from the alveoli to plasma and red blood cells) by increasing the partial pressure of O_2 in the alveoli. • However, high F_IO_2 can also result in excessive O_2 partial pressures can cause oxygen toxicity.

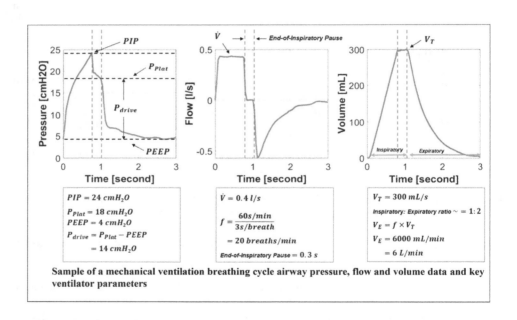

Sample of a mechanical ventilation breathing cycle airway pressure, flow and volume data and key ventilator parameters

These ventilator parameters show that a wide range of possible ventilation settings can be set for patient-specific purposes. Given an overwhelming number of possible combinations of mechanical ventilation settings, various protocols and strategies have been introduced for the support of patients with respiratory failure.

These methods have been applied separately and, in some cases, combined to improve the patient's condition. These methods include mechanical ventilation using low tidal volume (The Acute Respiratory Distress Syndrome Network 2000), optimising PEEP selection (Brower *et al* 2004, Mercat *et al* 2008, Briel *et al* 2010), minimising driving pressure (Amato *et al* 2015, Goligher *et al* 2021), monitoring lung recruitment using lung imaging method and several others (Gattinoni *et al* 2006). Each method offers different potential advantages (Gattinoni *et al* 2017, Pelosi *et al* 2021). However, different methods further complicate clinical decision-making and introduce significant variability in care within and between patients. Furthermore, non-optimal mechanical ventilation settings can potentially further exacerbate the patient condition. Thus, there is a need to titrate optimal settings to fit individual patients' needs in a way that is feasible, and does not encumber a clinical practitioner's daily routine.

An important complicating factor in setting mechanical ventilation is that it is not clinically practical to assess internal lung status regularly to optimise mechanical ventilation settings. Clinicians often 'drive' the therapy partly blind, which is another course of variability in care and outcome. Hence, there is a significant clinical, social and economic need to standardise mechanical ventilation treatment based on measurable, directly quantified patient-specific needs. In this effort, technologies have been developed to incorporate respiratory system models to understand better and to help set mechanical ventilation treatment.

9.3 Respiratory system models

9.3.1 Single-compartment lung model

We can describe human breathing and respiratory system physiology through mathematical modelling. One of the simplest models for the human respiratory system is the single-compartment lung model. Instead of modelling multiple bronchi branches or multiple alveolars (alveoli) in a complex computational model, we can lump all of them into a single-compartment. In this model, the human respiratory system is modelled as a balloon sealed over the end of a pipe as shown in figure 9.7. Mathematically, this simplified respiratory system can be modelled as a combination of an elastic component with a resistance component.

The elastic component (balloon) represents the physical lung, whereas the resistive component (pipe) models the airway. When the airflow ($\dot{V}$) enters the lung through a subject's airway, a pressure drop (ΔP_r) occurs due to the resistance component (R_{rs}). As for the lung compartment, the pressure in the lung (P_{el}), it is modelled as an expandable elastic compartment with volume (V) and elastic property (E_{rs}). Finally, the pressure measured at the airway opening (P_{aw}) can be determined as a sum of these two mechanics as shown in equations (9.1)–(9.3):

$$P_{aw} = \Delta P_r + P_{el}, \tag{9.1}$$

$$\Delta P_r = P_1 - P_2 = R_{rs}\dot{V}, \tag{9.2}$$

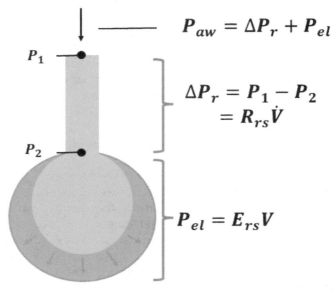

Airway pressure P_{aw}, Air flow, $\dot{V}$ measured
at the entrance of the lung compartment

$$P_{aw} = \Delta P_r + P_{el}$$

P_1

$$\Delta P_r = P_1 - P_2 = R_{rs}\dot{V}$$

P_2

$$P_{el} = E_{rs}V$$

Figure 9.7. Simplified respiratory system model with a combination of pipe and balloon mechanism.

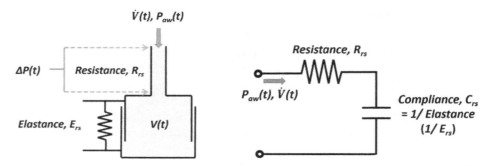

Figure 9.8. Schematic drawing for single-compartment linear lung model. (Left) Mechanical system and (right) electric circuit representation of the respiratory model.

$$P_{el} = E_{rs}V. \qquad (9.3)$$

The respiratory balloon pipe model can also be represented as a mechanical system or electrical circuit, as shown in figure 9.8. In the mechanical system, the elastic compartment balloon is replaced with a spring mechanism. As for the electrical circuit, airway resistance is replaced using a resistor, whereas the elastic compartment is replaced using a capacitor, where capacitance is the inverse of elastance.

To account for pressure equilibrium of the surrounding environment of the respiratory model, equation (9.1) must be added with an offset pressure, P_0 such that:

$$P_{aw}(t) = R_{rs}\dot{V}(t) + E_{rs}V(t) + P_0, \tag{9.4}$$

where in this case, P_{aw} is the airway pressure, t is time, R_{rs} is the respiratory system resistance, $\dot{V}$ is the airway flow, E_{rs} is the respiratory system elastance, V is the air volume of the lung compartment and P_0 is the offset pressure. This offset pressure is typically zero at atmospheric pressure. The value of P_0 will change if an external pressure is applied to the respiratory system, such as PEEP during mechanical ventilation treatment.

The model in equation (9.4) is known as the single-compartment linear lung model. It is the simplest form of respiratory mechanics and has been used in clinical studies. This single-compartment model can also be extended to include nonlinear components such as flow-dependent resistance Rohrer's equation (Bates 2009):

$$P_{aw}(t) = K_1\dot{V}(t) + K_2\dot{V}(t)\,|\,\dot{V}(t)\,| + E_{rs}V(t) + P_0, \tag{9.5}$$

where K_1 is the flow-independent term of the Rohrer equation for flow resistance and K_2 is the flow-dependent term of the Rohrer equation for flow resistance. The expression $|\dot{V}(t)|$ indicates absolute values of the flow. Adding the flow-dependent coefficients into the single-compartment model helps to describe the nonlinear pressure–flow relationships of endotracheal tubes at the flows encountered when a respiratory failure patient is under mechanical ventilation treatment.

Another method to further extend the respiratory mechanics model to capture nonlinear behaviours is through modification of the elastance component to a function of air volume, where E_{rs} increases with $V(t)$, such that (Bates 2009):

$$P_{aw}(t) = R_{rs}\dot{V}(t) + E_1V(t) + E_2(V(t))^2 + P_0. \tag{9.6}$$

9.3.2 Other compartment lung models

Viscoelasticity is a mechanical characteristic of biological tissues, and the human lungs are no exception. Thus, the human lung compartment model can also be described using a viscoelastic model. This model assumes that the alveolar tissues are viscoelastic rather than simply elastic as shown in figure 9.9. It has been extended with an elastance and a resistance component parallel to the main elastic alveolar compartment. This added mechanical property implies that the stress experienced by the lung tissue is not constant during a sustained constant strain. The pressure inside the lung compartment is not only a function of its volume but also depends on its volume history. When the lung compartment is maintained at a constant volume, the pressure in the lung decreases with time.

The lung model accounting for viscoelasticity is given by:

$$R_2\dot{P}_{aw}(t) + E_2P_{aw}(t) = R_1R_2\ddot{V}(t) + (R_2E_1 + E_2R_1 + E_2R_2)\dot{V}(t) + E_1E_2V(t), \tag{9.7}$$

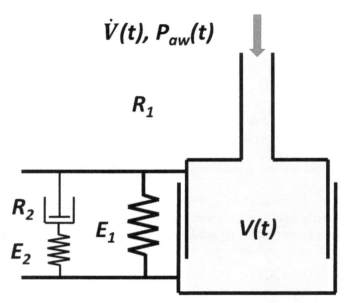

Figure 9.9. The viscoelastic lung model. The model consists of a typical airway with resistance, and the lung compartment consists of three viscoelastic elements.

where similar to the single-compartment models, P_{aw} is the airway pressure, t is the time, $\dot{V}$ is the airway flow, V is the air volume, R_1 denotes the major airway resistance, E_1 is the respiratory system elastance, and R_2 and E_2 are the resistance and elastance of the viscoelastic compartment, respectively.

Another alternative in modelling the human respiratory system is that we can include additional lung compartments in the model. For example, as the lung compartments in a human respiratory system can be separated into a left lung and a right lung, one possible model to better describe this physiology is the two-compartment lung model as shown in figure 9.10. The two-compartment model has progressed into a second-order linear differential equation with added complexity compared to the single-compartment model. This model is another representation of lung physiology and has been used to investigate lung heterogeneity in respiratory failure patients.

The mathematical model of the two-compartment model shown in figure 9.10 can be expressed as:

$$(R_1 + R_2)\dot{P}_{aw}(t) + (E_1 + E_2)P_{aw}(t)$$
$$= [R_1R_2 + R_c(R_1 + R_2)]\ddot{V}(t) \qquad (9.8)$$
$$+ [(R_c + R_2)E_1 + (R_c + R_1)E_2]\dot{V}(t) + E_1E_2V(t),$$

where the subscripts 1 and 2 denote the first and second compartments, R_1 is the airway resistance connecting compartment one, R_2 is the airway resistance for compartment two, $\dot{P}_{aw}$ is the rate of change of the airway pressure, t is time, E_1 is the

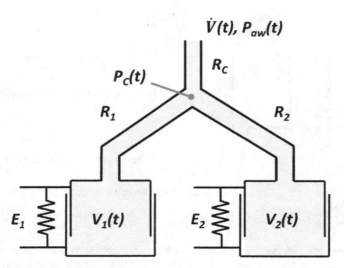

Figure 9.10. The two-compartment lung model consists of a common airway connecting to two lung compartments.

elastance for compartment one and E_2 is elastance for compartment two, P_{aw} is the airway pressure, R_c is the common respiratory system resistance connecting to both compartments, $\dot{V}$ is the airway flow acceleration, V is the airway flow, and finally, V is the total air volume of the lung compartment, with $V(t) = V_1(t) + V_2(t)$.

The viscoelastic model and the two-compartment model are higher-order compartment models. They are more complex and are capable of providing more physiological information about the respiratory failure patient's lung condition (Bates 2009, Ganzert *et al* 2009). The complexity of the lung models can be further extended, and the process of adding more compartments can be repeated, progressing into equations of higher order. While higher-order models are more descriptive, they also require more data measurements or risk issues of model identification (Docherty *et al* 2014). Thus, it is vital to balance model complexity and practicality.

9.3.3 Spontaneous breathing model

During mechanical ventilation, respiratory failure patients are sedated during full ventilation. The ventilator fully replaces the patient's work of breathing and eases patient recovery. During full mechanical ventilation, passive lung models such as single-compartment or multiple-compartment models can capture the mechanical behaviour of a respiratory system. However, as the patients slowly recover, patients on full mechanical ventilation will gradually regain their consciousness and begin to breathe spontaneously on top of the ventilation support.

When mechanically ventilated patients are breathing spontaneously, passive respiratory models such as the single-compartment model, viscoelastic model or two-compartment model cannot capture these active breathing mechanics. The models must be extended to include a functional component to capture these

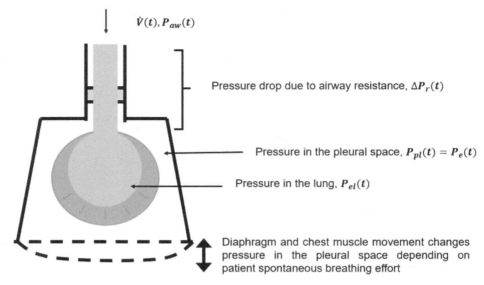

$\dot{V}(t), P_{aw}(t)$

Pressure drop due to airway resistance, $\Delta P_r(t)$

Pressure in the pleural space, $P_{pl}(t) = P_e(t)$

Pressure in the lung, $P_{el}(t)$

Diaphragm and chest muscle movement changes pressure in the pleural space depending on patient spontaneous breathing effort

Figure 9.11. Simple illustration of breathing mechanics during spontaneous breathing. Adapted from Chiew *et al* (2015). Copyright 2015 © PLOS.

spontaneous breathing efforts. Figure 9.11 illustrates a simplified mechanical model when a patient is breathing spontaneously.

In addition to the typical single-compartment model, the model includes an enclosure to encase the respiratory system. This enclosure represents the respiratory system's chest wall and diaphragm, creating an empty space to represent the pleural space between the chest wall and the single-compartment lung model. When a patient is breathing, the respiratory system diaphragm contracts downwards, and the chest wall expands. This combined movement creates a change in the pressure in the pleural space. The change in pressure in the pleural space, known as the pleural pressure, is usually negative, which causes the air from the surrounding environment to be inhaled into the lung during normal breathing. The pleural pressure is typically measured using an oesophageal balloon catheter. This catheter is inserted into the oesophageal tract to estimate the pressure change in the pleural space.

Aside from using an oesophageal balloon catheter, the pressure change in the pleural space can be modelled using an active pressure component, $P_e(t)$. Compared to the airway pressure $P_{aw}(t)$, the $P_e(t)$ is usually negative in value to simulate the pressure change within the pleural space. With this assumption, a single-compartment lung model can be further extended to include the active pressure component.

An example of a single-compartment lung model extended with $P_e(t)$ is given by:

$$P_{aw}(t) = R_{rs}\dot{V}(t) + E_{rs}V(t) + P_0 + P_e(t). \tag{9.9}$$

In the literature, the term P_e has been defined in different forms, such as a polynomial function (Redmond *et al* 2019), piecewise functions (Vicario *et al* 2015) or other forms of functions. An example of the piecewise functions used by Vicario *et al* (2015) is given by:

$$P_e(t) = \begin{cases} P_p \sin\left(\dfrac{\pi}{2t_p}t\right), & \text{for } 0 \leq t < t_p \\ P_p \sin\left(\dfrac{\pi(t + t_r - 2t_p)}{2(t_r - t_p)}\right), & \text{for } t_p \leq t < t_r \\ 0, & \text{for } t_r \leq t < t_N \end{cases} \tag{9.10}$$

where, t is time, t_p and t_r are the time samples at which the $P_e(t)$ reaches minimum peak (P_p), and return to 0. The polynomial function used by Redmond *et al* (2019) is given by:

$$P_e(t) = \begin{cases} 0, & \text{for } t < t_p \\ at^2 + bt + c, & \text{for } t_s \leq t < t_f \\ 0, & \text{for } t \geq t_f \end{cases} \tag{9.11}$$

where a, b and c are the shape and position of the quadratic effort function, t is time. t_s and t_f come from the roots of the quadratic function, indicating the start and finish of the patient breathing effort, respectively. While the models between Vicario *et al* (2015) and Redmond *et al* (2019) are different, their primary goal remains the same, which is to capture patients' spontaneous breathing efforts and better estimate the respiratory mechanics of the respiratory system.

9.3.4 Isotropic expansion and recruitment model

9.3.4.1 Isotropic expansion model

Most conventional respiratory system mechanics models describe lung expansion as an isotropic balloon-like system. These models assume the lung compartment is always open and expands with increasing inspiratory airway pressure and flow. One well-known isotropic expansion model is defined by Venegas *et al* (1998). It is used to describe a patient's lung compliance ($\Delta V/\Delta P$) on how much air can enter into the lung for a change of pressure. The authors used a sigmoidal equation to describe the patient static pressure–volume curve as shown in figure 9.12.

From this sigmoidal curve, an upper inflection point (UIP) and lower inflection point (LIP) can be defined using intersections of the three dashed red lines. The pressure at LIP (P_{LIP}) is the pressure point where lung volume begins to increase rapidly with increasing pressure, whereas the pressure at UIP (P_{UIP}) is the pressure point when the overall lung begins to overinflate. At this pressure, an increasing pressure only results in a relatively small amount of increased volume. The function that defines the sigmoidal shape of the patient static pressure–volume curve is known as the Venegas function and is given by:

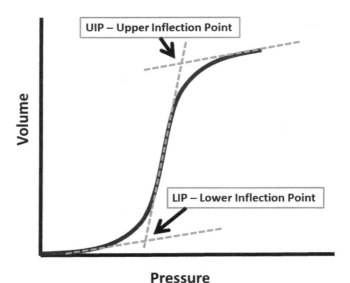

Pressure

Figure 9.12. A sigmoidal curve describing the isotropic expansion of the lung static pressure–volume curve. The curve defines three average compliances ($\Delta V/\Delta P$) with a tri-linear approximation of the pressure–volume curve. The intersections for the tri-linear approximation are the location of lower and upper inflection point.

$$V = a + \left[\frac{b}{1 + e^{-(P-c)/d}} \right], \tag{9.12}$$

where V is the inflation or absolute lung volume, P is pressure in the lung or transpulmonary pressure, and coefficients a, b, c, and d are other fitting parameters of the sigmoidal curve. The pressures P_{LIP} and P_{UIP} can be defined from the static pressure–volume curve, where the intersections between a tangent at the point of maximal compliance when $P = c$, meets the lower and upper asymptotes, with $P_{LIP} = c - 2d$ and $P_{LIP} = c + 2d$.

Note that the measured pressure and volume data from the static pressure–volume curve are pressure–volume data obtained during a specialised protocol. During this specialised protocol, there is no dynamic air movement or pressure difference due to the airway resistance. As a result, the pressure data in the static pressure–volume curve reflects the static pressure within the lung compartment without the airway resistance.

9.3.4.2 Recruitment model
The Venegas function fits the overall static pressure–volume curves relatively well but could not show the heterogeneous nature of a collapsed ARDS lung. Research and several in-vivo studies have suggested an alternate alveolar expansion theory other than the isotropic expansion theory. This theory is known as the recruitment theory (Hickling 1998, Schiller *et al* 2003). This theory describes the alveolar state as either opened or collapsed. Initially, all alveolar in the respiratory system is closed. During the respiration process, the alveolar will open and assume an alveolar

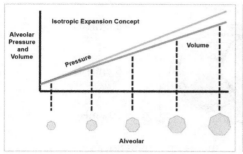 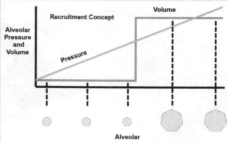

Figure 9.13. Different alveolar expansion theories during pressure increase. The light blue line is the pressure, and the red line represents the alveolar volume. (Left) The traditional theory describes the alveolar expansion as isotropic balloon-like. (Right) Recruitment theory shows that the alveolar is either open or close.

volume after a certain threshold pressure is reached. Once the alveolar is opened, it does not have significant volume change with increasing pressure. It is similar to an on-off switch to turn on the alveolar volume.

The comparison of a traditional expansion theory and the recruitment theory is shown in figure 9.13. In the traditional theory in figure 9.13 (left), the alveolar is always opened, and the volume of the alveolar increases as the pressure increases. As for recruitment theory in figure 9.13 (right), at the beginning, the alveolar is closed without assuming an alveolar volume. As the pressure increases, the alveolar is still closed until it reaches an alveolar opening pressure (threshold pressure). Once the alveolar pressure surpasses the threshold pressure, the alveolar assumes a constant volume. There is no increase in alveolar volume after that.

One of the earlier mathematical models describing the recruitment theory is presented by Hickling (1998). The model describes the lung as a collection of lung units, distributed in layers, with each layer subjected to a superimposed pressure. As the layer goes lower, the superimposed pressure increases. The increase in superimposed pressure will increase the lung unit opening pressure. The lung units at each layer have a distribution of lung units with opening pressure, as shown in figure 9.14.

During inspiration, the lung units are normally closed and can be opened (recruited) with positive pressure from mechanical ventilation. To open a lung unit, the pressure delivered by the mechanical ventilator must overcome an effective threshold opening pressure of the lung unit. Once the lung unit is recruited, it will assume a constant lung unit volume. As more and more lung units are being recruited, the combined lung unit volumes form the static pressure–volume curve. It is important to note that healthy, non-diseased lungs are typically always recruited. For a diseased lung, if the ventilator pressure is not able to overcome the threshold opening pressure, the lung units will remain closed. A sample of how a recruitment model can be modelled can be found in the codes for the chapter[1].

---

[1] Source code for this model (Chapter09a) is available at https://doi.org/10.1088/978-0-7503-4016-8.

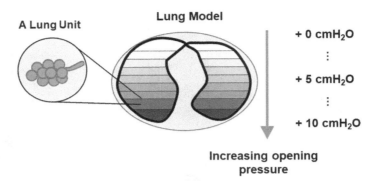

Figure 9.14. Lung units with the effect of superimposed pressure modified from Sundaresan *et al* (2011). Copyright © 2011, Sundaresan *et al*; licensee BioMed Central Ltd.

This recruitment concept provides new insight into lung physiology and can capture the internal heterogeneity observed in the ARDS lung. This concept has been adopted by a number of researchers and has shown potential in understanding respiratory failure physiology and to better guide mechanical ventilation (Sundaresan *et al* 2009, Chiew *et al* 2012, Schranz *et al* 2012b).

9.3.5 Gas exchange model

The models from earlier sections only account for the ventilation process, where they focused on capturing the mechanics of breathing, moving the air into and out of the lung, and the expansion of the lung compartment. Another critical aspect of respiratory system modelling is to model the gas exchange process. The gas exchange model attempts to capture the perfusion and diffusion process in the alveoli. Perfusion is the delivery of blood to the pulmonary capillaries, whereas diffusion is the movement of gases from the alveoli to plasma and red blood cells. As both perfusion and diffusion are closely connected, they are often modelled together to enable investigations of arterial oxygenation, pulmonary shunt or the change of oxygen diffusion resistance through the alveolar (Andreassen *et al* 1996, Rees *et al* 2002, Sundaresan *et al* 2010).

Before going in further into the model, it is important to understand a few basic terms used in the gas exchange model.

- *Physiological dead space* is the total volume of air in the respiratory system that does not take part in the gas exchange process. It comprises of anatomical dead space and alveolar dead space.
- *Anatomical dead space* is the total volume of the airways from the nose or mouth down to terminal bronchioles.
- *Alveolar dead space* is the difference between the physiologic dead space and the anatomic dead space. For a healthy subject, it is usually negligible. However, for a patient with respiratory failure, some alveoli are ventilated,

but they are not perfused. Thus, the gas exchange process does not occur in this dead space.

- *Effective alveoli* are the alveoli that are able to perform gas exchange effectively.
- *Pulmonary shunt* is a condition in which blood moves from the venous circulation to the arterial circulation without participating in gas exchange.

One known gas exchange model is the oxygen status model described by Andreassen *et al* (1996). This gas exchange model describes the alveolar dead space pulmonary shunt and effective alveoli (Sundaresan *et al* 2010). The model estimates the pulmonary hunt and oxygen diffusion resistance by measuring the variation of the fraction of inspired oxygen (F_IO_2) and arterial oxygen saturation (S_aO_2). The model is shown in figure 9.15, and it consists of 4 main components, (1) alveolar ventilation, (2) alveolar gas exchange, (3) shunt equation, (4) blood parameters, and (5) tissue oxygen consumption.

In this model, the net oxygen consumption by the alveoli (VO_2) is a function of F_IO_2, a fraction of expired oxygen (F_EO_2), respiratory frequency (f), tidal volume (V_T), and dead space volume (V_D). The V_D is the amount of air inspired into the lung

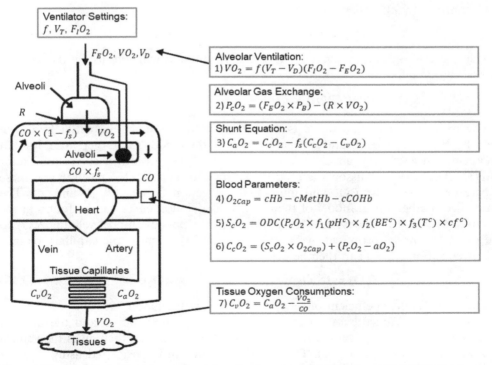

Figure 9.15. Gas exchange model reproduced from Sundaresan *et al* (2010). Copyright © 2011, Sundaresan *et al*; licensee BioMed Central Ltd.

that does not reach the alveoli, and it does not contribute to the gas exchange process. The net oxygen consumption is given by:

$$VO_2 = f(V_T - V_D)(F_IO_2 - F_EO_2). \tag{9.13}$$

Once the inspired air enters the alveolar compartments, the diffusion process begins. The oxygen diffuses across the alveolar membrane and enters the alveolar capillaries. The capillary partial pressure of oxygen (P_cO_2) is a function of the alveoli partial pressure, which is a function of the atmospheric pressure (P_B), minus the drop in partial pressure due to diffusion resistance (R). The P_cO_2 can be written as:

$$P_cO_2 = (F_EO_2 \times P_B) - (R \times VO_2). \tag{9.14}$$

After the oxygen has diffused into the alveolar capillaries through the alveolar wall, the high concentration of oxygen in the capillaries (C_cO_2) mixes with oxygen in the venous blood, which has a lower concentration (C_vO_2). The arterial oxygen concentration (C_aO_2) can then be evaluated, and it depends on the level of pulmonary shunt (f_s) using the following equation:

$$C_aO_2 = C_cO_2 - f_s(C_cO_2 - C_vO_2). \tag{9.15}$$

Next, the haemoglobin oxygen-carrying capacity (O_{2CAP}) is a function of blood parameters such as haemoglobin (cHb), methaemoglobin ($cMetHb$) and carboxyhaemoglobin ($cCOHb$), such that:

$$O_{2CAP} = cHb - cMetHb - cCOHb. \tag{9.16}$$

The oxygen saturation curve (S_cO_2) can then be calculated using the oxygen dissociation curve:

$$S_cO_2 = ODC(P_cO_2) \times f_1(pH^c) \times f_2(BE^c) \times f_3(T^c) \times cf^c. \tag{9.17}$$

The oxygen dissociation curve is a function of the capillary potential hydrogen (pH^c), base excess (BE^c) and the temperature of the blood (T^c). Other variables that can influence the oxygen dissociation curve are grouped into a correction factor (cf^c). The oxygen dissociation curve is then calculated by multiplying these parameters with the P_cO_2 and individual correction factors (f_1, f_2 and f_3). The detailed mathematical model of the oxygen dissociation curve can be found in the works by Siggard-Andersen et al (1984). Another possible model relating S_cO_2 to P_cO_2 is the model proposed by Severinghaus (1979). Finally, the capillary oxygen concentration (C_cO_2) can then be defined as:

$$C_cO_2 = (S_cO_2 \times O_{2CAP}) + (P_cO_2 \times \alpha O_2), \tag{9.18}$$

where αO_2 is the coefficient of oxygen solubility in the blood.

The net difference between the arterial oxygen concentration and the drop in oxygen consumption over cardiac output (CO) by the tissues then gives the venous oxygen concentration (C_vO_2). The cardiac output can be measured using thermodilution techniques (which will be explained in chapter 10), but it can also be estimated using (Andreassen et al 1996):

$$C_vO_2 = C_aO_2 - \frac{VO_2}{CO}. \tag{9.19}$$

To apply this model, firstly, the model requires a gas exchange analyser to measure the F_IO_2 and F_EO_2. Then, the S_aO_2 is estimated using the pulse oximeter. Respiratory frequency, f and tidal volume V_T are set in the ventilator, while the haemoglobin concentrations are measured by taking a blood sample. Using these measurements and an estimate of dead space, it is then possible to calculate shunt and diffusion resistance by solving equations (9.13)–(9.19).

9.4 Application of respiratory system models

9.4.1 Mechanical ventilation monitoring

Critically ill respiratory failure patients are typically admitted to the hospital intensive care for mechanical ventilation treatment. The patient vital signs are closely monitored 24 h a day as this information is necessary for clinical decision-making. Some essential clinical measurements are performed on the patient to understand the lung condition. For example, lung imaging such as x-rays, CT-scans are used for inspection of the lungs and help diagnose cancer, a build-up of fluids, or fibrosis (scar tissue). Other measurements, such as arterial blood gases, can provide information on the oxygenation level and carbon dioxide removal.

While the abovementioned measurements are helpful, some are not typically available in hospital intensive care due to invasive procedures, treatment disruptions and high costs. For example, a computerised tomography (CT) scan is regarded as the gold standard for understanding and treating respiratory failure patients. However, performing CT imaging for these patients is largely impractical. It is a costly and over-demanded hospital resource and exposes the patient to a further risk of lung injury (Pesenti et al 2001). Electrical impedance tomography is a non-invasive tool and has demonstrated a good correlation with CT findings (Zhao et al 2010). However, the limited availability of the EIT technology along with high cost and lack of trained personnel remain the main issues against its widespread application. Another imaging technique, using lung ultrasound for immediate patient bedside therapeutic decisions, requires mastery of its operation techniques (Lichtenstein 2014).

Hence, model-based research focuses on using bedside available clinical data to aid model-based method development and its application. Table 9.3 shows a list of measurements commonly used in model-based respiratory research. These measurements can be used together with respiratory system models to provide unique descriptions of the subject's disease progression and response to different mechanical ventilation treatments and drug therapies. Such data can give recommendations to the clinician to guide mechanical ventilation treatment and decision-making in real-time.

Table 9.3. Physiological measurements of the respiratory system.

Measurements	Measurement Device	Descriptions
Mechanical ventilation airway pressure, flow and other ventilatory parameters	Mechanical ventilator or other pressure or flow pneumotachometer	• Airway pressure is the pressure supplied to the patient during mechanical ventilation treatment. It reflects the airway pressure (P_{aw}) experienced by the whole respiratory system • Airway flow ($\dot{V}$) is the flow of air entering the patient's lung during mechanical ventilation. • Fraction of inspired oxygen (F_IO_2), breathing frequency (f), positive end-expiratory pressure (PEEP)
Oesophageal pressure	Oesophageal balloon catheter	• Oesophageal pressure (P_{eo}) is the pressure change within the mechanical ventilated patient pleural space. It is used to estimate patients breathing effort
Electrical diaphragmatic activity	Electrical diaphragmatic activity catheter	• It is a catheter inserted into the oesophageal tract to measure the diaphragm electrical signal. • This electrical signal represents the patients breathing demand and is used for signalling the ventilation triggering.
Arterial blood gases	Blood gas analyser	• Partial pressure of the arterial blood oxygen (P_aO_2)—is a measurement of oxygen pressure in arterial blood. • It is an indication of how well oxygen is able to move from the lungs to the blood. • Partial pressure of the arterial blood carbon dioxide (P_aCO_2)—an indicator of CO_2 production and removal • Oxygen saturation (S_aO_2)—the fraction of oxygen-saturated haemoglobin relative to total haemoglobin in the blood.
Peripheral oxygen saturation (SpO_2)	Pulse oximeter	• It is a continuous and non-invasive estimate of blood oxygen saturation.
End-tidal CO_2	Capnography devices	• End-tidal carbon dioxide ($ETCO_2$) is the level of CO_2 that is released at the end of expiration. $ETCO_2$ levels reflect the amount of CO_2 carried in the blood back to the lung and exhaled.
Cardiac outputs (CO)	Thermodilution method	• CO measurement is defined as the amount of blood (in litres) pumped by the heart in minutes.

9.4.2 Determining respiratory mechanics

9.4.2.1 Single-compartment model

One of the most clinically used respiratory models is none other than in its simplest form, the single-compartment lung model. Continuous airway pressure and flow data of the mechanically ventilated patient are used as the input for the single-compartment model to estimate the patient's respiratory mechanics. Specifically, respiratory system elastance (E_{rs}) is the reciprocal of compliance ($E_{rs} = 1/C_{rs}$), where it is a measure of the pressure required to inflate the lungs and airway resistance, R_{rs} is the resistance of the airway during ventilation. E_{rs} has been found to be higher in respiratory failure patients with moderate or severe respiratory failure when compared to those with healthy lungs. Similarly, R_{rs} is also much higher in subjects with COPD than those with normal lung and ARDS. Thus, identifying the values of respiratory mechanics can help diagnose a patient condition.

During mechanical ventilation, E_{rs} can be determined using an end-of-inspiratory pause method. The ventilator is first set in volume control mode to deliver a square flow profile with a set tidal volume (V_T). An end of inspiratory pause can be used to pause ventilation to obtain the plateau pressure (P_{plat}), which reflects the alveolar pressure experienced by the patient's lung. This P_{plat} can then be used to compute the (R_{rs}) and the elastance (E_{rs}) of the respiratory system. Figure 9.16 shows a sample of airway pressure with an end-of-inspiratory pause.

From the single-compartment model in equation (9.4), at the end-of-inspiratory pause, we can assume the $V(t) = V_T$, $P_{aw}(t) = P_{plat}$, P_0 can be assumed as set PEEP in the ventilator, and the $\dot{V}$ is zero as there is no flow involved. Equation (9.4) can be rewritten as:

$$P_{plat} = 0 + E_{rs}V_T + \text{PEEP}, \qquad (9.20)$$

$$E_{rs} = \frac{P_{plat} - \text{PEEP}}{V_T}. \qquad (9.21)$$

Similarly, with the end-of-inspiratory pause, the respiratory system resistance (R_{rs}) can be determined using the following equation:

$$R_{rs} = \frac{PIP - P_{plat}}{\dot{V}}. \qquad (9.22)$$

The peak inspiratory pressure is the maximum observed airway pressure, $PIP = \max(P_{aw}(t))$ and $\dot{V}$ is the maximum flow of the square flow profile.

The respiratory system E_{rs} and R_s can be determined using the end-of-inspiratory pause method. However, this method disrupts the routine ventilation treatment, and thus, it is not used regularly. The model-based method enables the respiratory system mechanics to be determined noninvasively without disrupting the ventilation treatment. The single-compartment model, with $P_{aw}(t)$ and $V(t)$ as input, can be rearranged to obtain the E_{rs} and R_s using the multiple linear regression method introduced in chapter 7. First, the air volume can be obtained through the integration of the $V(t)$ with time as shown below:

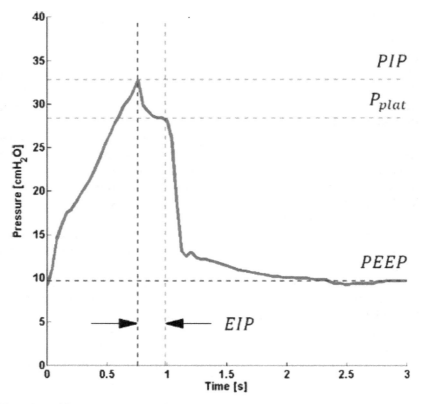

Figure 9.16. Airway pressure data with a short end of inspiratory pause (EIP) to obtain P_{plat}.

$$V(t) = \int_{t_0}^{t_f} \dot{V}(t)dt, \qquad (9.23)$$

where t_0 is the start of a breathing cycle and t_f is the end of the breathing cycle. We can assume that there is no intrinsic pressure, and P_0 can assume as the pressure value of PEEP. Thus, given $P_{\text{aw}}(t)$, PEEP, $\dot{V}(t)$ and $V(t)$ as the input, we can rearrange the single-compartment model to solve for R_{rs} and E_{rs} such that:

$$\begin{bmatrix} P_{\text{aw}}(t_1) \\ P_{\text{aw}}(t_2) \\ \vdots \\ P_{\text{aw}}(t_f) \end{bmatrix} = R_{\text{rs}} \begin{bmatrix} \dot{V}(t_1) \\ \dot{V}(t_2) \\ \vdots \\ \dot{V}(t_f) \end{bmatrix} + E_{\text{rs}} \begin{bmatrix} V(t_1) \\ V(t_2) \\ \vdots \\ V(t_f) \end{bmatrix} + \text{PEEP}, \qquad (9.24)$$

which can be rearranged to give:

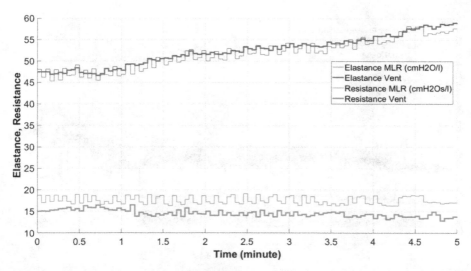

Figure 9.17. Comparison between respiratory mechanics estimated using multiple linear regression (MLR) method and ventilator end-of-inspiratory pause (Vent).

$$\begin{bmatrix} \dot{V}(t_1) & V(t_1) \\ \dot{V}(t_2) & V(t_2) \\ \vdots & \vdots \\ \dot{V}(t_f) & V(t_f) \end{bmatrix} \begin{bmatrix} R_{rs} \\ E_{rs} \end{bmatrix} = \begin{bmatrix} P_{aw}(t_1) - \text{PEEP} \\ P_{aw}(t_2) - \text{PEEP} \\ \vdots \\ P_{aw}(t_f) - \text{PEEP} \end{bmatrix}. \qquad (9.25)$$

Assuming that:

$$A = \begin{bmatrix} \dot{V}(t_1) & V(t_1) \\ \dot{V}(t_2) & V(t_2) \\ \vdots & \vdots \\ \dot{V}(t_f) & V(t_f) \end{bmatrix}, \quad \theta = \begin{bmatrix} R_{rs} \\ E_{rs} \end{bmatrix}, \quad b = \begin{bmatrix} P_{aw}(t_1) - \text{PEEP} \\ P_{aw}(t_2) - \text{PEEP} \\ \vdots \\ P_{aw}(t_f) - \text{PEEP} \end{bmatrix}, \qquad (9.26)$$

and if $A\theta = b$, we can solve R_{rs} and E_{rs} using:

$$\theta = (A^T A)^{-1} A^T b. \qquad (9.27)$$

The parameters R_{rs} and E_{rs} can thus be estimated via multiple linear regression without a need for disruptive measurements. A 5 min sample analysis of respiratory system mechanics calculated using multiple linear regression compared to an automated end-inspiratory pause is shown in figure 9.17. The sample Matlab code can be found together with chapter 9.[2]

---

[2] Source code for this model (Chapter09b) is available at https://doi.org/10.1088/978-0-7503-4016-8.

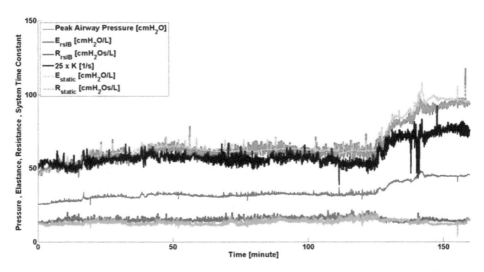

Figure 9.18. Continuous monitoring of respiratory parameters for an ARDS animal experiment adapted from van Drunen *et al* (2013). Copyright © 2013, van Drunen *et al*; licensee BioMed Central Ltd. E_{rsIB} and R_{sIB} are elastance and resistance obtained using regression, K is time constant, E_{static} and R_{static} are elastance and resistance from ventilator end-of-inspiratory pause. At the start of the experiment, at zero minute, a healthy animal is injected with oleic acid and slowly develops respiratory failure.

From figure 9.17, it can be seen the respiratory mechanics estimated using multiple linear regression yield very similar values to the values calculated using the ventilator end-of-inspiratory pause method. The difference between the two methods is likely due to insufficient time for the automated end-of-inspiratory pause. A longer end-of-inspiratory pause allows dynamic airway pressure dissipation and the pressure to reach static elastic equilibrium (Barberis *et al* 2003).

In the works by van Drunen *et al* (2013), they monitored breath-by-breath E_{rs} and R_{rs} continuously using a model-based method in experimental ARDS animal trials. They found that the E_{rs} and R_{rs} obtained using multiple linear regression results in similar E_{rs} and R_{rs} values when using a short end-of-inspiratory pause. In addition, they found that the E_{rs} were low when the animal's respiratory system was healthy. As experimentally induced ARDS begins to take place in the animal, the E_{rs} also increases as shown in figure 9.18. Their work suggested that continuous monitoring of respiratory mechanics of a mechanically ventilated patient can help with understanding the disease progression and how they respond to treatment.

In other studies, mechanically ventilated patients' respiratory elastance during PEEP titration has been monitored. These studies found that these elastances can be used to guide the selection of PEEP (Lambermont *et al* 2008, Carvalho *et al* 2007). These observations have also led to clinical trials investigating the feasibility of PEEP selection using respiratory system elastance (Pintado *et al* 2013).

Recently, Goligher *et al* (2021) also found that respiratory elastance plays a role in mechanically ventilated respiratory failure patients' mortality. Overall, these works have highlighted that determining the respiratory mechanics of mechanically ventilated respiratory failure patients, either through conventional methods or model-based methods, can be useful in improving mechanical ventilation treatment.

9.4.2.2 Viscoelastic model

The multiple linear regression method has also been used to solve more complex respiratory mechanics models, such as the viscoelastic model. Prior to inverse simulation on mechanical ventilation airway pressure and flow data, it is essential to ensure that the measured data (input to the model) contains information on the lung viscoelasticity. A typical mechanical ventilation airway pressure and flow waveform data may not be sufficient to estimate the viscoelastic model parameters E_1, E_2, R_1 and R_2. A specialised mechanical ventilation protocol is required, such as the end-of-inspiratory pause during square wave volume control mode (Ganzert *et al* 2009, Schranz *et al* 2012a).

Figure 9.19 shows a sample of simulated airway pressure and flow profile from a viscoelastic model with an end of inspiratory pause from one to four seconds to allow dynamic airway pressure dissipation elastic equilibrium.

If we wish to perform inverse simulation, equation (9.7) can be rearranged so that the left-hand side of the equation is left with $\dot{P}_{aw}(t)$, such that:

$$\dot{P}_{aw}(t) = \frac{-E_2}{R_2}P_{aw}(t) + R_2\ddot{V}(t) + \frac{(R_2E_1 + E_2R_1 + E_2R_2)}{R_2}\dot{V}(t) + \frac{E_1E_2}{R_2}V(t). \quad (9.28)$$

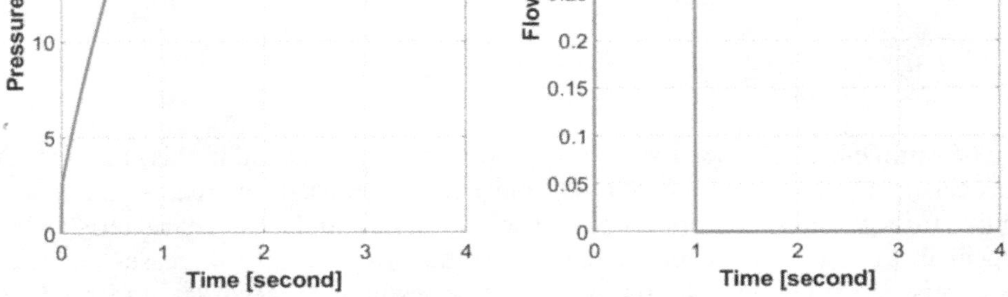

Figure 9.19. Airway pressure and flow data in a viscoelastic model. The parameters for the viscoelastic models are $E_1 = 25$ cmH$_2$O/l, $E_2 = 10$ cmH$_2$O/l, $R_1 = 15$ cmH$_2$Os/l, and $R_2 = 5$ cmH$_2$Os/l.

Equation (9.28) can then be integrated to yield:

$$\int_{t_0}^{t_e} \dot{P}_{aw}(t)dt = \frac{-E_2}{R_2} \int_{t_0}^{t_e} P_{aw}(t)dt + R_2 \int_{t_0}^{t_e} \ddot{V}(t)dt + \frac{(R_2 E_1 + E_2 R_1 + E_2 R_2)}{R_2}$$

$$\int_{t_0}^{t_e} \dot{V}(t)dt + \frac{E_1 E_2}{R_2} \int_{t_0}^{t_e} V(t)dt, \tag{9.29}$$

where t_0 is the start of the breathing cycle, and t_e is the end of the inspiratory pause. Rearranging the model in the matrix form results in:

$$P_{aw}(t) = \frac{-E_2}{R_2} \int_{t_0}^{t_e} P_{aw}(t)dt + R_2 \dot{V}(t) + \frac{(R_2 E_1 + E_2 R_1 + E_2 R_2)}{R_2} V(t) + \frac{E_1 E_2}{R_2} \int_{t_0}^{t_e} V(t)dt \tag{9.30}$$

$$\begin{bmatrix} P_{aw}(t_1) \\ P_{aw}(t_2) \\ \vdots \\ P_{aw}(t_e) \end{bmatrix} = \begin{bmatrix} \int_{t_0}^{t_1} P_{aw}(t_1)dt & \dot{V}(t_1) & V(t_1) & \int_{t_0}^{t_1} V(t_1)dt \\ \int_{t_0}^{t_2} P_{aw}(t_2)dt & \dot{V}(t_2) & V(t_2) & \int_{t_0}^{t_2} V(t_2)dt \\ \vdots & \vdots & \vdots & \vdots \\ \int_{t_0}^{t_e} P_{aw}(t_e)dt & \dot{V}(t_e) & V(t_e) & \int_{t_0}^{t_e} V(t_e)dt \end{bmatrix} \begin{bmatrix} A \\ B \\ C \\ D \end{bmatrix}, \tag{9.31}$$

where

$$A = \frac{-E_2}{R_2},$$

$$B = R_2,$$

$$C = \frac{(R_2 E_1 + E_2 R_1 + E_2 R_2)}{R_2}, \tag{9.32}$$

$$D = \frac{E_1 E_2}{R_2}.$$

The sample Matlab code for the above solution can be found in this chapter[3]. The viscoelastic model has increased parameters, and thus, it increases the model's ability to accurately capture all the airway pressure and flow characteristics that appear in the data. However, increased parameterisation also increases parameter trade-offs and potentially limits the parameter estimation accuracy and predictive

---

[3] Source code for this model (Chapter09c) is available at https://doi.org/10.1088/978-0-7503-4016-8.

capability of the model. Studies also found that different parameter identification approaches yielded different results affecting the accuracy of identified parameters (Schranz *et al* 2012a). Thus, it is important to ensure respiratory models are defined using physical measurements during conditions indicative of conditions induced by therapy.

9.4.3 Decision support system

9.4.3.1 Monitoring recruitment

During mechanical ventilation, the use of PEEP has been identified as a key ventilation parameter when treating ARDS patients. The objective of PEEP is to increase the level of oxygenation by increasing the number of recruited alveoli retained at a pressure higher than atmospheric pressure at the end of expiration. However, PEEP comes with risks of causing ventilation-induced lung injury (VILI) if an inappropriate PEEP is set. For example, higher PEEP recruits more alveoli but risks injuring healthy alveoli, whereas lower PEEP levels could cause cyclic opening and closing of alveoli, damaging them. Despite a considerable amount of research to evaluate the benefit of different PEEP levels, the level of appropriate PEEP over a given cohort has never been properly established.

To tackle this issue, the patient-specific static-compliance curves have been used to aid PEEP selection. For example, research has been conducted with the Venegas function model to identify the pressure at LIP and UIP. The locations of LIP and UIP provided a guideline for clinicians to set PEEP (Albaiceta *et al* 2008), where PEEP should be set at a pressure level between LIP and UIP. Patient-specific static-compliance curves have also been used for the recruitment models. The recruitment models enabled an estimation of the threshold pressure based on performing a model fitting the static-compliance curve to a Gaussian distribution curve, such as in figure 9.20. This Gaussian distribution mean represents the average of all lung units opening pressure, and the standard deviation (SD) represents the spread of the distribution. If a ventilation pressure is above this mean value, more than 50% of the lung units are opened (Hickling 1998, Sundaresan *et al* 2009).

In figure 9.21, the change in the mean and standard deviation of the recruitment model helps to capture the changes in the patient-specific static-compliance curve. As shown in figure 9.21 (left), an increase in mean with the same SD indicates a lung with higher lung units opening pressure. For a lung with both a higher mean and standard deviation, this indicates a more heterogeneous lung with a wide range of opening pressure (Chiew *et al* 2012).

These models, along with patient-specific static-compliance curves have provided unique insight into the patient's lung condition. However, they are not being practised clinically due to the challenges in obtaining a static-compliance curve. In particular, getting a static or quasi-static pressure–volume curve is difficult as they interrupt mechanical ventilation treatment routine. A static pressure–volume curve cannot be obtained via tidal ventilation. They required a specialised manoeuvre,

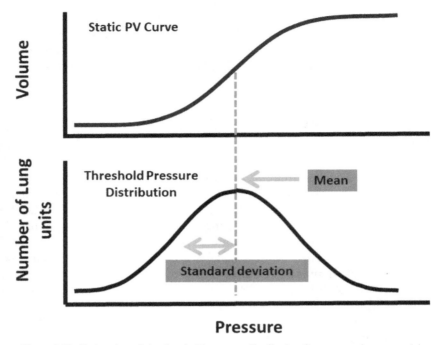

Figure 9.20. Estimation of the threshold pressure distribution from a recruitment model.

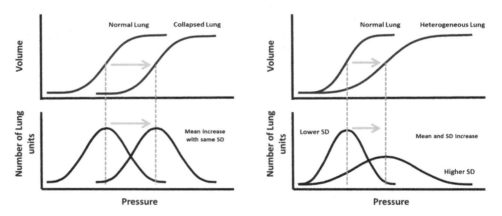

Figure 9.21. Effects of the mean and standard deviation (SD) of the recruitment model to signify different lung conditions. Adapted from Chiew *et al* (2012). Copyright © 2012, Chiew *et al*; licensee BioMed Central Ltd.

such as the super-syringe method (Janney 1959), inspiration occlusion (Ranieri *et al* 1994), or quasi-static low-flow ventilation (Schranz *et al* 2012b). These methods interrupt routine mechanical ventilation treatment and are thus not generally performed for mechanically ventilated patients.

9.4.3.2 Gas exchange and combined models

The pulmonary gas exchange model or other updated variations have been used extensively in the clinical environment. Specifically, the gas exchange model has been used as a non-invasive estimation of pulmonary gas exchange parameters. It has provided insight into the patient's gas exchange abnormalities due to heterogeneous diffusion and perfusion as well as clinical decision-making. Sundaresan *et al* (2010) incorporated the gas exchange model into a lung recruitment model to help in estimating cardiac output noninvasively. They have assessed the impact of mechanical ventilation PEEP on cardiac output, and it can potentially be used to assist in mechanical ventilation PEEP selection with respect to gas exchange and oxygenation. The model proposed by Andreassen *et al* (1996) has also been extended and implemented in clinical decision support systems (Rees *et al* 2002, 2022, Rees 2011). Further studies have also been carried out to develop a state-of-the-art mechanical ventilator for breathing support.

Das and Bates *et al* have developed a computer simulation model of lung pathophysiology. The model has been used to provide physiological information on the risk of ventilator-associated lung injury (Das *et al* 2013). They have also used the lung simulator model to evaluate a clinical protocol for recruitment manoeuvres in ARDS patients (Das *et al* 2015). In a more recent study, Scott *et al* (2020) presented a lung injury simulator that can accurately model the mechanism of a blast lung injury seen in military conflict. Overall, these models can be used to compute multiple scenarios to improve the understanding of the physiological process and investigate the effect of medical interventions during mechanical ventilation treatment.

Finally, while not covered in this chapter, there is also gas exchange modelling research into a different method of ventilation, such as modelling the extracorporeal membrane oxygenation (ECMO) (Zanella *et al* 2016). The model describes the ECMO machine's connection to the patients via their arteries and veins. The patient's blood is pumped from the body to an oxygenator that adds oxygen and removes carbon dioxide from the blood. The ECMO machine then pumps the blood back to the patient. Mathematical modelling of ECMO is found to be a useful teaching tool and a valuable decision-making aid for the management of this ventilation method that replaces the heart and lung functions.

9.5 Summary

In summary, various respiratory system models have been developed to provide a better understanding of respiratory failure patients' lung physiology and to guide mechanical ventilation treatment. Continuous data can be obtained from mechanically ventilated patients, and identification of respiratory mechanics can be performed in intensive care without disruption using model-based approaches. Ultimately, a correct selection of a suitable respiratory model and bedside parameters to monitor and interpret the model-based analysis is crucial for safe clinical decision-making in managing mechanical ventilation treatment for respiratory failure patients.

References

Albaiceta G M, Blanch L and Lucangelo U 2008 Static pressure–volume curves of the respiratory system: were they just a passing fad? *Curr. Opin. Crit. Care* **14** 80–6

Amato M B P *et al* 2015 Driving pressure and survival in the acute respiratory distress syndrome *New Engl. J. Med.* **372** 747–55

Andreassen S, Egeberg J, Schröter M P and Andersen P T 1996 Estimation of pulmonary diffusion resistance and shunt in an oxygen status model *Comput. Meth. Prog. Biomed.* **51** 95–105

Ashbaugh D, Boyd D, Petty T and Levine B 1967 Acute respiratory distress in adults *Lancet* **290** 319–23

Barberis L, Manno E and Guérin C 2003 Effect of end-inspiratory pause duration on plateau pressure in mechanically ventilated patients *Intensive Care Med.* **29** 130–4

Bates J H T 2009 *Lung Mechanics: An Inverse Modeling Approach* (New York: Cambridge University Press)

Bernard G R, Artigas A, Brigham K L, Carlet J, Falke K, Hudson L, Lamy M, Legall J R, Morris A and Spragg R 1994 Report of the American–European consensus conference on ARDS: definitions, mechanisms, relevant outcomes and clinical trial coordination *Intensive Care Med.* **20** 225–32

Briel M *et al* 2010 Higher vs lower positive end-expiratory pressure in patients with acute lung injury and acute respiratory distress syndrome: systematic review and meta-analysis *JAMA* **303** 865–73

Brower R G, Lanken P N, Macintyre N, Matthiay M A, Morris A, Ancukiewicz M, Schoenfeld D and Thompson B T 2004 Higher versus lower positive end-expiratory pressures in patients with the acute respiratory distress syndrome *N. Engl. J. Med.* **351** 327–36

Carvalho A, Jandre F, Pino A, Bozza F, Salluh J, Rodrigues R, Ascoli F and Giannela-Neto A 2007 Positive end-expiratory pressure at minimal respiratory elastance represents the best compromise between mechanical stress and lung aeration in oleic acid induced lung injury *Crit., Care* **11** R86

Chiew Y S, Chase J G, Lambermont B, Janssen N, Schranz C, Moeller K, Shaw G and Desaive T 2012 Physiological relevance and performance of a minimal lung model—an experimental study in healthy and acute respiratory distress syndrome model piglets *BMC Pulm. Med.* **12** 59

Chiew Y S, Pretty C, Docherty P D, Lambermont B, Shaw G M, Desaive T and Chase J G 2015 Time-varying respiratory system elastance: a physiological model for patients who are spontaneously breathing *PLoS One* **10** e0114847

Das A, Cole O, Chikhani M, Wang W, Ali T, Haque M, Bates D and Hardman J 2015 Evaluation of lung recruitment maneuvers in acute respiratory distress syndrome using computer simulation *Crit. Care* **19** 8

Das A, Menon P P, Hardman J G and Bates D G 2013 Optimisation of mechanical ventilator settings for pulmonary disease states *IEEE Trans. Biomed. Eng.* **60** 1599–607

Dasta J F, Mclaughlin T P, Mody S H and Piech C T 2005 Daily cost of an intensive care unit day: the contribution of mechanical ventilation *Crit. Care Med.* **33** 1266–71

Docherty P D, Schranz C, Chiew Y S, Möller K and Chase J G 2014 Reformulation of the pressure-dependent recruitment model (PRM) of respiratory mechanics *Biomed. Signal Process. Control* **12** 47–53

Esteban A *et al* 2002 Characteristics and outcomes in adult patients receiving mechanical ventilation: a 28-day international study *JAMA* **287** 345–55

Ferguson N D *et al* 2005 Airway pressures, tidal volumes, and mortality in patients with acute respiratory distress syndrome *Crit. Care Med.* **33** 21–30

Ferring M and Vincent J L 1997 Is outcome from ARDS related to the severity of respiratory failure? *Eur. Respir. J.* **10** 1297–300

Ganzert S, Moller K, Steinmann D, Schumann S and Guttmann J 2009 Pressure-dependent stress relaxation in acute respiratory distress syndrome and healthy lungs: an investigation based on a viscoelastic model *Crit. Care* **13** R199

Gattinoni L, Caironi P, Valenza F and Carlesso E 2006 The role of CT-scan studies for the diagnosis and therapy of acute respiratory distress syndrome *Clin. Chest Med.* **27** 559–70

Gattinoni L, Marini J J, Collino F, Maiolo G, Rapetti F, Tonetti T, Vasques F and Quintel M 2017 The future of mechanical ventilation: lessons from the present and the past *Crit. Care* **21** 183

Girard T D and Bernard G R 2007 Mechanical ventilation in ARDS *Chest* **131** 921–9

Goligher E C, Costa E L V, Yarnell C J, Brochard L J, Steward T E, Tomlinson G, Brower R G, Slutsky A S and Amato M P B 2021 Effect of lowering vt on mortality in acute respiratory distress syndrome varies with respiratory system elastance *Am. J. Respir. Crit. Care Med.* **203** 1378–85

Hasan A 2010 *Understanding Mechanical Ventilation: A Practical Handbook* (London: Springer)

Hickling K G 1998 The pressure–volume curve is greatly modified by recruitment. A mathematical model of ARDS lungs *Am. J. Respir. Crit. Care Med.* **158** 194–202

Janney C D 1959 Super-syringe *Anesthesiology* **20** 709–11

Kaier K, Heister T, Wolff J and Wolkewitz M 2020 Mechanical ventilation and the daily cost of ICU care *BMC Health Serv. Res.* **20** 267

Kollef M H and Schuster D P 1995 The acute respiratory distress syndrome *New Engl. J. Med.* **332** 27–37

Lambermont B, Ghuysen A, Janssen N, Morimont P, Hartstein G, Gerard P and D'orio V 2008 Comparison of functional residual capacity and static compliance of the respiratory system during a positive end-expiratory pressure (PEEP) ramp procedure in an experimental model of acute respiratory distress syndrome *Crit. Care* **12** R91

Lichtenstein D A 2014 Lung ultrasound in the critically ill *Ann. Intensive Care* **4** 1

Major V J, Chiew Y S, Shaw G M and Chase J G 2018 Biomedical engineer's guide to the clinical aspects of intensive care mechanical ventilation *Biomed. Eng. Online* **17** 169

Mercat A *et al* 2008 positive end-expiratory pressure setting in adults with acute lung injury and acute respiratory distress syndrome: a randomized controlled trial *JAMA* **299** 646–55

Mortelliti M P and Manning H L 2002 Acute respiratory distress syndrome *Am. Fam. Physician* **65** 1823–30

Pelosi P *et al* 2021 Personalised mechanical ventilation in acute respiratory distress syndrome *Crit. Care,* **25** 250

Pesenti A, Tagliabue P, Patroniti N and Fumagalli R *et al* 2001 Computerised tomography scan imaging in acute respiratory distress syndrome *Intens. Care Med.* **27** 631–9

Phua J *et al* 2009 Has mortality from acute respiratory distress syndrome decreased over time? A systematic review *Am. J. Respir. Crit. Care Med.* **179** 20–227

Pintado M-C, De Pablo R, Trascasa M, Milicua J-M, Rogero S, Daguerre M, Cambronero J-A, Arribas I and Sánchez-García M 2013 Individualized PEEP setting in subjects with ARDS: a randomized controlled pilot study *Respir. Care* **58** 1416–23

Ranieri V M, Giuliani R, Fiore T, Dambrosio M and Milic-Emili J 1994 Volume–pressure curve of the respiratory system predicts effects of PEEP in ARDS: 'occlusion' versus 'constant flow' technique *Am. J. Respir. Crit. Care Med.* **149** 19–27

Redmond D, Chiew Y S, Major V and Chase J G 2019 Evaluation of model-based methods in estimating respiratory mechanics in the presence of variable patient effort *Comput. Meth. Prog. Biomed.* **171** 67–79

Rees S E 2011 The Intelligent Ventilator (INVENT) project: the role of mathematical models in translating physiological knowledge into clinical practice *Comput. Meth. Prog. Biomed.* **104** S1–29

Rees S E, Kjærgaard S, Thorgaard P, Malczynski J, Toft E and Andreassen S 2002 The automatic lung parameter estimator (ALPE) system: non-invasive estimation of pulmonary gas exchange parameters in 10–15 minutes *J. Clin. Monit. Comput.* **17** 43–52

Rees S E, Spadaro S, Dalla Corte F, Dey N, Brohus J B, Scaramuzzo G, Lodahl D, Winding R R, Volta C A and Karbing D S 2022 Transparent decision support for mechanical ventilation using visualisation of clinical preferences *Biomed. Eng. Online* **21** 5

Mason R J, Broaddus V C, Martin T R, King T E, Schraunfagel D E, Murray J F and Nadel J A 2010 *Murray and Nadel's Textbook of Respiratory Medicine* (New York: Elsevier)

Rouby J J, Contantin J M, Girardi C, Zhang M and Qin L 2004 Mechanical ventilation in patients with acute respiratory distress syndrome *Anesthesiology* **101** 228–34

Schiller H J, Steingberg J, Halter J, McCann U, Dasilva M, Gatto L A, Carney D and Nieman G 2003 Alveolar inflation during generation of a quasi-static pressure/volume curve in the acutely injured lung *Crit. Care Med.* **31** 1126–33

Schranz C, Docherty P, Chiew Y S, Moller K and Chase J G 2012a Iterative integral parameter identification of a respiratory mechanics model *Biomed. Eng. Online* **11** 38

Schranz C, Docherty P, Chiew Y S, Chase J G and Moller K 2012b Structural identifiability and practical applicability of an alveolar recruitment model for ARDS patients *IEEE Trans. Biomed. Eng.* **59** 3396–404

Scott T E, Das A, Haque M, Bates D G and Hardman J G 2020 Management of primary blast lung injury: a comparison of airway pressure release versus low tidal volume ventilation *Intensive Care Med. Exp.* **8** 26

Severinghaus J W 1979 Simple, accurate equations for human blood O_2 dissociation computations *J. Appl. Physiol.* **46** 599–602

Siggard-Andersen O, Wimberley P D, Göthgen I and Siggard-Andersen M 1984 A mathematical model of the hemoglobin–oxygen dissociation curve of human blood and of the oxygen partial pressure as a function of temperature *Clin. Chem.* **30** 1646–51

Sundaresan A, Chase J, Hann C and Shaw G 2010 Cardiac output estimation using pulmonary mechanics in mechanically ventilated patients *Biomed. Eng. Online* **9** 80

Sundaresan A, Yuta T, Hann C E, Chase J and Shaw G M 2009 A minimal model of lung mechanics and model-based markers for optimising ventilator treatment in ARDS patients *Comput. Meth. Prog. Biomed.* **95** 166–80

Sundaresan A, Chase J, Shaw G M, Chiew Y S and Desaive T 2011 Model-based optimal PEEP in mechanically ventilated ARDS patients in the intensive care unit *Biomed. Eng. Online* **10** 64

The Acute Respiratory Distress Syndrome Network 2000 Ventilation with lower tidal volumes as compared with traditional tidal volumes for acute lung injury and the acute respiratory distress syndrome *N. Engl. J. Med.* **342** 1301–8

The ARDS Definition Task Force 2012 Acute respiratory distress syndrome: the berlin definition *JAMA* **307** 2526–33

van Drunen E, Chiew Y S, Chase J, Shaw G, Lambermont B, Janssen N, Damanhuri N and Desaive T 2013 Expiratory model-based method to monitor ARDS disease state *Biomed. Eng. Online* **12** 57

Venegas J G, Harris R S and SIMON B A 1998 A comprehensive equation for the pulmonary pressure–volume curve *J. Appl. Physiol.* **84** 389–95

Vicario F, Albanese A, Karamolegkos N, Wang D, Seiver A and Chbat N W 2015 Noninvasive estimation of respiratory mechanics in spontaneously breathing ventilated patients: a constrained optimisation approach *IEEE Trans. Biomed. Eng.* **63** 775–87

Ware L B and Matthay M A 2000 The acute respiratory distress syndrome *N. Engl. J. Med.* **342** 1334–49

Zambon M and Vincent J-L 2008 Mortality rates for patients with acute lung injury/ARDS have decreased over time *Chest* **133** 1120–27

Zanella A *et al* 2016 A mathematical model of oxygenation during venovenous extracorporeal membrane oxygenation support *J. Crit. Care* **36** 178–86

Zhao Z, Steinmann D, Frerichs I, Guttmann J and Moller K *et al* 2010 titration guided by ventilation homogeneity: a feasibility study using electrical impedance tomography *Crit. Care* **14** R8

Chapter 10

Cardiovascular system

10.1 The human cardiovascular system

Cardiovascular disease is the leading cause of death globally (Roth *et al* 2020). With an estimated 17.9 million people dying from this disease, it represents 32% of all global deaths in the year 2019. Cardiovascular disease appears to be more prevalent at advanced ages. However, it can develop at younger ages, leading to premature deaths. Thus, cardiovascular disease has an enormous impact on the socio-economics of the country. Not only does it affect the burden on healthcare systems, but it also significantly impacts the patients' quality of life, their productivity and that of their informal caregivers. Thus, it is important to understand cardiovascular system functions. In this chapter, we will learn more about the human cardiovascular system, understand the physiology and how to model the human cardiovascular system.

The human cardiovascular system is a complex system involving hydraulic interactions, nervous system responses and other biological influences. The cardiovascular system consists of three interrelated components, the blood, the heart, and blood vessels. Breaking down the term cardiovascular, 'cardio' is the heart, and 'vascular' means the blood vessels connecting the whole body. The cardiovascular system is a transport system for the blood, where the heart acts as a pump to deliver blood to the body (Betts *et al* 2013, Aaronson *et al* 2020). The system transports nutrients and oxygen-rich blood to the rest of the body and carries deoxygenated blood back to the lungs. The cardiovascular system essentially provides the 'hardware' for the transport system to keep blood continuously circulating to fulfil a critical homeostatic need. The human heart is no more than a transport system's pump, and the hollow blood vessels are the delivery routes.

10.1.1 Circulatory system

The human circulatory system comprises two main circuits, the pulmonary circuit and the systemic circuit, as shown in figure 10.1. In most illustrations of the

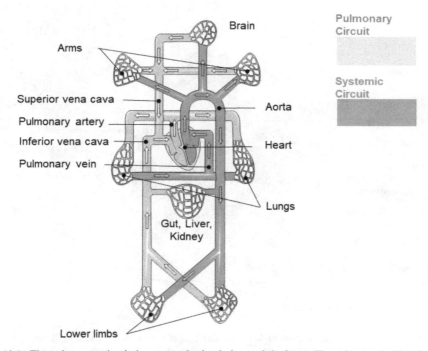

Figure 10.1. The pulmonary circulation, systemic circulation and the heart. The veins are depicted in blue to denote low oxygen blood, while the arteries with oxygen-rich blood are depicted in bright red. The arrows indicate the blood flow direction. Copyright © smart.servier.com. The figure was partly generated using Servier Medical Art, provided by Servier, licensed under a Creative Commons Attribution 3.0 unported license.

cardiovascular system, the veins are depicted in blue to denote oxygen-poor blood, while the arteries with oxygen-rich blood are depicted in bright red. In figure 10.1, the blood vessels that carry blood to and from the lungs form the pulmonary circulation. On the left side of this circuit, the heart receives oxygen-poor blood from body tissues and then pumps this blood to the lungs to pick up oxygen through diffusion between the alveoli and the capillaries. At the same time, the blood also carries the carbon dioxide from the body and eliminates it to the atmosphere during the breathing process. On the right side of the circuit, the heart receives oxygenated blood from the lungs and pumps this blood throughout the body to supply oxygen and nutrients to body tissues. The blood vessels that carry blood to and from all body tissues form the systemic circulation.

10.1.2 The anatomy and function of the heart

At the centre of the cardiovascular system is the human heart. The heart plays an important role in driving the blood circulation process and is divided into two distinct sections: the right and the left. The right heart supports the pulmonary circuit, while the left heart aids in the systemic circuit.

Figure 10.2 shows the cross-section of the human heart, where both the left and right heart consists of an atrium and a ventricle. The atria (the plural form of atrium)

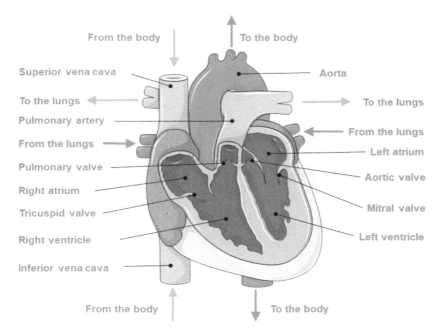

Figure 10.2. The human heart consists of four chambers: right atrium, left atrium, right ventricle and left ventricle. The blood flows into these chambers via four sets of valves: tricuspid valve, pulmonary valve, mitral valve, and aortic valve. Copyright © smart.servier.com. The figure was partly generated using Servier Medical Art, provided by Servier, licensed under a Creative Commons Attribution 3.0 unported license.

and ventricles are active elastic chambers that contract by increasing wall tension to pump blood. The atria and ventricles are contained within the pericardium. The pericardium is a thin and relatively stiff passive elastic sac that encapsulates the heart. During pumping, the atrium and ventricle walls thicken, swelling both inwards and outwards to reduce chamber volume. Nevertheless, the pericardium acts as an external constraint that limits the outward expansion of the heart. As such, the myocardium (or the heart muscle) primarily expands inwards, forcing blood out of the ventricle.

The right atrium and left atrium are the heart's receiving chambers. The right atrium receives oxygen-poor blood returning from the systemic circulation, while the left atrium receives oxygen-rich blood from the pulmonary circulation. The left and right ventricles are the two main pumping chambers that pump blood around the pulmonary and systemic circulations. The right ventricle pumps the oxygen-poor blood into the pulmonary circulation for gas exchange, while the left ventricle pumps the oxygen-rich blood into the systemic circulation. Using blood as the transport medium, the heart continuously propels oxygen, nutrients, waste, and many other substances into the interconnecting blood vessels that service body cells.

The heart valves are essential for heart function. They are one-way valves that allow blood to flow in one direction through the heart chambers. They are located at the inlets (tricuspid valve and mitral valve) and outlets (pulmonary valve and aortic valve) of the ventricles (see figure 10.2). During ventricular contraction, the ventricle inlet valves (tricuspid valve and mitral valve) close and the outlet valves (pulmonary valve and aortic valve) open. This allows blood to flow out of the heart and into the pulmonary and systemic circulations. During ventricle expansion, the outlet valves (pulmonary valve and aortic valve) close, and the inlet valves (tricuspid valve and mitral valve) open to allow blood to flow into the ventricles.

The pumping mechanism of the heart is regulated by an electrical conduction system that coordinates the contraction of the various chambers of the heart. This is shown in figure 10.3. The muscle contraction is an electrochemical mechanism that turns electrical impulses into muscle contraction. When the myocardial muscle cells are stimulated above a threshold, the muscle cell calcium channels open to allow positively charged calcium ions (Ca^{2+}) to enter the cells. These ions cause depolarisation in the cells, resulting in muscle contraction. After a short delay, the potassium channels in the cell open, resulting in a flow of potassium ions (K^+) out of the cell, causing repolarisation and relaxation of the myocardial cells. The myocardial cells then return to their resting state until the next stimulation.

This heart mechanism is initiated through an electrical pulse generated by the sinoatrial node, also known as the SA node. The SA node is a mass of specialised pacemaker cells in the heart's upper right chamber. Acting as a natural pacemaker, the SA node generates electrical impulses in the atria, causing them to contract and pump blood into the ventricles. This electrical impulse travels from the SA node to the atrioventricular node, also known as the AV node. The electrical impulse is slowed for approximately 0.1–0.2 s in the AV node before travelling down to the ventricles via the conduction pathway. This delay gives the atria sufficient time to

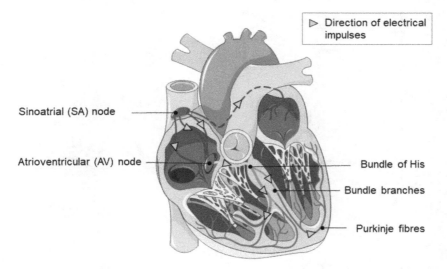

Figure 10.3. The human heart electrical conduction circuit. An electrical impulse is generated in the SA node before sending it to the AV node and the rest of the heart muscles. Copyright © smart.servier.com. The figure was partly generated using Servier Medical Art, provided by Servier, licensed under a Creative Commons Attribution 3.0 unported license.

eject blood into the ventricles before the ventricles contract fully. The electrical impulse travels from the AV node through the bundle of His to the Purkinje fibres of the ventricles. The bundle of His is a segment within the heart that connects the AV Node to the left and right bundle branches of the septal crest. The Purkinje Fibres are specialised electrical conduction fibres that spread the electrical impulse into the ventricle muscles. The electrical impulse signals the ventricles to contract and finally pump the blood out from the heart to the systemic and pulmonary circulations.

The electrical impulses produced during the heart cycle (or cardiac cycle) conduct throughout the body. These electrical impulses can be detected on the human skin surface using electrodes and recorded as an electrocardiogram (ECG). An example of an ECG measurement is shown in figure 10.4. On the ECG, the first wave is called the P-wave. It represents the conduction of electrical impulses through the atria. A short flat line follows the P-wave, indicating that the electrical impulses are being transferred to the ventricles. The next wave is called the QRS-complex, which depicts the spread of electrical activity throughout the ventricular myocardium. The T-wave indicates that the ventricles are returning to their resting state, thus ending the heart cycle. In some instances, a U-wave may be observed after the T-wave. U-waves are thought to represent the repolarisation of the Purkinje fibres. Interpretation of the ECG signal can provide useful information on the heart condition and performance to the medical worker to have a good clinical diagnosis of cardiac disease.

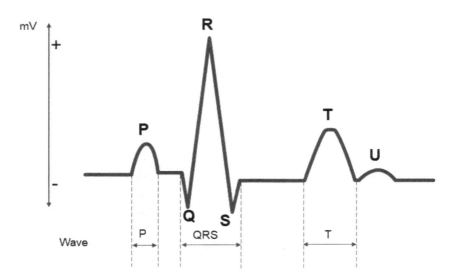

Figure 10.4. Electrocardiogram (ECG) measurement during a cardiac cycle, with the location of P-wave, QRS-complex, T-wave and U-wave. Copyright © smart.servier.com. The figure was partly generated using Servier Medical Art, provided by Servier, licensed under a Creative Commons Attribution 3.0 unported license.

10.2 Cardiac cycle

The cardiac cycle refers to the series of heart relaxation and contraction from the start of one heartbeat to the next. The relaxation and contraction representing one full cardiac cycle can be divided into four stages. The relaxation phase is known as the diastole, and it consists of a short relaxation stage followed by a filling stage. The contraction phase is known as the systole, and it consists of a contraction stage followed by a ventricular ejection stage. During a cardiac cycle, each heart chamber experiences pressure change that results in the movement of blood from one chamber to another, as well as from the heart to the entire body. The blood from the whole body returns to the heart again before the next cardiac cycle.

10.2.1 Stages of a cardiac cycle

10.2.1.1 Diastole—relaxation stage

At the start of the relaxation stage, both the aortic and pulmonary valves are closing, and the heart is still contracted. At this point, the mitral valve and tricuspid valves remain closed, and the ventricles start to relax by keeping a constant volume. This ventricular relaxation at a constant volume creates a pressure decrease within the ventricles. The state of the valves during the relaxation stage is illustrated in figure 10.5.

10.2.1.2 Diastole—filling stage

At the beginning of the filling stage, the tricuspid valves and mitral valves open as the ventricular pressure drops. The openings of the valve enable blood in the atria to flow into the ventricles. This rapid blood flow marks the beginning of the early filling phase. As blood accumulates in the ventricles, pressure in the ventricle chambers increases. This increase causes the pressure difference between the atria and the ventricles to be gradually compensated, and causes the blood flow from the atria to the ventricles to rapidly slow down. At some point, blood flow becomes near zero,

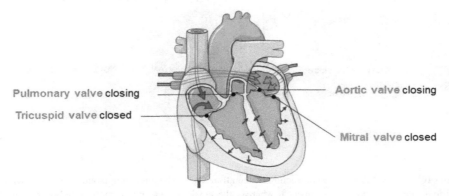

Pulmonary valve closing

Tricuspid valve closed

Aortic valve closing

Mitral valve closed

Figure 10.5. Relaxation. All heart valves are closed. Copyright © smart.servier.com. The figure was partly generated using Servier Medical Art, provided by Servier, licensed under a Creative Commons Attribution 3.0 unported license.

marking the phase of diastasis. Figure 10.6 shows the filling stage, where the tricuspid and mitral valves are opened, with blood flowing from the atria into the ventricles.

At the end of the ventricular filling, the atria contract. The contraction of the atria pushes the remaining blood into the ventricles, as shown in figure 10.7. Throughout the whole filling process, the aortic and pulmonary valves remain closed, preventing any backflow of blood. Shortly after atrial contraction, ventricular contraction initiates, causing the mitral valves and the tricuspid valves (collectively known as the atrioventricular valves) to close, marking the end of the filling phase.

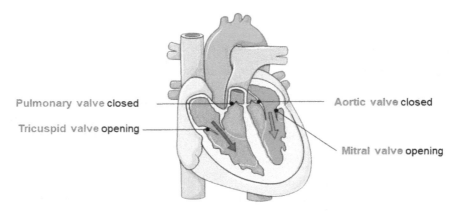

Figure 10.6. Start of filling. The tricuspid and mitral valves are opened, with blood flowing from the atria into the ventricles. The pulmonary and aortic valves remain closed. Copyright © smart.servier.com. The figure was partly generated using Servier Medical Art, provided by Servier, licensed under a Creative Commons Attribution 3.0 unported license.

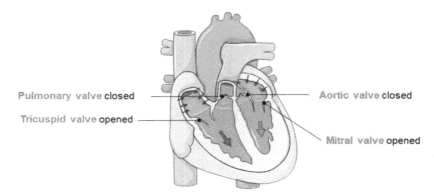

Figure 10.7. Active filling. The contraction of the atrial pushes the remaining blood into the ventricles. The tricuspid and mitral valves are opened, whereas the aortic valves and pulmonary valves remain closed. Copyright © smart.servier.com. The figure was partly generated using Servier Medical Art, provided by Servier, licensed under a Creative Commons Attribution 3.0 unported license.

10.2.1.3 Systole—contraction stage

After the blood has filled the ventricles, ventricular contraction continues. During ventricular contraction, all four heart valves are closed, meaning that the ventricular volume remains constant. This phase is termed the contraction stage and is illustrated in figure 10.8.

10.2.1.4 Systole—ejection stage

At the end of the cardiac cycle is the ejection stage. Further ventricles contraction increases the ventricular pressure, and this causes the aortic and pulmonary valves to open. The opening of the aortic and pulmonary valves allows the ejection of blood into the aorta and pulmonary arteries. This phase is called ejection and is shown in figure 10.9. Blood flows into the arteries until pressures in the arteries become larger

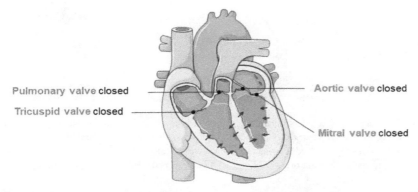

Figure 10.8. Contraction with all heart valves closed. Copyright © smart.servier.com. The figure was partly generated using Servier Medical Art, provided by Servier, licensed under a Creative Commons Attribution 3.0 unported license.

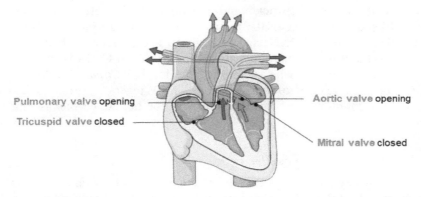

Figure 10.9. Ejection stage. The pulmonary and aortic valves are opened to allow blood flow into the pulmonary and systemic circuits. Copyright © smart.servier.com. The figure was partly generated using Servier Medical Art, provided by Servier, licensed under a Creative Commons Attribution 3.0 unported license.

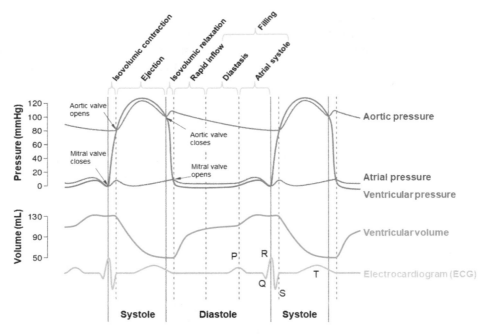

Figure 10.10. A sample of Wiggers diagram together with an electrocardiogram showing the cardiac cycle events occurring in the left ventricle. Copyright © adh30, revised work by DanielChangMD who revised original work of DestinyQx; Redrawn as SVG by xavax Creative Commons Attribution-ShareAlike 4.0 International https://en.wikipedia.org/wiki/Wiggers_diagram#/media/File:Wiggers_Diagram_2.svg.

than the pressures in the ventricles. At this point, the aortic and pulmonary valves close, marking the end of the ejection phase. The cardiac cycle then continues with the next relaxation stage, which is the beginning of the next cardiac cycle.

These four stages of a cardiac cycle can be described with reference to the pressure and volume in the left ventricle, and pressures in the left atrium and aorta. Figure 10.10 shows a sample of the pressure and volume graph of the atrial, aortic and ventricle together with an electrocardiogram. This pressure and volume graph is also known as the Wiggers diagram, named after Professor Carl J Wiggers; a pioneer in cardiovascular research who established the journal *Circulation Research* published by the American Heart Association. The Wiggers diagram (Mitchell and Wang 2014) is commonly used in the studies of the human cardiovascular system pressure and volume.

10.2.2 Key parameters of a cardiac cycle

There are a few key parameters that define a cardiac cycle, such as cardiac period, heart rate, end-diastolic volume, end-systolic volume, stroke volume, stroke volume index, cardiac output and cardiac index. The descriptions of these cardiac cycle parameters are presented in table 10.1, along with a sample cardiac cycle figure as an illustration.

Table 10.1. Sample cardiac cycle and the key parameters. (Figure Copyright © adh30, revised work by DanielChangMD who revised original work of DestinyQx; Redrawn as SVG by xavax Creative Commons Attribution-ShareAlike 4.0 International https://en.wikipedia.org/wiki/Wiggers_diagram#/media/File: Wiggers_Diagram_2.svg.

Sample cardiac cycle

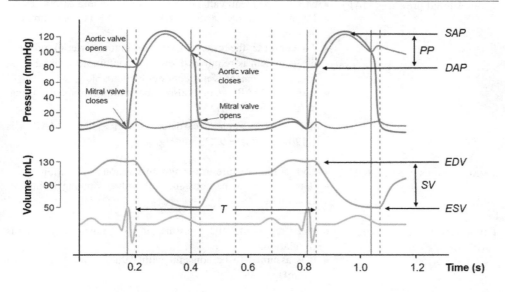

Parameters	Descriptions
Cardiac period (T)	• T is the time interval separating two heart beats. • From the sample cardiac cycle above, T is approximately 0.65 s.
Heart rate (HR)	• HR is the inverse of the cardiac period, i.e., HR $= 1/T$ • It is also known as the cardiac frequency. • In the sample cardiac cycle, HR $= 1/0.65 = 1.54$ Hz, or $1.54 \times 60 = 92.4$ beats per minute (BPM).
Systolic arterial pressure (SAP)	• The maximum arterial pressure throughout a cardiac cycle that occurs during systole is the systolic arterial pressure (SAP). • SAP is approximately 120 mmHg in the sample cardiac cycle.
Diastolic arterial pressure (DAP)	• During diastole, the arterial pressure reaches its minimum. • This minimum pressure value is the diastolic arterial pressure (DAP). • The DAP is approximately 80 mmHg in the sample cardiac cycle.

Arterial pulse pressure (PP)	• PP is the difference between the maximum and minimum arterial pressure, i.e., PP = SAP − DAP. • In the sample cardiac cycle, the arterial PP = 120 − 80 = 40 mmHg.
Mean arterial pressure (MAP)	• MAP is the mean value of arterial pressure in a cardiac cycle. • From the sample cardiac cycle, the MAP is approximately 96 mmHg. • To compute the exact MAP, continuous arterial pressure measurement is required. However, continuous arterial pressure measurement is not commonly available. • Hence, MAP can also be approximated using: $MAP = \frac{1}{3}SAP + \frac{2}{3}DAP$. • In the sample cardiac cycle, the MAP is $\frac{1}{3}(120) + \frac{2}{3}(80) = 93.33$ mmHg.
Central venous pressure (CVP)	• CVP is the pressure in the systemic venous circulation. • It is assumed to be constant with values ranging from 8 to 12 mmHg.
Pulmonary venous pressure (PVP)	• PVP represents the pressure in the pulmonary venous circulation. • It is assumed to be constant with values ranging from 5 to 6 mmHg.
End-diastolic volume (EDV)	• EDV is the volume of a ventricle at the end of diastole. This is when the ventricular volume reaches a maximum during a cardiac cycle. • In the sample cardiac cycle, the left ventricular EDV is approximately 130 ml.
End-systolic volume (ESV)	• ESV is the volume of a ventricle at the end of systole, which is the minimum ventricular volume during a cardiac cycle. • In the sample cardiac cycle, the left ventricular ESV is approximately 50 ml.
Stroke volume (SV) and stoke volume index (SVI)	• SV is defined as the volume of blood ejected by a ventricle at each cardiac cycle, i.e., SV = EDV − ESV. • The SV in the sample cardiac cycle is approximately 130 − 50 = 80 ml. • The stroke volume index (SVI) is the ratio of SV to the body surface.
Cardiac output (CO) and cardiac index	• CO is the average blood flow exiting the heart in a cardiac cycle and is given by CO = SV/T.

(Continued)

Table 10.1. (*Continued*)

Sample cardiac cycle	
	• In the sample cardiac cycle, CO = 80/0.65 = 123.07 ml s^{-1}, or 7.38 L min^{-1}. • The cardiac index (CI) is defined as the ratio of CO to the body surface area.
Systemic vascular resistance (SVR)	• SVR is the resistance to blood flow exerted by the systemic vasculature given by SVR = $\frac{\text{MAP} - \text{CVP}}{\text{CO}}$. • In the sample cardiac cycle, assuming CVP = 10 mmHg, SVR = $\frac{93.33 - 10}{123.07}$ = 0.68 mmHg·s/ ml. • From the expression above, SVR is the ratio of the driving force for blood flow, defined as the pressure difference between the beginning and end of the systemic circulation to the resulting flow. • The lower the SVR is, the easier it is for blood to flow through the systemic vasculature.
Pulmonary vascular resistance (PVR)	• PVR is the pulmonary counterpart of SVR.

10.2.3 The cardiac cycle pressure–volume diagram

The pressure–volume diagram of the cardiac cycle is often used by health professionals as an indicator to diagnose patient conditions. From the pressure–volume diagram, health professionals can derive various properties of the heart to analyse the heart's performance. A sample pressure–volume diagram is shown in figure 10.11.

Two important metrics of the pressure–volume diagram are: (1) the lines plotting the end-systolic pressure–volume relationship (ESPVR), and (2) the end-diastolic pressure–volume relationship (EDPVR). These lines represent the heart muscle contractility (ESPVR) and compliance (EDPVR). These relationships help to approximate the shape of the pressure–volume diagram from a given EDV and ESV. Aside from the two lines, the area enclosed by the pressure–volume diagram represents the external work (stroke work) done to the artery by the heart. The slope or arterial elastance (E_A) reflects the arterial load imposed on the ventricle. Finally, the general characteristics of the pressure–volume diagram are the same for both left and right ventricles.

10.2.4 The cardiac output

One of the most important parameters in cardiovascular system heath monitoring is the cardiac output during a cardiac cycle. Cardiac output (CO) can be determined as

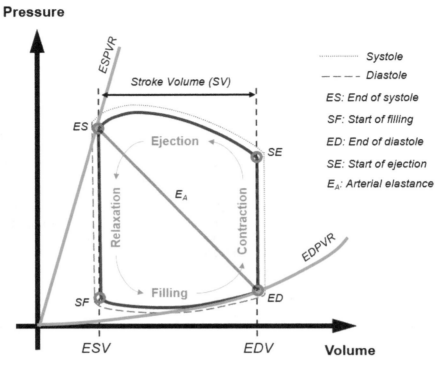

Figure 10.11. A sample of a ventricular pressure–volume diagram during a cardiac cycle. ESPVR: end-systolic pressure–volume relation, EDPVR: end-diastolic pressure–volume relation, ESV: end-systolic volume, EDV: end-diastolic volume.

the product of heart rate and stroke volume (CO = HR × SV) or stroke volume divided by cardiac period (CO = SV/T). The cardiac output is essentially the amount of blood pumped by the heart per minute. Cardiac output for a healthy individual will adjust to meet the metabolic demands, ensuring sufficient oxygen and nutrient supply to the cells of the body. However, changes in cardiac output can be an indication of cardiovascular disease. Specifically, an increase in cardiac output can be associated with cardiovascular disease that can occur during infection and sepsis (Greer 2015). In contrast, a decrease in cardiac output can be associated with cardiomyopathy (Weber *et al* 1985), cardiogenic shock (Vahdatpour *et al* 2019) and hypovolemia (Kreimeier 2000). Cardiac output is determined by four main factors: preload, contractility, afterload and heart rate (HR). These factors describe the heart's ability as a pump.

10.2.4.1 Preload
Preload is the stretching of the heart muscle fibres before heart contraction. It indicates the heart's ability to fill up. A larger preload will generate a larger contraction force, resulting in a larger stroke volume. The effect of preload on stroke

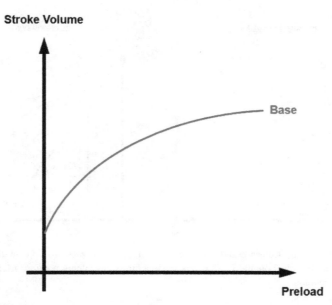

Figure 10.12. A Frank–Starling curve for stroke volume versus preload.

volume is often represented using the Frank–Starling curve shown in figure 10.12. As preload increases, the stroke volume increases. However, at a certain point, an increase in preload will no longer lead to an increase in stroke volume. Beyond this point, any further increase in preload will not increase further the cardiac output.

Preload is estimated from end-diastolic ventricular pressure. For the right ventricle, the preload is measured by the central venous pressure. For the left ventricle, preload is measured by the pulmonary artery pressure, which is typically not available due to the requirement of invasive procedures to obtain its measurement. In clinical settings, the values of end-diastolic volume and/or end-diastolic pressure are often used as surrogates to represent preload, replacing the x-axis preload in the Frank–Starling curve. End-diastolic volume represents the ventricular volume just before contraction. Therefore, it can be associated with the stretching of the muscle fibres at that moment.

Figure 10.13 shows the effects of changing preload on the ventricular pressure–volume diagram, where blue colour indicates a base pressure–volume diagram and red shows the effects of decreased and increased preload. In this example, preload can be represented by the ventricle end-diastolic volume. The ventricular contractility and afterload are kept constant. It is seen that a decrease in preload (or EDV) causes a decrease in stroke volume and systolic pressure in the ventricle. Stroke volume decreases because end-diastolic volume decreases more than the baseline end-diastolic volume. The opposite effects are seen when the preload is increased.

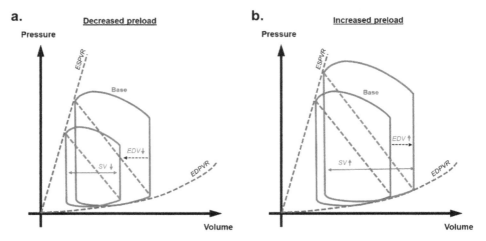

Figure 10.13. Effect of (a) decreased and (b) increased preload on the pressure–volume diagram. SV: stroke volume, EDV: end-diastolic volume, ESPVR: end-systolic pressure–volume relation, EDPVR: end-diastolic pressure–volume relation.

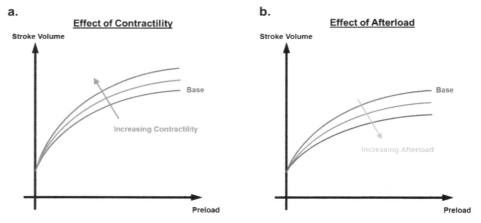

Figure 10.14. Effect of (a) contractility and (b) afterload towards Frank–Starling stroke volume–preload curve.

10.2.4.2 Contractility

Contractility is the heart muscle's ability to generate force. A larger contractility will have a larger contraction force being generated. Thus, a larger contractility will also result in a larger stroke volume. An increase in contractility will thus move the Frank–Starling curve upwards, as shown in figure 10.14(a).

The gold standard measure of contractility is end-systolic elastance (E_{es}) (Chen *et al* 2001) represented by the slope of the ESPVR in figure 10.11. This relationship defines the maximum pressure that can be produced by the ventricle for a given unit

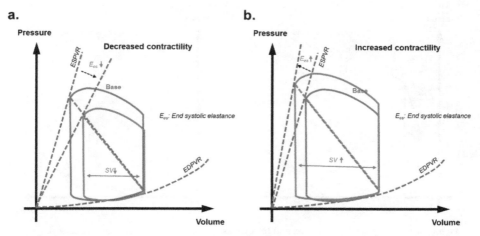

Figure 10.15. Effect of (a) decreased and (b) increased contractility on the pressure–volume diagram.

of volume for any one heartbeat. The end-systolic elastance can be considered as a constant over a normal range of loading conditions for a given inotropic state, and thus, can be represented by the following relationship:

$$E_{es} = \frac{P_{es}}{V_{es} - V_d}, \tag{10.1}$$

where P_{es} and V_{es} are the end-systolic pressure and end-systolic volume in the ventricle and V_d is the unstressed volume. The effects of E_{es} on the ventricle's pressure–volume diagram is shown in figure 10.15. A decrease in contractility leads to a drop in the systolic pressure and stroke volume, and an increase in contractility will result in an increase in systolic pressure and stroke volume.

10.2.4.3 Afterload

The afterload is another important factor that determines cardiac output. It is the resistance that the ventricle must overcome to eject blood into circulation. This resistance is caused by everything located downstream of the ventricle; for example, the ventricular–arterial valve and the pressure of the blood in the arteries. At a given preload and contractility, a larger afterload will result in a lower stroke volume. Thus, increasing afterload will see the Frank–Starling curve moving downwards, as shown in figure 10.14(b). Overall, a low afterload implies less work is required to achieve a given blood flow.

Effective arterial elastance (E_A) is the gold standard clinical measure of afterload (Naeije *et al* 2014). It is defined as:

$$E_A = \frac{P_{es}}{SV}. \tag{10.2}$$

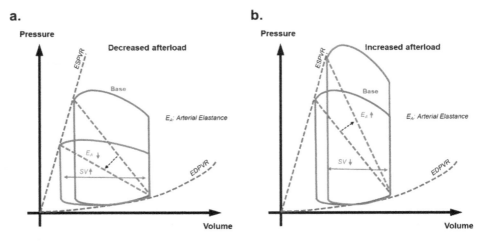

Figure 10.16. Effect of (a) decreased and (b) increased afterload on the pressure–volume diagram.

Changes in E_A can be used to analyse the effects of afterload on the ventricular pressure–volume diagram, as illustrated in figure 10.16. A decrease in E_A will see an increase in stroke volume and a decrease in systolic pressure, whereas an increase in E_A causes an increase in systolic pressure and a decrease in stroke volume. Note that the effective arterial elastance is not the same as the mechanical elastance property of the arteries (i.e., their stiffness).

10.2.4.4 Heart rate
The heart rate is perhaps the simplest determinant of cardiac output to visualise. The faster the heart beats, the more blood can be pumped over a particular period. The previous three factors, i.e., preload, contractility and afterload, determine the stroke volume, which is the volume of blood ejected at each heartbeat. The heart rate determines the total volume pumped per minute based on the number of times the heart beats every minute. Thus, if the heart rate is too slow or too fast, the cardiac output can be impaired.

10.2.4.5 The cyclist analogy for cardiac output
Understanding the applicability and practical relevance of each factor is important when interpreting cardiac output values. In an analogy presented by Jean-Louis Vincent (Vincent 2008), he relates the cardiac output and its four factors to a cyclist pedalling a bicycle, namely the cyclist's speed (cardiac output), tailwind (preload), cyclist's muscles (contractility), road condition (afterload) and cycling cadence (heart rate).

The cardiac output can be related to the speed of the cyclist, with an increase in speed representing a higher cardiac output. Preload can be compared with a tailwind allowing the cyclist to move faster without any additional muscle effort. A difference between this analogy and the speed of the cyclist is that the latter will continue to increase as the speed of the wind increases. In the heart, a preload value will eventually be reached with no further cardiac output increase (see figure 10.12). Contractility can be represented as the cyclist flexing his/her muscles and pushing harder on the pedals. This effort will result in the cyclist moving faster or having a higher cardiac output.

Afterload can be represented by the condition of the road. Cycling on a smooth road compared to on a narrow, bumpy road is easier, and thus the cyclist's speed can increase significantly for any given muscle effort. As such, in the sense of cardiac output, reducing afterload can increase cardiac output, especially in conditions where contractility is impaired.

Finally, heart rate can be related to cycling cadence, the rate of a cyclist pedalling. Higher cadence means an increase in cyclist speed. However, a cyclist who pedals too fast for too long will get tired and be unable to maintain the rate of pedalling, resulting in slowing down. Thus, there is an optimal rate of pedalling: too fast, and the cyclist will tire too quickly and must slow down; too slow, and the cyclist will not move fast enough to cover the required distance.

10.3 Cardiovascular disease and circulatory shock

10.3.1 Cardiovascular disease

Cardiovascular diseases are disorders that affect heart functions and blood vessels. In most cases, the root cause of cardiovascular disease is due to behavioural risk factors such as an unhealthy diet, lack of physical activity, and the use of alcohol and tobacco. These may have an effect of increasing an individual's blood pressure, high blood sugar level (glucose), overweight and obesity. The following are some of the common cardiovascular diseases.

- *Myocardial infarction (heart attack)*—A myocardial infarction, more often known as a heart attack, is a condition in which a portion or the whole heart muscle is cut off from the oxygen supply. In most cases, the blood flowing into the heart is hindered by a build-up of plague in the coronary arteries (also known as atherosclerosis). Blood clots form around the plaque, narrowing the arterial walls and subsequently reducing or completely blocking the blood flow. The muscle is depleted of oxygen and stops working, causing a heart attack.
- *Stroke*—A stroke is a problem with blood flow to the brain rather than the heart. However, it is considered a cardiovascular disease because it centres around blood circulation. There are two types of strokes, ischemic and haemorrhagic strokes. Ischemic strokes account for more than 80% of all strokes. They occur because of a blockage in a blood vessel that delivers blood and oxygen to the brain. Parts of the brain can suffer damage or die off due to a lack of blood and oxygen. Haemorrhagic stroke occurs when blood from an artery suddenly begins bleeding into the brain. This could be due to blockages, vascular malformation, or abnormal growth of brain blood vessels.

- *Heart arrhythmia*—An arrhythmia is when the heart is beating at an abnormal rhythm. The rhythm can be too slow (bradycardia), too fast (tachycardia), or at an irregular tempo. Without a proper rhythm, the heart may not be able to pump sufficient blood to deliver oxygen and nutrients to the body. Arrhythmia can occur due to various reasons such as other cardiovascular diseases, imbalance electrolytes, heart tissue injury, medication, problems with heart electrical signals, stress or intake of alcohol, tobacco, or caffeine.
- *Heart valve disease*—For a patient with heart valve disease, the heart valves do not function properly, causing the blood flow through the heart to be disrupted. Stenosis is a condition where there the valves do not open enough to allow blood to flow through. Regurgitation occurs when the heart valves do not close completely, causing the backflow of the blood. Heart valve disease could be due to old age, infection, or other cardiovascular disease risk factors, or it is present at birth (congenital heart disease).

Most cardiovascular diseases can be prevented by addressing behavioural risk factors, such as diet and exercise. Thus, detecting cardiovascular disease in an early stage is important in the management and treatment of cardiovascular disease. Treatments for cardiovascular disease are mostly surgical; they include coronary artery bypass, balloon angioplasty, valve repair and replacement, heart transplant, artificial heart operations, pacemakers, prosthetic valves, or patches for closing holes in the heart. There are also pharmacotherapy or drug therapies for treating cardiovascular diseases.

10.3.2 Circulatory shock

In intensive care, circulatory shock is a common cardiovascular condition that affects up to one-third of the patients admitted to the ICU (Cecconi *et al* 2014). It is a circulatory failure that results in inadequate cellular oxygen utilisation. The patients risk severe cellular dysoxia, multiple organ failure, and death if not treated. Causes of circulatory shock can be categorised into four main pathophysiological mechanisms: (a) distributive, (b) cardiogenic, (c) hypovolemia, and (d) obstructive (Standl *et al* 2018). Each mechanism reflects an abnormality in a different part/function of the cardiovascular system.

- *Distributive shock*—Distributive shock is a dysfunction in the cardiovascular capillary system and its regulatory functions. It is the most common form of cardiovascular dysfunction in the ICU (Vincent and De Backer 2013). This dysfunction is mostly caused by bacterial infection, where high levels of toxins in the blood trigger the body's inflammatory response. This inflammatory response affects vascular regulation, leading to abnormalities in the microcirculation, affecting the ability of the systemic circulatory system to exchange nutrients and oxygen and return the blood back to the heart. Patients with distributive dysfunction are treated with fluid resuscitation (Gyawali *et al* 2019).

- *Cardiogenic shock*—Cardiogenic shock is the second largest cause of cardiovascular dysfunction in the ICU (Vincent and De Backer 2013). It is caused by severe impairment of the myocardial performance, such as ventricular septal rupture and valve regurgitation, myocardial ischemia that results in diminished cardiac output, end-organ hypoperfusion, and hypoxia. Treatment includes coronary artery bypass grafting, a heart transplant or percutaneous circulatory assist devices to support the heart function (Vahdatpour *et al* 2019).
- *Hypovolemia*—Hypovolemia refers to the state of low extracellular fluid volume in the patient (Vincent and De Backer 2013). This condition is often found in intensive care patients who are suffering from severe haemorrhages. The cardiovascular system is significantly compromised due to the loss of blood volume in the circulatory system, decreasing the preload and stroke volume. Hypovolemia is managed through intravenous fluid resuscitation and vasopressor support.
- *Obstructive shock*—Obstructive shock is a rare form of circulatory shock in the ICU (Vincent and De Backer 2013). It is caused by the inability to produce adequate cardiac output due to physical obstruction of blood flow into or out of the heart. Examples of obstructive shock include tension pneumothorax, pulmonary embolism, pulmonary or systemic hypertension, and congenital or acquired outflow obstructions. Obstruction in the circulatory system leads to an increase in afterload. Treating the cause of obstructive shock such as decompressing lung pressure, surgical removal of embolism or clot etc (Standl *et al* 2018).

These circulatory shocks are common in the ICU, and they may lead to changes in the cardiovascular system physiology and subsequently reduce the stroke volume and cardiac output of patients. Hence, the ability to monitor and accurately interpret the reasons for changes in cardiovascular system physiology as well as stroke volume and cardiac output in intensive care is of great importance. Modelling the cardiovascular system can potentially provide insight into the patient's condition and propose potential treatment.

10.4 Cardiovascular system modelling

The human cardiovascular system can be modelled differently depending on the purpose, such as to improve physiological understanding of the cardiovascular system interaction or to provide decision support in a clinical environment. As such, cardiovascular system models (CVS models) of different complexities can be developed. Most approaches in modelling the human cardiovascular system are through a three-dimensional, multi-compartments, finite element approach. These approaches involve breaking down the cardiovascular system function in greater detail and utilising FEM to simulate their functions. These models consist of millions of degrees of freedom and are often good at providing education and insight into the understanding of the human cardiovascular system. Nevertheless, these models are computationally expensive and require high-powered workstations for simulation and application. In addition, these models require significant clinical data and assumptions during the development phase.

At the other end of the spectrum lies a simpler approach, which is to group model parameters and make assumptions to simplify the model as much as possible, while still attempting to simulate the essential dynamics. This approach generates the physiological lumped parameter CVS models. The lumped parameter models are comparatively simpler and can be simulated without the need for high computation power (Shimizu *et al* 2018). They focus more on capturing the macro-physiological trends rather than accurately reproducing the cardiovascular system physiology. They provide the opportunity to guide bedside treatment in real-time.

In the following section, we will look at the development of two lumped CVS models. There are a few important mechanics that must be considered during the modelling of the human cardiovascular system.

10.4.1 Fundamental concepts in modelling the cardiovascular system

Before we introduce the CVS model, it is important to understand some fundamental concepts during the development of a lumped parameter CVS model. These concepts include (1) chamber pressure–volume relationship, (2) time-varying elastance, (3) blood vessel pressure–flow relationship, (4) valve opening and closing mechanism, (5) blood flow inertia, and (6) no blood loss in the CVS model. Using these fundamental concepts, various forms and complexities of CVS models can be developed.

10.4.1.1 Chamber pressure–volume relationship

In a lumped parameter CVS model, a passive elastic element can be used to account for the deformable properties of the large vessels, namely the arteries and veins. The pressure–volume relationship of a chamber describes the relationship between the blood volume inside the chamber and the pressure exerted by the chamber:

$$P(t) = EV_s(t), \tag{10.3}$$

where P is the pressure within a chamber, t is time, E is the elastance of the chamber (its stiffness) and V_s is the stressed volume within the chamber.

In an actual physiological condition, the cardiovascular system takes a certain blood volume to fill the cardiovascular system to the point where its presence exerts a force on the vessel walls. This blood volume is known as the unstressed volume. Any volume above this level is the stressed volume, which will exert an increasing degree of pressure on the vessel walls. The total stressed blood volume, TV_s is defined as the total pressure-generating blood volume in the circulation and has the potential to be used as an index of fluid responsiveness.

10.4.1.2 Time-varying elastance

Another important concept is the time-varying elastance of the heart chamber. The heart, which consists of the ventricles and atria, contracts and relaxes to pump blood around the body. In lumped CVS models, the heart is an active chamber, where it can generate a pressure increase through contraction. Consequently, the pressure generated by the chamber does not solely depend on the volume inside of the chamber but also depends on the time when an electrical impulse triggers the contraction. As such, the elastance term for the heart chamber is time-varying and can be represented by a driver function, i.e., a function that generates cardiac muscle activation. The driver function is a major determinant of cardiovascular dynamics (Hann *et al* 2011). The pressure–volume relationship within the heart can thus be written as:

$$P_h(t) = e(t)E_h V_{s,\,h}(t),\tag{10.4}$$

where P_h is the pressure in the heart, $V_{s,\,h}(t)$ is the heart stressed blood volume, E_h is the elastance of the heart, and $e(t)$ is the driver function (Suga *et al* 1973).

The driver function $e(t)$ can be derived in many different forms, and they typically describe the different shapes of the function (Hann *et al* 2011). Figure 10.17 shows an example of the driver function modified from Stevenson *et al* (2012).

Examples of driver functions can be found in the works of Smith *et al* (2004) and Hann *et al* (2005), where they used a Gaussian function to represent the driver function:

$$e(t) = \sum_{i=1}^{N} A_i e^{-B_i(t-C_i)^2},\tag{10.5}$$

where A_i, B_i, C_i and N are parameters that define the shape of the driver function. Some sample driver function parameters are $N = 1$, $A_1 = 1$, $B_1 = 80\ \mathrm{s}^{-1}$, $C_1 = 0.27\ \mathrm{s}$ (Hann *et al* 2005).

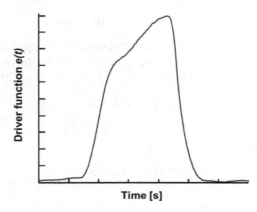

Figure 10.17. An example of a driver function modified from Stevenson *et al* (2012). Copyright © 2012, Stevenson *et al*; licensee BioMed Central Ltd.

Pironet *et al* (2015b, 2016a) proposed a simple driver function using a modulus operation as shown in the equations below:

$$e(t) = \exp\left[-W\left((t \times \bmod(T)) - \frac{T}{2}\right)^2\right],$$ (10.6)

where W dictates the width of the Gaussian function, T is the cardiac period, t is the time, and mod is the modulo operator. There are also other works that used piecewise functions (Stevenson *et al* 2012). These functions may provide a better representation of the shape of the driver function.

10.4.1.3 Blood vessel pressure–volume relationship

Next, a relationship between the resistance and the blood flow within the blood vessel is required. As such, blood flow and pressure in the blood vessel can be related to the resistance, R of the blood vessel. The pressure upstream of the vessel is $P_{up}(t)$, while the downstream pressure is $P_{down}(t)$. The blood flow $Q(t)$ can then be described as:

$$Q(t) = \frac{P_{up}(t) - P_{down}(t)}{R}.$$ (10.7)

10.4.1.4 Mechanics of valve opening and closing

In the cardiovascular system, another important concept that must be taken into consideration is the mechanism of valve opening and closing. As such, blood can only flow through the valve when the upstream pressure of the valve is higher than the downstream pressure. If $P_{down}(t)$ is higher than $P_{up}(t)$, no blood can flow through the valve. Thus, blood flowing through a valve can be described using a piecewise function, i.e.:

$$Q(t) = \begin{cases} \dfrac{P_{up}(t) - P_{down}(t)}{R}, & \text{if } P_{up}(t) > P_{down}(t) \\ 0, & \text{otherwise} \end{cases}.$$ (10.8)

Equation (10.8) can also be modelled by replacing every appearance of a flow $Q(t)$ that is controlled by a valve with $H[Q(t)]Q(t)$, where the notation $H[]$ denotes the Heaviside function, such that (Hann *et al* 2005, Paeme *et al* 2011):

$$H(t) = \begin{cases} 0, & \text{if } t \le 0 \\ 1, & \text{if } t > 0 \end{cases}.$$ (10.9)

Thus, equation (10.8) can be written as:

$$Q(t) = H[Q(t)]Q(t).$$ (10.10)

10.4.1.5 Blood flow inertia

The next concept is the consideration of blood flow inertia. This consideration implies that blood in the cardiovascular system will continue to flow for some time, even if the pressure difference between upstream and downstream reaches zero, due to inertia. Thus, the blood flow in equation (10.7) can be rewritten as:

$$Q(t) = \frac{P_{up}(t) - P_{down}(t)}{R} - \frac{L}{R}\frac{dQ(t)}{dt}, \tag{10.11}$$

where L is the inertia. The term $-\frac{L}{R}\frac{dQ(t)}{dt}$ implies that blood will keep on flowing for some time, even if the pressure difference between upstream and downstream reaches zero. The closing and opening mechanisms of the valve can also be adapted to take the blood's inertia into account, as in equation (10.8) (Paeme *et al* 2011).

10.4.1.6 No blood loss in the cardiovascular system volume

Finally, within the CVS model, the continuity equation states that there can be no loss of matter. In lumped CVS models, this implies that there is no loss of volume or blood within the chamber, such that:

$$\frac{dV(t)}{dt} = Q_{in}(t) - Q_{out}(t), \tag{10.12}$$

or if we consider only the stressed blood volume within a chamber, i:

$$\frac{dV_{s,\,i}(t)}{dt} = Q_{in,\,i}(t) - Q_{out,\,i}(t). \tag{10.13}$$

Summing equation (10.13) for all chambers of the CVS model will result in:

$$\sum_i \frac{dV_{s,\,i}(t)}{dt} = \sum_i Q_{in,\,i}(t) - \sum_i Q_{out,\,i}(t) = 0. \tag{10.14}$$

The total stressed blood volume for all i chambers can thus be considered as a constant, where:

$$TV_s = \sum_i V_{s,\,i}, \tag{10.15}$$

where TV_s represents a model-based equivalent of total stressed blood volume. For most of the time, TV_s is a constant (Spiegel 2016). However, this assumption of total stressed volume as constant may not be true for larger models due to the sympathetic nervous actions, time-dependent vascular properties, fluid exchange through the capillaries, haemorrhage and other factors.

10.4.2 Simple cardiovascular system models

One simple form of the CVS model is a model with the least parameters, where it is divided into blocks of Windkessel-like circuits (Westerhof *et al* 2009). The circuits separate the pressure–volume and the fluid flow properties of each section of the cardiovascular system into different model components. These models can be found in the works of Danielsen and Ottesen (2001), Parlikar and Verghese (2005) and Zenker *et al* (2007). The following CVS model was derived from the works of

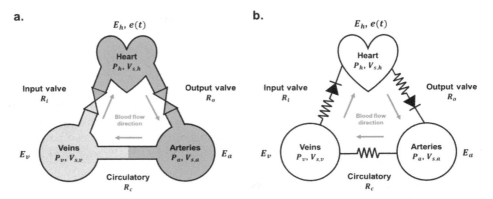

Figure 10.18. The three-chamber CVS model is represented as (a) a mechanical circuit, or (b) an electrical circuit equivalent.

Pironet *et al* (2019) and Cushway *et al* (2022), where they depicted the cardiovascular system as a three-chamber model.

This simple model assumes the cardiovascular system to consist of three elastic chambers, namely the heart, arteries and veins. This is shown in figure 10.18, where figure 10.18(a) shows the mechanical circuit of the three-chambers model and figure 10.18(b) shows the electrical circuit equivalent of the three-chambers CVS model. The first chamber represents the heart (h), the second chamber represents the arteries (a), and the third chamber represents the veins (v). All three chambers are linked by blood vessels with resistance components. Note that this model only includes the systemic circuit and does not consider the pulmonary circuit.

The mathematical equations for the three-chamber CVS model are listed as follows. First, we have the pressure–volume relationship of each chamber:

$$P_a(t) = E_a V_{s,\,a}(t), \tag{10.16}$$

$$P_v(t) = E_v V_{s,\,v}(t), \tag{10.17}$$

$$P_h(t) = e(t) E_h V_{s,\,h}(t), \tag{10.18}$$

where P is pressure, V_s is the stressed blood volume and E is the elastance. The subscripts a, v and h represent the arteries, veins and heart chambers, respectively. $e(t)$ is the driver function. Note that the arterial elastance E_a is not the same as the effective arterial elastance E_A introduced in section 10.2.4.

The blood flow through the input and output valves can be modelled using the simple valve model:

$$Q_i(t) = \begin{cases} \dfrac{P_v(t) - P_h(t)}{R_i}, & \text{if } P_v(t) > P_h(t) \\ 0, & \text{otherwise} \end{cases}, \tag{10.19}$$

$$Q_o(t) = \begin{cases} \frac{P_h(t) - P_a(t)}{R_o}, & \text{if } P_h(t) > P_a(t) \\ 0, & \text{otherwise} \end{cases}. \tag{10.20}$$

The input valve resistance is denoted as R_i, and the output valve resistance is R_o. As for the blood flow in the circulatory $Q_c(t)$, it is written as:

$$Q_c(t) = \frac{P_a(t) - P_v(t)}{R_c}, \tag{10.21}$$

where R_c denotes the circulatory resistance. Note that the blood flow in equation (10.21) did not include the term for blood flow inertia. The blood flow equations can be modified to include the terms in equation (10.11) to include blood flow inertia, but were excluded from this chapter for simplicity.

The continuity equation gives the rate at which the stressed volumes of the chambers change, which results in:

$$\frac{dV_{s,h}(t)}{dt} = Q_i(t) - Q_o(t), \tag{10.22}$$

$$\frac{dV_{s,a}(t)}{dt} = Q_o(t) - Q_c(t), \tag{10.23}$$

$$\frac{dV_{s,v}(t)}{dt} = Q_c(t) - Q_i(t), \tag{10.24}$$

$$\frac{dV_{s,h}(t)}{dt} + \frac{dV_{s,a}(t)}{dt} + \frac{dV_{s,v}(t)}{dt} = 0. \tag{10.25}$$

The total stressed volume contained in the CVS model, $V_{s,3}$ is a constant, i.e.:

$$V_{s,h}(t) + V_{s,a}(t) + V_{s,v}(t) = V_{s,3}. \tag{10.26}$$

The model can be initiated using a driver function $e(t)$ and the initial conditions for $V_{s,h}$, $V_{s,a}$ and $V_{s,v}$. Details of the three-chamber model simulation are presented in section 10.5.2.

10.4.3 Six-chamber cardiovascular system model

A more complex CVS model is the six-chamber model (Smith *et al* 2004). The model divides the cardiovascular system into six blood reservoirs representing the main haemodynamic components of the circulation. The six-chamber model uses fundamental theories similar to the three-chamber model. It expands the model from three to six chambers by describing the single heart chamber as two chambers to capture the physiology of the left and right ventricles; the artery chamber is separated into systemic and pulmonary arteries; the vein chamber is separated into systemic and pulmonary veins. Both systemic and pulmonary circulations are included in the model. An illustration of the six-chamber model is shown in figure 10.19.

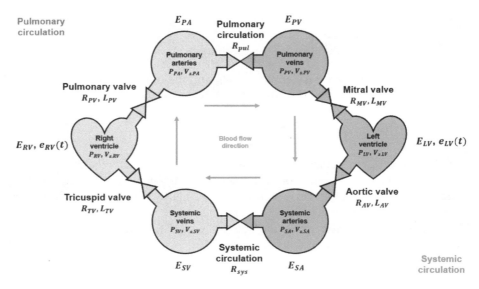

Figure 10.19. Representation of the six-chamber CVS model.

The six-chamber model and its variation have been studied by numerous researchers including Smith *et al* (2004), Szabó *et al* (2004), Hann *et al* (2005), Paeme *et al* (2011), Stevenson *et al* (2012), Revie *et al* (2013b), Pironet *et al* (2016a) and Chase *et al* (2018). They have been used to represent the cardiac and circulatory state of the cardiovascular system in a variety of pathological, physiological, and clinical conditions. The model equations for the six-chamber model are depicted in the works of Pironet *et al* (2015b, 2016a). For the systemic arteries and veins chambers, the pressure–volume relationships are given by:

$$P_{SA}(t) = E_{SA} V_{s,SA}(t), \tag{10.27}$$

$$P_{SV}(t) = E_{SV} V_{s,SV}(t), \tag{10.28}$$

where P_{SA}, E_{SA} and $V_{s,SA}$ denote the systemic arterial pressure, elastance and stressed volume at the systemic arteries chamber, respectively, while P_{SV}, E_{SV} and $V_{s,SV}$ are the systemic venous pressure, elastance and stressed volume at the systemic veins chamber, respectively.

Similarly, the pressure–volume relationship of the pulmonary arteries and veins chambers are given by:

$$P_{PA}(t) = E_{PA} V_{s,PA}(t), \tag{10.29}$$

$$P_{PV}(t) = E_{PV} V_{s,PV}(t), \tag{10.30}$$

where P_{PA}, E_{PA} and $V_{s,PA}$ are the pulmonary arterial pressure, elastance and stressed volume at the pulmonary arteries chamber, respectively, and P_{PV}, E_{PV} and $V_{s,PV}$

denote the pulmonary venous pressure, elastance and stressed volume at the pulmonary veins chamber, respectively.

The six-chamber model consists of two active chambers, the left and right ventricles. The relationship between pressure and volume in these chambers is modulated by driver functions. The pressure–volume relationships for the active chambers are written as:

$$P_{LV}(t) = e_{LV}(t)E_{LV}V_{s,LV}(t), \tag{10.31}$$

$$P_{RV}(t) = e_{RV}(t)E_{RV}V_{s,RV}(t), \tag{10.32}$$

where P_{LV}, E_{LV} and $V_{s,LV}$ denote the pressure, elastance, and stressed volume in the left ventricle, respectively, and $e_{LV}(t)$ is the driver function for the left ventricle. The equivalent right ventricular quantities are denoted using the subscript of RV, where P_{RV}, E_{RV}, $V_{s,RV}$ and $e_{RV}(t)$ are respectively the pressure, elastance, stressed volume and driver function for the right ventricle.

Next, blood flow in the systemic, $Q_{sys}(t)$ and pulmonary, $Q_{pul}(t)$ circulations are given by:

$$Q_{sys}(t) = \frac{P_{SA}(t) - P_{SV}(t)}{R_{sys}}, \tag{10.33}$$

$$Q_{pul}(t) = \frac{P_{PA}(t) - P_{PV}(t)}{R_{pul}}, \tag{10.34}$$

where R_{sys} and R_{pul} denote the resistance of the systemic and pulmonary circulations, respectively.

In the case of the valve law, the model assumes that there is only flow when the pressure difference across the valve is positive. Thus, the flow through the valves can be written as:

$$Q_{AV}(t) = \begin{cases} \frac{P_{LV}(t) - P_{SA}(t)}{R_{AV}}, & \text{if } P_{LV}(t) > P_{SA}(t) \\ 0, & \text{otherwise} \end{cases}, \tag{10.35}$$

$$Q_{TV}(t) = \begin{cases} \frac{P_{SV}(t) - P_{RV}(t)}{R_{TV}}, & \text{if } P_{SV}(t) > P_{RV}(t) \\ 0, & 0, \text{ otherwise} \end{cases}, \tag{10.36}$$

$$Q_{PV}(t) = \begin{cases} \frac{P_{RV}(t) - P_{PA}(t)}{R_{PV}}, & \text{if } P_{RV}(t) > P_{PA}(t) \\ 0, & \text{otherwise} \end{cases}, \tag{10.37}$$

$$Q_{MV}(t) = \begin{cases} \frac{P_{PV}(t) - P_{LV}(t)}{R_{PV}}, & \text{if } P_{PV}(t) > P_{LV}(t) \\ 0, & \text{otherwise} \end{cases}. \tag{10.38}$$

where Q and R are the blood flow rate and flow resistance, respectively. The subscripts AV, TV, PV and MV represent the aortic valve, the tricuspid valve, the pulmonary valve and the mitral valve, respectively. These valves and their positions within the six-chamber model are shown in figure 10.19.

Finally, the volume change in each chamber is given by the difference between the blood flow, in and out of the respective chamber. The sum of the volume changes in all chambers is zero, where there is no loss of blood volume within the CVS model. They can be represented using the following equations:

$$\frac{dV_{s,LV}(t)}{dt} = Q_{MV}(t) - Q_{AV}(t), \tag{10.39}$$

$$\frac{dV_{s,SA}(t)}{dt} = Q_{AV}(t) - Q_{sys}(t), \tag{10.40}$$

$$\frac{dV_{s,SV}(t)}{dt} = Q_{sys}(t) - Q_{TV}(t), \tag{10.41}$$

$$\frac{dV_{s,RV}(t)}{dt} = Q_{TV}(t) - Q_{PV}(t), \tag{10.42}$$

$$\frac{dV_{s,PA}(t)}{dt} = Q_{PV}(t) - Q_{pul}(t), \tag{10.43}$$

$$\frac{dV_{s,PV}(t)}{dt} = Q_{pul}(t) - Q_{MV}(t), \tag{10.44}$$

$$\frac{dV_{s,LV}(t)}{dt} + \frac{dV_{s,SA}(t)}{dt} + \frac{dV_{s,SV}(t)}{dt} + \frac{dV_{s,RV}(t)}{dt} + \frac{dV_{s,PA}(t)}{dt} + \frac{dV_{s,PV}(t)}{dt} \tag{10.45}$$
$$= 0.$$

The total stressed volume contained in the six-chamber CVS model can be obtained by integrating equation (10.45), yielding:

$$V_{s,LV} + V_{s,SA} + V_{s,SV} + V_{s,RV} + V_{s,PA} + V_{s,PV} = V_{s,6}. \tag{10.46}$$

The six-chamber CVS model is comparatively more descriptive than the three-chamber model as it considers the pulmonary circuit. Additional considerations can be included to further extend the model to better represent the human cardiovascular system. For example, the CVS model can be extended via the inclusion of the atria, ventricular interaction between the septum and the pericardium, or the influence of the thoracic pressure on the cardiovascular system (Smith *et al* 2005). These extensions also increase model complexity, which may result in model parameter identification problems. Clinically, the model may not be practical due to insufficient data.

10.4.3.1 Consideration of blood flow inertia

The six-chamber model depicted by Pironet *et al* (2015b, 2016a) (see equations (10.27)–(10.46)) did not include blood flow inertia consideration for simplicity. If we wish to include the effect of blood flow inertia, equations (10.35)–(10.46) for the blood flow through the valves can be extended to include the term $-\frac{L}{R}\frac{dQ(t)}{dt}$.

10.4.4 Electrocardiogram models

Aside from modelling the physiological cardiovascular system, there are also attempts to perform signal modelling for the cardiovascular system on the electro-cardiogram signal. Signal modelling describes a signal with respect to an underlying structure to help understand the signal's fundamental behaviour (Goodwin 1998). Modelling the cardiovascular electrical signal or the cardiac conductivity has shown to be helpful to clinicians in clinical diagnostics. As electrocardiogram models attempt to capture the shape of the ECG without the need for a physiological mechanism, we will not be covering these models in this chapter. You may explore some of these models as follows:

- Mukhopadhyay and Sircar (1996) presented an amplitude-modulated sinus-oidal signal model to model the ECG signal parametrically.
- McSharry *et al* (2003) presented a model that can generate realistic ECG signals. The model is based on three coupled ordinary differential equations.
- Ryzhii and Ryzhii (2014) proposed a model of the cardiac conduction system, which includes modelling of the natural pacemakers and heart muscles.
- Quiroz-Juárez *et al* (2019) developed a model that generates electrocardio-gram signals based on a discretised reaction-diffusion system to produce a set of three nonlinear oscillators that simulate the main pacemakers in the heart.

10.5 Application of the human cardiovascular system

10.5.1 Measurements for cardiovascular system

Cardiovascular dysfunction originates from different parts of the cardiovascular system; however, the common consequence of these dysfunctions is the reduction in the ability of the heart to pump enough blood to the body tissues. Accurate identification of the model parameters, namely stroke volume and cardiac output relies on measurements of the circulatory system. The following are some key measurements for the cardiovascular system. Some measurements are invasive, as they require surgical insertion of a sensor in the cardiovascular system.

10.5.1.1 Flow-volume and pressure measurements
- *Aortic flow probe*—An ultrasonic aortic flow probe is used to measure the blood flow rate within the aorta. This ultrasound flow probe is surgically clamped onto the aorta for blood flow measurement. It utilises soundwaves propagating through blood in motion to determine flow, which is integrated over the systolic period to estimate the beat-to-beat stroke volume.

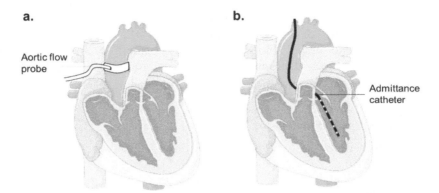

Figure 10.20. Example of cardiovascular system pressure and flow sensors placement, (a) aortic flow probe and (b) admittance catheter. Copyright © smart.servier.com. The figure was partly generated using Servier Medical Art, provided by Servier, licensed under a Creative Commons Attribution 3.0 unported license.

Figure 10.20(a) shows the aortic flow probe clamped onto the aorta for flow measurements. This sensor is mainly used in animal studies.

- *Admittance catheters*—Admittance catheters use the relationship between conductance changes within the ventricle with changes in ventricular blood volume for estimating stroke volume (Wei *et al* 2007). The catheter consists of excitation electrodes, voltage recording electrodes, and a pressure sensor for obtaining pressure–volume information within the ventricle. It is surgically placed into the ventricle and measures the changes in voltage at the recording electrodes from the electric field produced by the excitation electrode. The placement of the admittance catheter is shown in figure 10.20(b).

- *Echocardiography machine*—Echocardiography uses the Doppler principle to determine flow velocity and cross-sectional area of the aorta to produce an estimate of stroke volume. The echocardiograph is placed on the patient's chest during measurement. A systematic review by Wetterslev *et al* (2016) showed that the Doppler echocardiography has a mean error of ±32% when compared to thermodilution technique (explained below). Nevertheless, the main advantage of echocardiography is that it is non-invasive, which adds no further risks to the patient. However, this technique may have high errors and is impractical for obtaining continuous stroke volume.

- *Pulmonary artery catheter*—Pulmonary artery catheter (also known as the Swan-Ganz catheterisation) is used to monitor the blood flow and pressures in the heart (Bootsma *et al* 2022a, 2022b). It allows direct, simultaneous measurement of pressures in the right atrium, right ventricle, pulmonary artery, and the filling pressure of the left atrium using the transducer in the catheter. It is different from other pressure catheters, where it has a balloon at its tip, which helps to correctly position the catheter in the pulmonary artery. The pulmonary artery catheter also contains two temperature sensors

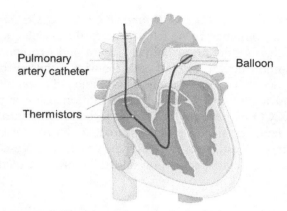

Figure 10.21. Pulmonary artery catheter. Copyright © smart.servier.com. The figure was partly generated using Servier Medical Art, provided by Servier, licensed under a Creative Commons Attribution 3.0 unported license.

(thermistors) for the measurement of cardiac output through thermodilution. This is shown in figure 10.21.

- *Sphygmomanometer*—The sphygmomanometer is a blood pressure monitor for measuring systolic and diastolic arterial pressure. The device consists of an inflatable rubber cuff, which is wrapped around the upper arm and is connected to an apparatus that records pressure, such as a mercury column, or a dial (an aneroid manometer or digital monitor) (Muniyandi *et al* 2022). At each heartbeat, blood pressure increases to the systolic level, and in between beats, it drops to the diastolic level. As the cuff is inflated with air until blood flow in the arm stops, a stethoscope is placed against the skin at the crook of the arm. As the cuff deflates, the first sound heard marks the systolic pressure; as the release continues, a dribbling noise is heard, which marks the diastolic pressure.

10.5.1.2 Cardiac output measurement
- *Thermodilution*—Thermodilution is a method to calculate cardiac output using the two thermistors located in a pulmonary artery catheter. One thermistor is placed at the upstream of the heart (right atrium), and another downstream (pulmonary artery), such as shown in figure 10.21 (Bootsma *et al* 2022a, 2022b, Isakow and Schuster 2006). Before thermodilution, the baseline blood temperature upstream and downstream of the heart is measured. To estimate cardiac output, ice-cold saline is injected at the upstream. The cold saline subsequently reaches the downstream thermistor, and the drop in downstream temperature is measured. The downstream temperature will eventually return to baseline at a rate that is proportional to the blood flow, which can be used to calculate cardiac output.

- *Pulse index Continuous Cardiac Output (PiCCO)*—PiCCO is a cardiac output monitor that combines a model of the cardiovascular system and transpulmonary thermodilution technique (Litton and Morgan 2012). It consists of three components, an arterial catheter with a thermistor near its tip, an injection device that connects to the distal lumen of a standard central venous catheter and a monitor. Unlike thermodilution using a pulmonary artery catheter, PiCCO requires ice-cold saline to be injected into both sides of the heart. The temperature drop is measured at the thermistor located at the femoral artery to estimate the cardiac output. The ice-cold saline travels through the pulmonary circulation and therefore, is called transpulmonary thermodilution.

10.5.1.3 Electrical signal of the heart

- *Electrocardiogram (ECG)*—The ECG is a recording of the electrical activity of the heart at rest. It provides information about the heart rate and rhythm. It is a non-invasive test to detect abnormal heart rhythms that may potentially indicate heart problems. ECG can also indicate pathological changes even before structural/physical changes in the heart can be detected by other methods (Stern 2006). ECG comprises four or more electrodes that are placed on the chest or at the four extremities (at the right and left arm, right and left leg). The recording of an ECG is of great value for cardiologists and continues to provide vital information in cardiovascular system monitoring.

10.5.2 Simulation of cardiovascular system model

Forward simulation of cardiovascular models can provide useful information for the understanding of the heart's function. In the following example, we forward simulate the three-chamber model by solving equations (10.16)–(10.26) using Picard's iteration to obtain stroke volume and cardiac output. The steps involved are summarised below:

Step 1: Set initial parameters t, E_a, E_v, E_h, R_i, R_o, R_c, T and estimate $V_{s\,3}$.

Step 2: Decide on a driving function $e(t)$.

Step 3: Set the initial guesses for $Q_i(t)$, $Q_o(t)$ and $Q_c(t)$ as ones for the duration of the cardiac period to initiate Picard's iteration.

Step 4: Set the initial stressed volume for each chamber, $V_{s,a}(0)$, $V_{s,v}(0)$ and $V_{s,h}(0)$.

Step 5: Perform iterations for the following:

Step 5a: Integrate equations (10.22)–(10.24) to solve for $V_{s,a}(t)$, $V_{s,v}(t)$ and $V_{s,h}(t)$:

$$V_{s,a}(t) = V_{s,a}(0) + \int_0^t \left(Q_o(t) - Q_c(t)\right)dt$$

$$V_{s,v}(t) = V_{s,v}(0) + \int_0^t \left(Q_c(t) - Q_i(t) \right) dt$$

$$V_{s,h}(t) = V_{s,h}(0) + \int_0^t \left(Q_i(t) - Q_o(t) \right) dt$$

Step 5b: Obtain pressure $P_a(t)$, $P_v(t)$ and $P_h(t)$ using equations (10.16)–(10.18).

Step 5c: Recalculate $Q_i(t)$, $Q_o(t)$ and $Q_c(t)$ using equations (10.19)–(10.21).

Step 6: Repeat *Step 5* until $P_a(t)$, $P_v(t)$ and $P_h(t)$ converge.

Step 7: Display the blood pressure, flow and volume for each chamber.

In addition to the forward simulation procedure, we can perform model-based estimation of the key parameters in a cardiac cycle, such as those presented in table 10.1 using built-in Matlab functions as below.

For SAP, it is defined as the maximum arterial pressure P_a, such that:

$$\text{SAP} = \max(P_a). \tag{10.47}$$

For DAP, it is the minimum arterial pressure:

$$\text{DAP} = \min(P_a). \tag{10.48}$$

For arterial PP, it is the difference between the maximum and minimum arterial pressure:

$$\text{PP} = \text{SAP} - \text{DAP}. \tag{10.49}$$

For the mean arterial pressure (MAP), it is the mean value of arterial pressure in a cardiac cycle:

$$\text{MAP} = \text{mean}(P_a). \tag{10.50}$$

For EDV and ESV, we can assume the stressed volume of the heart $V_{s,h}(t)$ to be the blood volume at the ventricles. If we have the measures of unstressed volume, the actual volume of the heart chamber can be estimated using:

$$V_h = V_{u,h}(t) + V_{s,h}(t), \tag{10.51}$$

where, $V_{u,h}(t)$ and $V_{s,h}(t)$ are the unstressed volume (can be assumed as a constant without the loss of blood) and stressed volume in the heart chamber, respectively. Denoting t_{EF} and t_{EE} as the time at the end of filling (end of diastole) and at the end of ejection (systole), respectively, EDV and ESV can be calculated using:

$$\text{EDV} = V_{s,h}(t_{EF}) + V_{u,h}, \tag{10.52}$$

$$\text{ESV} = V_{s,h}(t_{EE}) + V_{u,h}. \tag{10.53}$$

The change of cardiac volume or stroke volume is thus:

$$SV = EDV - ESV,$$
$$= SV = V_{s,h}(t_{EF}) + V_{u,h} - V_{s,h}(t_{EE}) - V_{u,h}, \quad (10.54)$$

which can be further expressed as:

$$SV = \Delta V_h = \Delta V_{s,h} = V_{s,h}(t_{EF}) - V_{s,h}(t_{EE}). \quad (10.55)$$

The model-based equivalent of cardiac output, CO can then be determined using:

$$CO = \frac{\Delta V_{s,h}}{T}. \quad (10.56)$$

Note that not all parameters can be estimated from the three-chamber model. For example, as the model did not consider the pulmonary circuit, we will not be able to estimate the pulmonary venous pressure (PVP).

Figure 10.22 shows a sample of simulation results for the three-chambers model. This model uses the parameters in table 10.2 and a driver function $e(t)$ from equation (10.5) (Pironet *et al* 2019). This driver function contains only two parameters and was chosen for its simplicity. The use of a more complex driver function will yield a more realistic cardiac pressure curve.

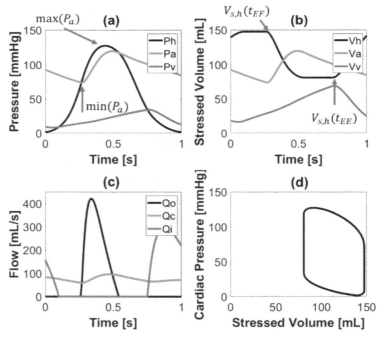

Figure 10.22. Forward simulation of the three-chamber CVS model: (a) Blood pressures in the heart (P_h), arteries (P_a) and veins (P_v); (b) stressed volumes in the heart (V_h), arteries (V_a) and veins (V_v); (c) blood flows through the output valve (Q_o), circulatory (Q_c) and input valve (Q_i); (d) pressure–volume diagram for the heart chamber.

Table 10.2. Three-chamber CVS model parameters.

Parameter	Descriptions	Units	Value
T	Cardiac period	s	1.0
t	Time	s	0:0.01:1.0
E_h	Heart elastance	mmHg ml^{-1}	1.5
E_a	Arterial elastance	mmHg ml^{-1}	1.0
E_v	Venous elastance	mmHg ml^{-1}	0.5
R_i	Input valve resistance	mmHg s ml^{-1}	0.05
R_o	Output valve resistance	mmHg s ml^{-1}	0.05
R_c	Circulatory resistance	mmHg s ml^{-1}	1
$V_{s,3}$	Total stressed volume	ml	250
$e(t)$	Driver function	$e(t) = \exp\left[-W((t \times \mathrm{mod}(T)) - \frac{T}{2})^2\right],\ W = 20\mathrm{s}^{-2}$	

The model-based cardiac cycle parameters can be calculated using the pressure and volume waveform values obtained from the forward simulation as follows:

$$\mathrm{SAP} = \max(P_a) = 119.5 \text{ mmHg}$$
$$\mathrm{DAP} = \min(P_a) = 73.6 \text{ mmHg}$$
$$\mathrm{PP} = \mathrm{SAP} - \mathrm{DAP} = 45.9 \text{ mmHg}$$
$$\mathrm{MAP} = \mathrm{mean}(P_a) = 96.1 \text{ mmHg}$$

The stroke volume (SV) and cardiac output (CO) can be calculated from the values obtained based on the heart stressed volume waveform in figure 10.21 (top right), such that:

$$\mathrm{SV} = V_{s,h}(t_{EF}) - V_{s,h}(t_{EE}) = 147.4 - 80.7 = 66.7 \text{ ml}$$
$$\mathrm{CO} = \frac{\Delta V_{s,h}}{T} = \frac{66.7}{1} = 66.7 \text{ ml/s.}$$

From figure 10.22, one may observe that the model simulation does not fully replicate the dynamics of the pressure, flow and volume waveform of a typical Wiggers diagram shown in figure 10.10. This is because the three-chamber model is a simplified model of the cardiovascular system, and thus, several effects and dynamics are neglected. These include the absence of the pulmonary circuit and the exclusion of blood flow inertia, as mentioned in section 10.3. However, in terms of bedside clinical application, the simplicity enables parameter identification to be performed (Pironet et al 2019). For instance, the three-chamber model has been used to determine conditions in experimental animal trials as well as potentially provide decision support during fluid resuscitation (Pironet et al 2015a, 2016b). A sample of the Matlab code for the three-chamber model forward simulation can be found in this chapter[1].

---

[1] Source code for this model (Chapter10a) is available at https://doi.org/10.1088/978-0-7503-4016-8.

10.5.3 Six-chamber cardiovascular system model

The steps to forward simulate the six-chamber CVS model follow those employed for the three-chamber model, as outlined in section 10.5.2. The main difference between the six-chamber model and the three-chamber model is that the former has more parameters to be initiated due to the inclusion of the pulmonary circuit. As more chambers are involved, we will need to estimate the stressed volumes in all chambers at the start of the simulation.

The simulation results for the six-chamber model using the parameters presented in table 10.3 are shown in figure 10.23. The parameters used for forward simulation of the six-chamber CVS model are shown in table 10.3. A sample of the Matlab code for the six-chamber model is attached[2].

The additional considerations of the six-chamber model allow it to simulate better the cardiovascular system dynamics when compared to the three-chamber model. The six-chamber model and its extension models are one of the more common CVS models that have been used and researched. It has been used particularly to simulate different

Table 10.3. Parameter values of the six-chamber CVS model obtained from Paeme *et al* (2011) and Revie (2013). Adapted from Paeme *et al* (2011) Copyright © 2011, Paeme *et al*; licensee BioMed Central Ltd.

Parameter	Descriptions	Unit	Value
T	Cardiac period	s	0.6
t	Time	s	0:0.01:0.60
E_{LV}	Left ventricle elastance	mmHg ml^{-1}	2.8798
E_{RV}	Right ventricle elastance	mmHg ml^{-1}	0.5850
E_{SA}	Systemic arteries elastance	mmHg ml^{-1}	0.6913
E_{SV}	Systemic veins elastance	mmHg ml^{-1}	0.0059
E_{PA}	Pulmonary arteries elastance	mmHg ml^{-1}	0.3690
E_{PV}	Pulmonary veins elastance	mmHg ml^{-1}	0.0073
R_{sys}	Systemic circulatory resistance	mmHg s ml^{-1}	1.0889
R_{pul}	Pulmonary circulatory resistance	mmHg s ml^{-1}	0.1552
R_{AV}	Aortic valve resistance	mmHg s ml^{-1}	0.0180
R_{TV}	Tricuspid valve resistance	mmHg s ml^{-1}	0.0237
R_{PV}	Pulmonary valve resistance	mmHg s ml^{-1}	0.0055
R_{MV}	Mitral valve resistance	mmHg s ml^{-1}	0.0158
L_{AV}	Aortic valve inertia	mmHg s^2 ml^{-1}	1.2189×10^{-4}
L_{TV}	Tricuspid valve inertia	mmHg s^2 ml^{-1}	8.0093×10^{-5}
L_{PV}	Pulmonary valve inertia	mmHg s^2 ml^{-1}	1.4868×10^{-4}
L_{MV}	Mitral valve inertia	mmHg s^2 ml^{-1}	7.6968×10^{-5}
$V_{s,6}$	Total stressed volume	ml	1500
$e_{LV}(t)$	Left ventricle driver function	$e_{LV}(t) = \exp\left[-W((t \times \mathrm{mod}(T)) - \frac{T}{2})^2\right]$, $W = 80 \text{ s}^{-2}$	
$e_{RV}(t)$	Right ventricle driver function	$e_{RV}(t) = \exp\left[-W((t \times \mathrm{mod}(T)) - \frac{T}{2})^2\right]$, $W = 80 \text{ s}^{-2}$	

---

[2] Source code for this model (Chapter10b) is available at https://doi.org/10.1088/978-0-7503-4016-8.

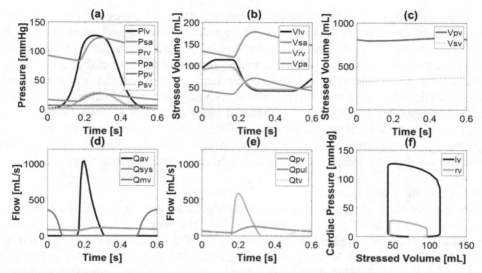

Figure 10.23. Forward simulation of the six-chamber CVS model. (a) Blood pressures for all six chambers, left ventricle (P_{lv}), systemic arteries (P_{sa}), right ventricle (P_{rv}), pulmonary arteries (P_{pa}), pulmonary venous (P_{pv}) and systemic venous (P_{sv}). (b) Stressed volumes in the left ventricle (V_{lv}), systemic arteries (V_{sa}), right ventricle (V_{rv}) and pulmonary arteries (V_{pa}). (c) Stressed volumes in the pulmonary venous (V_{pv}) and systemic venous (V_{sv}), respectively. (d) Blood flow through the aortic valve (Q_{av}), systemic circulatory (Q_{sys}) and mitral valve (Q_{mv}). (e) Blood flow through pulmonary valve (Q_{pv}), pulmonary circulatory (Q_{pul}) and tricuspid valve (Q_{tv}). (e) Pressure–volume diagram for the left ventricle (lv) and right ventricle (rv).

types of cardiovascular system dysfunction encountered in patients who are critically ill. For example, myocardial dysfunction, valvular disorders and circulatory shocks, and their impact on cardiovascular system function can potentially be simulated (Smith *et al* 2004, 2007, Revie *et al* 2013a, Kosta *et al* 2017, Szabó *et al* 2004). The effect of CVS model parameters on the pressure–volume diagram can also be simulated to provide a better understanding of the cardiovascular system physiology and response to treatment.

10.5.4 Other applications of the cardiovascular system model

Aside from model simulation to provide a better understanding of cardiovascular system physiology of cardiac dysfunction, response to treatment, or to guide treatment, CVS models have been applied in the controls and testing in surgical applications of cardiac devices. For example, testing, development and controls of the total artificial heart and artificial pacemakers.

10.5.4.1 Total artificial heart

The total artificial heart is a mechanical pump that is surgically installed to provide blood circulation and replace diseased or damaged heart ventricles (Cook *et al* 2015). It has been used in end-stage biventricular heart failure as a bridge to heart transplantation. However, with an increasing global burden of cardiovascular disease and congestive heart failure, it has been used as an alternative treatment for patients who are unable to receive a heart transplant.

The total artificial heart replaces the heart ventricle functions, where it pumps blood out of the heart to the lungs via the pulmonary arteries and other parts of the body via the aorta. A power source and controller are connected to the artificial heart from outside of the body for power and control of the artificial heart pumping mechanism. The artificial heart also has four mechanical valves that mimic the work of the aortic valve, tricuspid valve, pulmonary valve and mitral valve. CVS models have been used for testing the total artificial heart (Khalil *et al* 2010, Cappon *et al* 2021). Works have been undertaken to simulate the cardiovascular system condition and how the total artificial heart would respond to patient conditions. This enables better control of the pump as well as better human–device interaction.

10.5.4.2 Artificial pacemakers

CVS models have also been applied in the development and control of artificial pacemakers. The heart's natural pacemaker, i.e., the sinus node, produces electrical impulses to stimulate the heart to beat. However, if these impulses are disrupted, an artificial pacemaker can be used to aid the subject (Wood and Ellenbogen 2002). A pacemaker is a device placed under the skin in the chest to help control the subject's heartbeat more regularly in cases of arrhythmia. This is shown in figure 10.24.

A pacemaker comprises two parts:

- *Pulse generator*—The generator houses the power supply (battery), the electrical circuit and the controller that regulates the rate of electrical impulses sent to the heart.
- *Leads* (*electrodes*)—The electrodes are placed in a heart chamber(s) to deliver the electrical impulses to the heart.

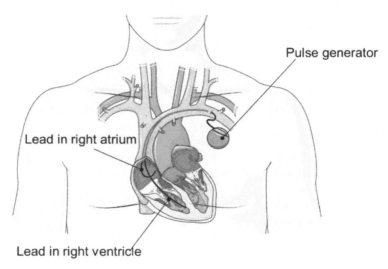

Figure 10.24. Artificial pacemaker consists of two main parts, (a) pulse generator and (b) leads. Copyright © smart.servier.com. The figure was partly generated using Servier Medical Art, provided by Servier, licensed under a Creative Commons Attribution 3.0 unported license.

These devices can be implanted permanently to correct a slow or irregular heartbeat or, in some people, to help treat heart failure. They can also be used after a heart attack, surgery, or medication overdose to temporarily treat a slow heartbeat. Many mathematical models of cardiac pacemaking cells have been developed for the control of pacemakers. For example, Purkinje cell models, sinoatrial node cell models and atrioventricular node cell models (Li *et al* 2013). These models potentially provide better control and regulate the electrical signal generator.

10.6 Summary

The human cardiovascular system is a complex interactive system. Modelling the human cardiovascular system has shown potential in capturing a wide range of cardiovascular system dynamics that could be of direct use in the clinical environment. In particular, the models may potentially be used to provide a better understanding of the complex interaction between the physiological response during the treatment of cardiovascular dysfunction. Studies and investigations need to be carried out to explore further developments in the model structure and governing equations, enabling more specific and subtle dynamics to be captured while being clinically applicable.

References

Aaronson P I, Ward J P and Connolly M J 2020 *The Cardiovascular System at a Glance* 5th edn (Hoboken, NJ: Wiley)

Betts J G, Young K A, Wise J A, Johnson E, Poe B, Kruse D H, Korol O, Johnson J E, Womble M and Desaix P 2013 *Anatomy and Physiology* (Houston, TX: OpenStax) retrieved from https://perlego.com/book/695138/anatomy-and-physiology-pdf

Bootsma I T, Boerma E C, De Lange F and Scheeren T W L 2022a The contemporary pulmonary artery catheter. Part 1: placement and waveform analysis *J. Clin. Monit. Comput.* **36** 5–15

Bootsma I T, Boerma E C, Scheeren T W L and De Lange F 2022b The contemporary pulmonary artery catheter. Part 2: measurements, limitations, and clinical applications *J. Clin. Monit. Comput.* **36** 17–31

Cappon F, Wu T, Papaioannou T, Du X, Hsu P-L and Khir A W 2021 Mock circulatory loops used for testing cardiac assist devices: a review of computational and experimental models *Int. J. Artif. Organs* **44** 793–806

Cecconi M *et al* 2014 Consensus on circulatory shock and hemodynamic monitoring. Task force of the European Society of Intensive Care Medicine *Intensive Care Med.* **40** 1795–815

Chase J G *et al* 2018 Next-generation, personalised, model-based critical care medicine: a state-of-the art review of in silico virtual patient models, methods, and cohorts, and how to validation them *Biomed. Eng. Online* **17** 24

Chen C-H, Fetics B, Nevo E, Rochitte C E, Chiou K-R, Ding P-A, Kawaguchi M and Kass D A 2001 Noninvasive single-beat determination of left ventricular end-systolic elastance in humans *J. Am. Coll. Cardiol.* **38** 2028–34

Cook J A, Shah K B, Quader M A, Cooke R H, Kasirajan V, Rao K K, Smallfield M C, Tchoukina I and Tang D G 2015 The total artificial heart *J. Thorac. Dis.* **7** 2172–80

Cushway J, Murphy L, Chase J G, Shaw G M and Desaive T 2022 Physiological trend analysis of a novel cardio-pulmonary model during a preload reduction manoeuvre *Comput. Methods Programs Biomed.* **220** 106819

Danielsen M and Ottesen J T 2001 Describing the pumping heart as a pressure source *J. Theor. Biol.* **212** 71–81

Goodwin M M 1998 Signal models and analysis-synthesis ed M M Goodwin *Adaptive Signal Models: Theory, Algorithms, and Audio Applications* (Boston, MA: Springer)

Greer J 2015 Pathophysiology of cardiovascular dysfunction in sepsis *BJA Educ.* **15** 316–21

Gyawali B, Ramakrishna K and Dhamoon A S 2019 Sepsis: the evolution in definition, pathophysiology, and management *SAGE Open Med.* **7** 2050312119835043

Hann C E, Chase J G and Shaw G M 2005 Efficient implementation of non-linear valve law and ventricular interaction dynamics in the minimal cardiac model *Comput. Methods Programs Biomed.* **80** 65–74

Hann C E *et al* 2011 Patient specific identification of the cardiac driver function in a cardiovascular system model *Comput. Methods Programs Biomed.* **101** 201–7

Isakow W and Schuster D P 2006 Extravascular lung water measurements and hemodynamic monitoring in the critically ill: bedside alternatives to the pulmonary artery catheter *Am. J. Physiol.* **291** L1118–31

Khalil H A, Kerr D T, Schusterman M A, Cohn W E, Frazier O H and Radovancevic B 2010 Induced pulsation of a continuous-flow total artificial heart in a mock circulatory system *J. Heart Lung Transplant.* **29** 568–73

Kosta S, Negroni J, Lascano E and Dauby P C 2017 Multiscale model of the human cardiovascular system: description of heart failure and comparison of contractility indices *Math. Biosci.* **284** 71–9

Kreimeier U 2000 Pathophysiology of fluid imbalance *Crit. Care* **4** S3–7

Li P, Lines G T, Maleckar M M and Tveito A 2013 Mathematical models of cardiac pacemaking function *Front. Phys.* **1** 20

Litton E and Morgan M 2012 The PiCCO monitor: a review *Anaesth. Intensive Care* **40** 393–408

McSharry P E, Clifford G D, Tarassenko L and Smith L A 2003 A dynamical model for generating synthetic electrocardiogram signals *IEEE Trans. Biomed. Eng.* **50** 289–94

Mitchell J R and Wang J-J 2014 Expanding application of the Wiggers diagram to teach cardiovascular physiology *Adv. Physiol. Educ.* **38** 170–5

Mukhopadhyay S and Sircar P 1996 Parametric modelling of ECG signal *Med. Biol. Eng. Comput.* **34** 171–4

Muniyandi M, Sellappan S, Chellaswamy V, Ravi K, Karthikeyan S, Thiruvengadam K, Selvam J M and Karikalan N 2022 Diagnostic accuracy of mercurial versus digital blood pressure measurement devices: a systematic review and meta-analysis *Sci. Rep.* **12** 3363

Naeije R, Brimioulle S and Dewachter L 2014 Biomechanics of the right ventricle in health and disease (2013 Grover Conference series) *Pulm. Circ.* **4** 395–406

Paeme S *et al* 2011 Mathematical multi-scale model of the cardiovascular system including mitral valve dynamics. Application to ischemic mitral insufficiency *Biomed. Eng. Online* **10** 86

Parlikar T A and Verghese G C 2005 A simple cycle-averaged model for cardiovascular dynamics *2005 Conf. Proc. IEEE Eng. Med. Biol. Soc. (17–18 January)* 5490–94

Pironet A, Dauby P C, Chase J G, Docherty P D, Revie J A and Desaive T 2016a Structural identifiability analysis of a cardiovascular system model *Med. Eng. Phys.* **38** 433–41

Pironet A, Dauby P C, Chase J G, Kamoi S, Janssen N, Morimont P, Lambermont B and Desaive T 2015a Model-based stressed blood volume is an index of fluid responsiveness *IFAC-PapersOnLine* **48** 291–6

Pironet A, Dauby P C, Morimont P, Janssen N, Chase J G, Davidson S and Desaive T 2016b Model-based decision support algorithm to guide fluid resuscitation *IFAC-PapersOnLine* **49** 224–9

Pironet A, Desaive T, Chase J G, Morimont P and Dauby P C 2015b Model-based computation of total stressed blood volume from a preload reduction manoeuvre *Math. Biosci.* **265** 28–39

Pironet A, Docherty P D, Dauby P C, Chase J G and Desaive T 2019 Practical identifiability analysis of a minimal cardiovascular system model *Comput. Methods Programs Biomed.* **171** 53–65

Quiroz-Juárez M A, Jiménez-Ramírez O, Vázquez-Medina R, Breña-Medina V, Aragón J L and Barrio R A 2019 Generation of ECG signals from a reaction-diffusion model spatially discretized *Sci. Rep.* **9** 19000

Revie J A, Stevenson D, Chase J G, Pretty C J, Lambermont B C, Ghuysen A, Kolh P, Shaw G M and Desaive T 2013a Evaluation of a model-based hemodynamic monitoring method in a porcine study of septic shock *Comput. Math. Methods Med.* **2013** 505417

Revie J A, Stevenson D J, Chase J G, Hann C E, Lambermont B C, Ghuysen A, Kolh P, Shaw G M, Heldmann S and Desaive T 2013b Validation of subject-specific cardiovascular system models from porcine measurements *Comput. Methods Programs Biomed.* **109** 197–210

Revie J A M 2013 Model-based cardiovascular monitoring in critical care for improved diagnosis of cardiac dysfunction *PhD Thesis* (New Zealand: University of Canterbury)

Roth G A, Mensah G A, Johnson C O, Addolorato G, Ammirati E, Baddour L M and Barengo N C *et al* 2020 Global burden of cardiovascular diseases and risk factors, 1990–2019: update from the GBD 2019 study *J. Am. Coll. Cardiol.* **76** 2982–3021

Ryzhii E and Ryzhii M 2014 A heterogeneous coupled oscillator model for simulation of ECG signals *Comput. Methods Programs Biomed.* **117** 40–9

Shimizu S, Une D, Kawada T, Hayama Y, Kamiya A, Shishido T and Sugimachi M 2018 Lumped parameter model for hemodynamic simulation of congenital heart diseases *J. Physiol. Sci.* **68** 103–11

Smith B W, Andreassen S, Shaw G M, Jensen P L, Rees S E and Chase J G 2007 Simulation of cardiovascular system diseases by including the autonomic nervous system into a minimal model *Comput. Methods Programs Biomed.* **86** 153–60

Smith B W, Chase J G, Nokes R I, Shaw G M and Wake G 2004 Minimal haemodynamic system model including ventricular interaction and valve dynamics *Med. Eng. Phys.* **26** 131–9

Smith B W, Chase J G, Shaw G M and Nokes R I 2005 Experimentally verified minimal cardiovascular system model for rapid diagnostic assistance *Control Eng. Prac.* **13** 1183–93

Spiegel R 2016 Stressed vs. unstressed volume and its relevance to critical care practitioners *Clin. Exp. Emerg. Med.* **3** 52–4

Standl T, Annecke T, Cascorbi I, Heller A R, Sabashnikov A and Teske W 2018 The nomenclature, definition and distinction of types of shock *Dtsch. Arztebl. Int.* **115** 757–68

Stern S 2006 Electrocardiogram *Circulation* **113** e753–6

Stevenson D, Revie J, Chase J G, Hann C E, Shaw G M, Lambermont B, Ghuysen A, Kolh P and Desaive T 2012 Algorithmic processing of pressure waveforms to facilitate estimation of cardiac elastance *Biomed. Eng. Online* **11** 28

Suga H, Sagawa K and Shoukas A A 1973 Load independence of the instantaneous pressure–volume ratio of the canine left ventricle and effects of epinephrine and heart rate on the ratio *Circ. Res.* **32** 314–22

Szabó G, Soans D, Graf A, Beller C J, Waite L and Hagl S 2004 A new computer model of mitral valve hemodynamics during ventricular filling *Eur. J. Cardiothroac. Surg.* **26** 239–47

Vahdatpour C, Collins D and Goldberg S 2019 Cardiogenic shock *J. Am. Heart Assoc.* **8** e011991

Vincent J-L 2008 Understanding cardiac output *Crit. Care* **12** 174

Vincent J-L and De Backer D 2013 Circulatory shock *New Engl. J. Med.* **369** 1726–34

Weber K T, Janicki J S and Maskin C S 1985 Pathophysiology of cardiac failure *Am. J. Cardiol.* **56** B3–7

Wei C, Valvano J W, Feldman M D, Nahrendorf M, Peshock R and Pearce J A 2007 Volume catheter parallel conductance varies between end-systole and end-diastole *IEEE Trans. Biomed. Eng.* **54** 1480–9

Westerhof N, Lankhaar J-W and Westerhof B E 2009 The arterial Windkessel *Med. Biol. Eng. Comput.* **47** 131–41

Wetterslev M, Møller-Sørensen H, Johansen R R and Perner A 2016 Systematic review of cardiac output measurements by echocardiography vs. thermodilution: the techniques are not interchangeable *Intens. Care Med.* **42** 1223–33

Wood M A and Ellenbogen K A 2002 Cardiac pacemakers from the patient's perspective *Circulation* **105** 2136–8

Zenker S, Rubin J and Clermont G 2007 From inverse problems in mathematical physiology to quantitative differential diagnoses *PLoS Comput. Biol.* **3** e204

Chapter 11

Ethics and biosafety

11.1 Introduction

In the preceding chapters, we have demonstrated how computational modelling can be used to simulate various biophysical and physiological problems pertaining to healthcare. *In silico* experiments carried out using these mechanistic and physiological models are highly beneficial to the development of healthcare due to their cheaper overall cost and shorter experimentation time. Moreover, these models allow better control of the variables of interest and the outputs can provide information that may not be retrievable from human and animal experimentation. In chapter 1, we have also pointed out that computational models bypass the need for human and animal ethics approval. Although this is the case, the principles and concepts related to the issue of ethics should neither be neglected nor taken lightly. This is because the predictions made using computational models, be they mechanistic or physiological, are only reliable if they can be validated or verified against clinical experimental results. On a larger scale, developments (treatments, drug delivery, etc) that are based partly or entirely on the outcome of computational model predictions must undergo various clinical trials to determine their safety before massive rollout. These clinical trials must obtain human ethics approval and require familiarity with the concepts of biosafety to ensure safe conduct and handling of the laboratory experiments and clinical trials. Hence, this chapter aims to provide readers with an overview of the role of human ethics in clinical research and the importance of biosafety when handling biological materials.

11.2 Human ethics

11.2.1 Clinical research

As pointed out in section 11.1, all clinical research or trials must obtain human ethics approval before they can proceed. So, what is clinical research? According to the World Health Organisation, a clinical trial is (WHO 2023):

'Any research study that prospectively assigns human participants or groups of humans to one or more health-related interventions to evaluate the effects on health outcomes.'

The United States National Institute of Health defines a clinical trial as (NIH 2017):

'A research study in which one or more human subjects are prospectively assigned to one or more interventions (which may include placebo or other control) to evaluate the effects of those interventions on health-related biomedical or behavioural outcomes.'

In the two definitions above, the word 'intervention' includes the administration of drugs, cells and other biological products to the human body, surgical and radiologic procedures, installation and/or administration of medical devices inside/to the human body, behavioural treatment, process-of-care changes, preventive care etc.

Clinical research is an important part of healthcare development. Outcomes from clinical research can inform researchers if a new treatment, drugs, or medical device, i.e., the 'intervention', is effective, and more importantly, safe for humans. Clinical research can be divided into four trial phases, namely phase I, phase II, phase III, and phase IV trials. A phase I trial is usually carried out in a small group of test subjects (<100) with emphasis placed on determining the safety and side effects of a particular treatment. Phase II trial involves a larger group of test subjects (100–300) with emphasis placed on the effectiveness of the treatment in addition to safety and side effects. A phase III trial is carried out among different populations, usually with the tested treatment in combination with other treatments. The number of subjects can approach 3000. Phase III trial will determine if the treatment gets approval from the relevant authorities. A phase IV trial is carried out after approval from phase III, where the treatment's effectiveness and safety are monitored in large, diverse populations. Phase IV trials can extend over several years to the risks of any long-term side effects.

11.2.2 Ethics in clinical research (trials)

The nature of clinical research meant that a few individuals (test subjects) are exposed to risk for the benefit of the society. As such, concerns arise over the potential exploitation and/or abuse of the test subjects to manipulate the outcome of the research for the benefit (usually financially) of some of the individuals or groups involved (Grady 2012). Ethics in clinical research is thus necessary and compulsory to prevent the exploitation of test subjects and manipulation of research outcome. In general, ethics in clinical research addresses the conditions that are deemed acceptable for the exposure of test subjects to risks for the benefit of the society (Sanmukhani and Tripathi 2011). In other words, ethics helps researchers decide what is right and wrong, good and bad, and what should and should not be done in clinical research (Varkey 2021).

According to the Belmont report[1], the three principles of ethical clinical research are:

(1) Respect for person:

Respect for person entails two ethical convictions. The first conviction requires every individual or test subject to be treated as autonomous agents. Autonomous agents in this context are individuals with the capacity to make informed and personal decisions about the healthcare services they receive (Leo 1999). The second conviction states that individuals who are not autonomous agents or with diminished autonomy must always be protected until they gain full autonomy.

(2) Beneficence and non-malfeasance:

There are two complementary regulations concerning beneficence and non-malfeasance in ethical clinical research, namely (1) to do no harm and (2) to maximise possible benefits and minimise potential harm. According to the second principle of ethical clinical research, an experiment or a trial should be carried out only if the expected benefits justify the risks involved. The welfare of the test subjects including the rights, safety and well-being must be placed at utmost priority and should take precedence over the interests of science and society.

(3) Justice:

Justice in the context of clinical research implies that all test subjects must be treated fairly. This extends to the selection of test subjects, which must be fair and not purposefully biased to elicit a targeted outcome. Furthermore, test subjects should not benefit (financially or otherwise) from the subsequent applications of the research as this may lead to skewed or fabricated responses from the test subjects.

11.2.3 The seven requirements of ethical research

Although the Belmont report establishes three principles for ethical clinical research, questions remain on what makes a clinical research ethical. There is often misconception that obtaining informed consent from the test subject constitutes ethical research. While informed consent is an important part of ethical clinical research, this alone does not make the research ethical. To address this issue, Emanuel *et al* (2000) proposed a framework consisting of seven requirements that define ethical clinical research. The seven requirements are:

(1) Societal/scientific value:

Ethical clinical research must have either societal or scientific value to it. This means that the intervention that is being trialled must have the capacity to improve the health and well-being of the society and increase the scientific knowledge in that area. This requirement in ethical clinical research protects test subjects from being exposed to unnecessary risks and harm that contribute zero values to both the society and science.

---

[1] The Belmont report is a report written by the National Commission for the Protection of Human Subjects of Biomedical and Behavioural Research published in 1979. It documents the ethical principles and guidelines involving research on human subjects.

(2) Scientific validity:

This requirement is tied to the first requirement. Scientific validity ensures that there are merits or justifications to the research that is to be carried out. This is important to ensure accurate and reproducible test results.

(3) Fair subject selection:

This requirement ensures that the subjects are selected fairly to prevent outcomes that are biased and inaccurate. Subjects are also not selected because of 'convenience' and should not have invested interest in the outcome and benefits of the research.

(4) Favourable risk–benefit ratio:

This requirement is important in ethical clinical research to: (i) minimise risks to the test subjects, (ii) enhance benefits to the test subjects, and (iii) balance out the benefits and the risks to the test subjects and/or the society.

(5) Respect for subjects:

All test subjects must be respected during the clinical research, from the time they are recruited, throughout the period of testing and even after the trials conclude. Respect for subjects entails the following: (i) subjects' privacy and confidentiality are protected, (ii) opportunities for early withdrawal early without any penalties, (iii) subjects' health and well-being are monitored and protected, (iv) subjects are informed of latest development, (v) subjects are informed of the outcomes and if relevant, their contributions recognised, (vi) subjects are compensated for any injuries inflicted due to the clinical trials.

(6) Informed consent:

Subjects must agree to participate in the clinical research voluntarily. In this regard, they must be informed of all the risks and benefits that are involved. If the subjects are also existing patients, then they must also be made aware of other treatment alternatives other than the one that is being trialled.

(7) Independent review board:

All clinical research study must be reviewed and approved by an independent review board (IRB). An IRB is an independent body whose members are from the medical, scientific, and non-scientific community. The responsibility of the members of IRB is to protect the rights, safety, and well-being of the test subjects. An important task of IRB is to review the risk–benefit ratio of the study (see requirement (4) above) to ensure that the clinical research has a favourable risk–benefit ratio.

11.3 Biosafety

According to the United States Centre for Disease Control and Prevention (CDC), biosafety is:

'The discipline addressing the safe handling and containment of infectious microorganisms and hazardous biological materials.'

Institutions from other countries have their own definition of biosafety. For instance, in Malaysia, the Ministry of Environment and Water defines biosafety as:

'Efforts to reduce and eliminate potential risks arising from the use of modern biotechnology or Living Modified Organism (LMO) and its products in order to safeguard human, plant and animal health, the environment and biological diversity.'

It is clear from the two definitions above that biosafety is not limited to only a specific field. Instead, different areas of study have different biosafety definitions; hence, different biosafety protocols. In clinical research (and medicine), biosafety involves the handling of biological materials including but not limited to medical wastes, organs, and tissues. Biosafety is important to protect not only the researchers and healthcare workers, but also the test subjects (patients) and the public. A complete guide and protocol for handling biological materials has been set by the World Health Organisation[2]. Hence, only a general overview of the important considerations related to biosafety will be presented in this section.

11.3.1 Biosafety in healthcare and medicine

Biosafety protocols in healthcare and medicine are prepared to address four different risk groups, as per the guideline set by the World Health Organisation:

11.3.1.1 Risk group 1
Biological materials under risk group 1 are unlikely to cause harm to humans and animals. Risks to the individual and the community are minimal. Some examples include non-pathogenic *Escherichia coli* and *Bacillus thuringiensis*.

11.3.1.2 Risk group 2
Biological materials under risk group 2 carries moderate individual risk. Community risk is low, however. Exposure to these can cause diseases to individuals but are unlikely to lead to an outbreak among the community. Effective treatment and preventive measures are available to limit the spread of the infection. Examples of biological materials under risk group 2 include *Streptococcus pneumonia* and *Salmonella choleraesuis*.

11.3.1.3 Risk group 3
Biological materials under risk group 3 carries high individual risk. Community risk remains low. Although these materials can cause serious diseases among humans and/or animals, they do not spread from an infected person to another. Effective treatment and preventive measures are available. Examples of biological materials under risk group 3 include HIV, H1N1 virus and SARS.

11.3.1.4 Risk group 4
Biological materials under risk group 4 have the highest risk to both individual and the community. They usually cause serious harm to the humans and/or animals and

---

[2] https://www.who.int/publications/i/item/9241546506

can spread readily among individuals and within the community. Unlike those in risk groups 2 and 3, effective treatment and preventive measures are not available to handle infections from risk groups 4. Examples of biological materials under risk group 4 include the Ebola virus, the Nipah virus and the Marburg virus.

11.3.2 Biosafety levels

The World Health Organisation sets four biosafety levels to handle the four risk groups presented in section 11.3.1.

11.3.2.1 Biosafety levels 1 and 2
Biosafety levels 1 and 2 are the most basic of the biosafety levels. Basic teaching and research laboratories, and laboratories that offer health and diagnostic services are categorised under biosafety levels 1 and 2. Health clinics and hospitals are designed and must operate to a minimum biosafety level 2. The protocols of biosafety levels 1 and 2 typically involve proper code of practice, proper laboratory design and facilities, adequate laboratory equipment, installation of health and medical surveillance, provision of training to personnel involved, proper waste handling and availability of safety procedures to tackle chemical, fire, electrical, radiation and equipment hazards. The workspace of biosafety level 1 is typically a standard open workbench. On the other hand, biosafety level 2 requires both open workbenches and Class I biosafety cabinets[3] (BSC).

11.3.2.2 Biosafety level 3
Biosafety level 3 is designed for handling biological materials under risk group 3. It includes all the elements of biosafety levels 1 and 2. laboratories designed under biosafety level 3 aims for containment of the biological material inside the laboratory. As such, there will be two entry levels, where the user can decontaminate before leaving the laboratory. Furthermore, self-closing doors are compulsory and access to biosafety level 3 laboratories are restricted and controlled. Laboratories offering specialised diagnostic and research services that handle biological materials under risk group 3 must be designed under this biosafety level. Specialised protective equipment must be worn by all personnel inside the laboratory. Class I BSC are provided and if necessary, Class II BSC must also be available.

11.3.2.3 Biosafety level 4
Laboratories under biosafety level 4 are designed for maximum containment of biological materials under risk group 4. It satisfies all the requirement of biosafety level 3 and includes additional safety features such as airlock entry, shower exit and specialised waste disposal unit. Handling of biological materials must be carried out inside a Class III BSC. Double ended autoclaves that are installed through the wall and proper air filtering system are also requirements under biosafety level 4.

---

[3] A biosafety cabinet is a laboratory workspace that is enclosed and ventilated. It provides a safe working environment for handling biological materials at the required biosafety level (Kruse *et al* 1991).

Development of a level 4 biosafety laboratory usually requires the approval of the World Health Organisation.

11.4 Summary

In this chapter, we have provided readers with an overview of the requirements for human ethics in clinical research trials and some underlying principles of biosafety. This chapter is not meant to be a complete guide to clinical research ethics and protocols of biosafety. A complete coverage of these topics extends beyond the scope of this book and interested readers may refer to the sources listed in the references. Although this book focuses primarily on model-based approaches and their applications in healthcare, we find it apt to introduce readers to the importance of clinical research ethics and biosafety. This is because model validation and experimental trials, both of which involve components of ethics and biosafety, are natural progression from simulation-based research work.

References

Emanuel E, Wendler D and Grady C 2000 What makes clinical research ethical? *JAMA* **283** 2701–11

Grady C 2012 Ethical principles in clinical research ed J I Gallin and F P Ognibene *Principles and Practice of Clinical Research* (London: Academic)

Kruse R H, Puckett W H and Richardson J H 1991 Biological safety cabinetry *Clin. Microbiol. Rev.* **4** 207–41

Leo R J 1999 Competency and the capacity to make treatment decisions: a primer for primary care physicians *Prim. Care Comapnion J. Clin. Psychiatry* **1** 131–41

NIH 2017 *NIH's Definition of a Clinical Trial* https://grants.nih.gov/policy/clinical-trials/definition.htm

Sanmukhani J and Tripathi C B 2011 Ethics in clinical research: the Indian perspective *Indian J. Pharm. Sci.* **73** 125–30

Varkey B 2021 Principles of clinical ethics and their application to practice *Med. Princ. Pract.* **30** 17–28

WHO 2023 International Clinical Trials Registry Platform (ICTRP) https://who.int/clinical-trials-registry-platform

IOP Publishing

Model-Based Approaches in Biomedical Engineering

Ean Hin Ooi and Yeong Shiong Chiew

Appendix A

Review on heat transfer

A.1 Fundamentals of heat transfer

Heat transfer is the transport of heat or thermal energy through space due to the presence of a temperature gradient. Heat transfer can occur with and without the presence of a medium, and the mode of heat transfer varies depending on the medium through which heat transfer occurs. There are three modes of heat transfer, namely conduction, convection and radiation. Each of the three modes will be presented separately next.

A.2 Heat conduction

Heat conduction is heat transfer that occurs through a solid or a stationary fluid, although with the latter, the process is more commonly referred to as heat diffusion. In solids, heat is conducted through the vibrations of atom lattices, which help to transfer heat from the more energetic particles to the less energetic particles. The mechanism is slightly different in liquids and gases since the molecules are no longer held in place. In liquids and gases, heat conduction occurs due to random molecular motion, where the collision of molecules transfer energy in the form of heat from one molecule to another.

Heat conduction is governed by Fourier's law, which states that the rate of heat conduction (q) is proportional to the temperature difference (ΔT) and cross-sectional area (A), and inversely proportional to the length of the domain (L):

$$q \propto -A\frac{\Delta T}{L}. \tag{A.1}$$

The negative sign preceding the right-hand side implies that heat flows from points of high temperature to low temperature. The negative also eliminates the negative due to $\Delta T = T_2 - T_1 < 0$, since $T_2 < T_1$, as shown in figure A.1.

Introducing the constant or proportionality and equating the left-hand and right-hand sides, one arrives at:

A-1

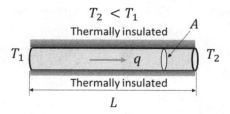

Figure A.1. Heat conduction through a cylindrical solid.

$$q = -kA\frac{\Delta T}{L} \text{ or } q" = \frac{q}{A} = -k\frac{\Delta T}{L}, \tag{A.2}$$

where $q"$ (W m^{-2}) is the rate of heat conduction per unit area (also known as the heat flux) and k (W (m·K)$^{-1}$) is the thermal conductivity, which is a material property that quantifies the ability of a material to conduct heat. Medium with a larger k can conduct heat more efficiently than one with a smaller k.

Taking the differential form of equation (A.2) and writing it for heat conduction in the x-, y- and z-directions, one obtains:

$$q_x" = -k\frac{\partial T}{\partial x}, \quad q_y" = -k\frac{\partial T}{\partial y}, \quad q_z" = -k\frac{\partial T}{\partial z}, \tag{A.3}$$

or

$$\mathbf{q}" = -k\nabla T. \tag{A.4}$$

Equations (A.3) and (A.4) imply that heat flow is a vector and depends on the spatial temperature gradient. A larger temperature gradient in a particular direction can induce greater heat conduction in that direction.

A.3 Heat convection

Heat convection occurs only in liquid and gas. The mechanisms by which heat is transferred via convection are through random molecular motion (also known as diffusion) and bulk motion of fluid. The term convection usually refers to the aggregated effect of both diffusion and bulk motion, while heat transfer solely by bulk motion is referred to as advection. Contribution from advection is typically orders of magnitude greater than diffusion; hence, the term convection is also sometimes used to describe the advection process only.

Two types of heat convection exist, namely natural convection and forced convection. The former occurs when fluid motion that drives the convection process is driven by buoyancy. Buoyancy is caused by differences in the density of air at different temperatures. Hot fluid has a lower density that causes it to rise, while cold fluid, which has a higher density, descends. The rise and fall of the fluid induce a circulation that carries with it heat via natural convection. This is shown in figure A.2(a). Forced convection occurs when there is an external force that drives the movement of fluid. For instance, a fan blowing onto a hot surface induces forced

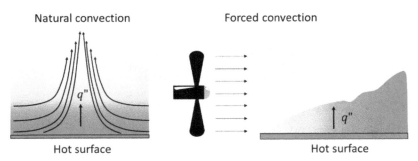

Figure A.2. Comparison between natural and forced convection.

Table A.1. A summary of some of the values of h.

Mechanism	h (W (m^2 K)$^{-1}$)
Free convection	
Gases	2–25
Liquids	50–1000
Forced convection	
Gases	25–250
Liquids	100–20 000

convection between the surface and the air. This is shown in figure A.2(b). Forced convection induces stronger heat transfer than natural convection.

The rate of heat transfer via convection from a solid surface to the surrounding fluid and vice versa can be estimated using Newton's cooling law:

$$q = hA(T - T_\infty), \tag{A.5}$$

where h (W (m^2 K)$^{-1}$) is the convection heat transfer coefficient, A is the surface area where heat convection occurs, T is temperature of the surface and T_∞ is the temperature of the fluid. The convection heat transfer coefficient controls the degree of heat transfer between the solid and the fluid, which varies depending on factors such as the geometry of the surface and the nature of the fluid flow. Table A.1 summarises some of the values of h obtained from Incropera *et al* (2006). Liquids and forced convection generally yield larger values of h than gases and natural convection, respectively.

A.4 Heat radiation

Unlike conduction and convection, radiation does not require a medium to transmit heat. Instead, heat is transmitted via electromagnetic waves. A typical example of heat radiation is the heat gained from the Sun, which are propagated through vacuum before reaching the Earth. Heat radiation can occur in solid, liquid and gas.

In fact, any object/medium that is at a temperature above absolute zero (0 K) will emit some form of radiation.

The rate of heat radiation over a unit area (W m^{-2}) from a surface is known as the surface emissive power, E:

$$E = \varepsilon \sigma T^4, \tag{A.6}$$

where ε is the surface emissivity, σ is the Stefan–Boltzmann constant (5.67×10^{-8} W m^{-2} K^{-4}) and T is the absolute temperature (K) of the surface. The surface emissivity is a rate constant that determines the amount of heat radiated from a surface. It has a value between 0 and 1. A value of $\varepsilon=1$ indicates the largest possible surface emissive power, which is a theoretical limit that represents the case of ideal radiation:

$$E_b = \sigma T^4. \tag{A.7}$$

An object with surface emissive power equivalent to equation (A.7) is known as a blackbody. Emission from a non-blackbody will always follow equation (A.7), such that $E < E_b$.

When describing heat radiation, one must account for both the emission from the surface and the emission incident from its surroundings, E_{surr}. The net rate of heat radiation is thus given by:

$$q" = E - E_{surr}, \tag{A.8}$$

which upon substituting the expressions from equation (A.7), gives:

$$q" = \varepsilon \sigma (T^4 - T_{surr}^4), \tag{A.9}$$

where T_{surr} is the surrounding temperature. When evaluating equation (A.9), the temperatures T and T_{surr} must be expressed in K and not in °C.

The term T^4 in equation (A.9) indicates that the expression is nonlinear. In some circumstances, it may be more convenient to express the net radiation heat exchange in the form of:

$$q" = h_{rad} \sigma (T - T_{surr}), \tag{A.10}$$

where h_{rad} is the heat radiation coefficient given by:

$$h_{rad} = \varepsilon \sigma (T + T_{surr})(T^2 + T_{surr}^2). \tag{A.11}$$

A.5 Heat diffusion equation

The equation describing the spatio-temporal temperature distribution inside a domain can be estimated by solving the heat diffusion equation, which in a 3D space, is given by:

$$\rho c \frac{\partial T}{\partial t} = k \left(\frac{\partial^2 T}{\partial x^2} + \frac{\partial^2 T}{\partial y^2} + \frac{\partial^2 T}{\partial z^2} \right) + \dot{q}, \tag{A.12}$$

Table A.2. Thermal boundary conditions that complement the heat equation.

Condition	Expression	Remarks
Prescribed temperature (Dirichlet)	$T = T_0$	• Sets the temperature at a given boundary to the value T_0. • Typically used for modelling constant temperature or inflow with a fixed temperature.
Prescribed heat flux (Neumann)	$\mathbf{q} \cdot \mathbf{n} = q_0$	• Sets the heat flux at a given boundary to the value q_0.
Zero heat flux	$\mathbf{q} \cdot \mathbf{n} = 0$	• Sets the heat flux at a given boundary to zero. • Typically used to model boundaries that are thermally insulated.
Outflow	$\mathbf{q} \cdot \mathbf{n} = 0$	• Typically used to describe conditions at the far-end boundary where mass is transported out of the solution domain by fluid.

where ρ, c and k are the density (kg m^{-3}), specific heat (J (kg·K)$^{-1}$) and thermal conductivity of the domain material, t (s) is time, T (K) is temperature, (x, y, z) are the coordinates in the 3D space and $\dot{q}$ is the rate of volumetric heat generation inside the domain. If the domain is fluid and heat convection is involved, then equation (A.12) becomes:

$$\rho c \frac{\partial T}{\partial t} + \rho c (\mathbf{v} \cdot \nabla T) = k\left(\frac{\partial^2 T}{\partial x^2} + \frac{\partial^2 T}{\partial y^2} + \frac{\partial^2 T}{\partial z^2}\right) + \dot{q}, \qquad (A.13)$$

where v is the velocity vector of the flow inside the fluid domain. The second term on the left-hand side of equation (A.13) represent the contribution to heat transfer due to convection.

Equations (A.12) and (A.13) can be solved to obtain the spatio-temporal distribution of temperature inside a given domain subject to prescribed initial-boundary conditions. Table A.2 summarises some of the boundary conditions that can be applied.

Reference

Incropera F P, DeWitt D P, Bergman T L and Lavine A S 2006 *Fundamentals of Heat and Mass Transfer* 6th edn (Hoboken, NJ: Wiley)

CPSIA information can be obtained
at www.ICGtesting.com
Printed in the USA
BVHW020214240423
662834BV00003B/10